Physical Activity, Aging and Sports

Volume III:

Toward Healthy Aging - International Perspectives

Part 1. Physiological and Biomedical Aspects

Physical Activity, Aging and Sports

Volume III:

Toward Healthy Aging - International Perspectives

Part 1. Physiological and Biomedical Aspects

Editors

Sara Harris
Center for the Study of Aging
Albany, New York

Pertti Era, Ph.D.
Department of Health Sciences, University of Jyväskylä, Jyväskylä, Finland; *Post-Doctoral Fellow,* Institute of Preventive Medicine, Kommune Hospital, Copenhagen, Denmark

Harri Suominen, Ph.D.
Department of Health Sciences
University of Jyväskylä
Jyväskylä, Finland

Willard S. Harris, M.D.
Chief Medical Service, James A. Haley Veterans' Hospital; *Professor and Associate Chairman,* Department of Internal Medicine, University of South Florida, Tampa, Florida

Center for the Study of Aging—Albany, New York, USA

Printed in the United States of America.

Published by the Center for the Study of Aging
706 Madison Avenue
Albany, New York 12208

Library of Congress Cataloguing in Publication Data (in process)

Main entry under title:

Physical Activity, Aging and Sports
Volume III: Toward Healthy Aging - International Perspectives
Part 1. Physiological and Biomedical Aspects

ISBN 0-937829-06-4 (v.III)
ISBN 0-937829-05-6 (Series)

Dedicated to Albert J. Abrams

(1914-1993)

President of the Center for the Study of Aging since 1989, Albert J. Abrams was a pioneer in the field of aging whose leadership spanned almost half a century. Founder of the National Council on the Aging, secretary of the Desmond Committee, developer of public policy for many national government and state agencies and groups, a key person in the establishment nationwide of senior citizen centers, Albert Abrams had a tremendous influence on the development of aging programs in the United States and throughout the world.

Contributors

Marjatta Ahonen, P.T., Chief Physiotherapist, Department of Physical Medicine and Rehabilitation, Malmi Hospital, Helsinki, Finland.

Katsumi Asano, Ph.D., Professor, Institute of Health and Sport Sciences, University of Tsukuba, Tsukuba, Japan.

Greg Atkinson, B.Sc. (Hon), Research Fellow, School of Human Sciences, Liverpool John Moores University, Liverpool, United Kingdom.

Alberto Ayalon, Ph.D., Biomechanics Department, The Zinman College of Physical Education, The Wingate Institute, Israel.

David Ben-Sira, Ph.D., Head, Biodynamic Department, The Zinman College of Physical Education, The Wingate Institute, Israel.

Jose Botella, M.B., Ch.B., Honorary Clinical Research Fellow, University Department of Geriatric Medicine, Royal Free Hospital School of Medicine, London, United Kingdom.

Maryse Boulard, P.Dt., M.Sc., Research Agent, Department of Physiology, Faculty of Medicine, Université de Montréal, Montreal, Canada.

Wiebo H. Brouwer, Ph.D., Experimental Clinical Neuro-Psychologist, Department of Psychology, Traffic Research Centre, University of Groningen, The Netherlands.

Laura Capranica, M.Sc., Research Assistant, Physiology Laboratory, Physical Education Institute of Rome, Italy.

Adam Coldwells, B.Sc. (Hon), Research Assistant, School of Human Sciences, Liverpool John Moores University, Liverpool, United Kingdom.

Achim Conzelmann, Research and Teaching Assistant, Institute of Sport Science, University of Tubingen, Germany.

Guido Curri, M.D., Full Professor and Chief, Department of Geriatry and Gerontology, University of Trieste, Trieste, Italy.

Giorgio Delbello, M.D., Researcher, Department of Normal Human Morphology, University of Trieste, Trieste, Italy.

.Giuseppe DeVito, M.D., Sport Medicine Specialist, Research Assistant, Physiology Laboratory, Human Physiology Institute, University La Sapienza, Rome, Italy.

John Eisman, Ph.D., F.R.A.C.P., Professor of Medicine, University of New South Wales; Staff Endocrinologist, St. Vincent's Hospital, Sydney; and Head, Bone and Mineral Research Division, Garvan Institute of Medical Research, Sydney, Australia.

Pertti Era, Ph.D., Researcher, Department of Health Sciences, University of Jyväskylä, Jyväskylä, Finland; and Post-Doctoral Fellow, Institute of Preventive Medicine, Kommune Hospital, Copenhagen, Denmark.

Timo Erkinjuntti, M.D., Ph.D., Memory Research Unit, Department of Neurology, University of Helsinki, Helsinki, Finland.

Roger A. Fielding, Ph.D., Clinical Assistant Professor of Health Sciences, Sargent College of Allied Health Professions, Boston University, Boston, Massachusetts; and Scientist III, USDA Human Nutrition Research Center on Aging, Tufts University, Boston, Massachusetts.

Francesco Figura, M.D., Full Professor of Human Physiology, Faculty of Medicine, University of L'Aquila, Italy.

Jerome L. Fleg, M.D., Senior Investigator, Laboratory of Cardiovascular Science, Gerontology Research Center, NIA, Baltimore, Maryland.

Vadim E. Fraifeld, M.D., Ph.D., Former Junior Scientific Researcher, Clinical Radiology Laboratory, Institute of Gerontology, Kiev, Ukraine; Presently Scientific Researcher, Clinical Radiology Laboratory, Ben-Gurion University, Negev, Israel.

Lesly Germain, M.D., F.R.C.S.(C), Orthopaedic Surgeon, Hôpital Notre-Dame and Head of Orthopaedics and Physiotherapy Departments, Hôpital Saint-Michel, Montreal, Canada.

Carolyn A. Greig, M.Sc., Ph.D., Lecturer in Human and Applied Physiology, University Department of Geriatric Medicine, Royal Free Hospital School of Medicine, London, United Kingdom.

Sara Harris, Executive Director, Center for the Study of Aging of Albany, New York; Recording Secretary, Council on Geriatric Cardiology.

Willard S. Harris, M.D., Chief, Medical Service, James A. Haley Veterans' Hospital; Professor and Associate Chairman, Department of Internal Medicine, University of South Florida, Tampa, Florida.

Yoko Hayakawa, M.S., Doctoral Program, Health and Sport Sciences, University of Tsukuba, Tsukuba, Japan.

Simon A. Henderson, B.Sc., M.D., Senior Registrar, Department of Orthopaedic Surgery, The Queens University of Belfast, Northern Ireland.

Mitsuru Higuchi, M.D., Head, Laboratory of Health Evaluation, Division of Health Promotion, National Institute of Health and Nutrition, Tokyo, Japan.

Teruo Hiyama, M.D., Director, Division of Cardiology, Higashi Toride Hospital, Ibaraki-ken, Japan.

Andrée Imbach, Ph.D., Professor, Department of Physiology, Faculty of Medicine, Université de Montréal, Montreal, Canada.

Keiko Ishii, R.D., Division of Health Promotion, National Institute of Health and Nutrition, Tokyo, Japan.

Takashi Kato, M.D., Professor Emeritus, Department of Public Health, Aichi Medical University, Nagakute, Japan.

Paul Kelly, M.D., F.R.A.C.P. Staff Endocrinologist, St. Vincent's Hospital, Sydney; and Research Physician, Bone and Mineral Research Division, Garvan Institute of Medical Research, Sydney, Australia.

Hyun Soo Kim, Ph.D., Department of Science of Living, Osaka City University, Osaka, Japan.

Yasuo Kimura, Ed.D., Physical Education Assistant, Laboratory for Exercise Physiology, School of Education, Waseda University, Tokyo, Japan.

Fumio Kobayashi, M.D., Associate Professor, Department of Health and Psychosocial Medicine, Aichi Medical University, Nagakute, Japan.

Shuhei Kobayashi, M.D., Director, National Institute of Health and Nutrition, Tokyo, Japan.

Michiko Koda, M.S., Laboratory of Exercise Physiology and Biomechanics, Faculty of Education, The University of Tokyo, Tokyo, Japan.

Olli Korhonen, M.D., Specialized Physician, Institute of Occupational Health, Vantaa, Finland.

Oleg V. Korkushko, M.D., Professor, Doctor of Medical Sciences, Head of Department of Clinical Physiology and Pathology of Internal Organs, Institute of Gerontology, Kiev, Ukraine.

Minoru Kubota, B.L., Professor, School of Human Sciences, Waseda University, Saitama, Japan.

Yasuhito Kumazaki, M.S., Master Program of Health and Sport Sciences, University of Tsukuba, Tsukuba, Japan.

Koen A.P.M. Lemmink, M.Sc., Department of Human Movement Sciences, University of Groningen, The Netherlands.

François Lessard, M.D., F.R.C.P.(C), Lecturer, Faculty of Medicine, Université de Montréal, and Head of Clinical Biochemistry, Hôpital Saint-Luc, Montreal, Canada.

Colette Lortie, P.Dt., Research Nutritionist, Department of Physiology, and Lecturer, Department of Nutrition, Faculty of Medicine, Université de Montréal, Montreal, Canada.

Yoshiyuki Matsuura, Ph.D., Professor, Department of Physical Education, Chukyo Women's University, Chukyo, Japan.

Kazimiera Milanowska, M.D., Professor, Head of the Rehabilitation Department, Institute of Orthopaedic Surgery and Rehabilitation, Academy of Medicine, Posnan, Poland.

M. Miyashita, Ph.D., Professor, Faculty of Education, The University of Tokyo, Tokyo, Japan.

Niamh M. Murphy, M.A., Exercise Science PE Officer, Physical and Health Education Unit, The Queens University of Belfast, Northern Ireland.

M. Mutoh, M.D., Professor, Faculty of Education, The University of Tokyo, Tokyo, Japan.

Yael Netz, Ph.D., Gerontological Studies, The Zinman College of Physical Education, The Wingate Institute, Israel.

Tuula Nurminen, Dr.P.H., Chief, Section of Statistics, Department of Epidemiology and Biostatistics, Finnish Institute of Occupational Health, Helsinki, Finland.

Toshiki Ohta, M.D., Director, Division of Health Promotion, National Institute of Health and Nutrition, Tokyo, Japan.

Lorenzo Pascazio, M.D., Researcher, Department of Geriatry and Gerontology, University of Trieste, Trieste, Italy.

Daniel Picard, M.D., M.Sc., F.R.C.P.(C), Associate Professor of Radiology and Nuclear Medicine Specialist, Faculty of Medicine, Université de Montréal and Hôpital Saint-Luc, Montreal, Canada.

Nicholas Pocock, M.D., F.R.A.C.P., Staff Nuclear Medicine Physician and Deputy Director, Department of Nuclear Medicine, St. Vincent's Hospital, Sydney, Australia.

Concetta Pulejo, A.P., Associate Professor, Physical Education Institute of Rome, Italy.

Ilmari Pyykkö, M.D., Associate Professor, University Hospital, Helsinki, Finland.

Thomas Reilly, B.A., M.Sc., Ph.D., Professor and Director, School of Human Sciences, Liverpool John Moores University, Liverpool, United Kingdom.

Piet Rispens, M.D., Ph.D., Professor, Human Movement Sciences; Chairman, Department of Human Movement Sciences, University of Groningen, The Netherlands.

Marc A. Rogers, Ph.D. Assistant Professor, Department of Kinesiology, University of Maryland, College Park, Maryland.

Gastone Sabbadini, M.D., Researcher, Department of Geriatry and Gerontology, University of Trieste, Trieste, Italy.

Pierre Sabouret, M.D., Lecturer, Orthopaedic Surgeon and Sport Medicine Specialist, Faculty of Medicine, Université de Montréal and Hôpital Saint-Luc, Montreal, Canada.

Amira Sagiv, R.N., Nursing School, Carmel Hospital, Haifa, Israel.

Michael Sagiv, Ph.D., Head, Sports Medicine and Rehabilitation Division, The Zinman College of Physical Education, The Wingate Institute, Israel.

Elina Saloheimo, M.D., Physiatrist, Head, Department of Physical Medicine and Rehabilitation, Maria Hospital, Helsinki, Finland.

Seija Salovaara, R.N., Head Nurse, Department of Rehabilitation, Malmi Hospital, Helsinki, Finland.

Philip Sambrook, M.D., F.R.A.C.P., Associate Professor, Staff Rheumatologist and Gerontologist, St. Vincent's Hospital, Sydney; and Senior Research Physician, Bone and Mineral Research Division, Garvan Institute of Medical Research, Sydney, Australia.

Konstantin G. Sarkisov, M.D., Ph.D., Deputy Director of the Institute of Gerontology AMSU, Kiev, Ukraine; Head of the Scientific Group on Microcirculation and Microhaemorheology.

Dawn A. Skelton, B.Sc., Postgraduate Student, University Department of Geriatric Medicine, Royal Free Hospital School of Medicine, London, United Kingdom.

Juhani Smolander, Ph.D., Specialized Researcher, Institute of Occupational Health, Vantaa, Finland.

Jeannie Crane Sykes, Ph.D., R.D., Coordinator of Preventive Medicine Curriculum, Moses H. Cone Memorial Hospital Family Practice Residency Training Program, Greensboro, North Carolina.

Harri Suominen, Ph.D., Docent, Department of Health Sciences, University of Jyväskylä, Jyväskylä, Finland.

Halina Szwarc, M.D., F.A., Professor, Medical Centre for Postgraduate Education, Warsaw; Academy of Physical Education, Warsaw.

Masaki Takeda, M.S., Doctoral Program, Health and Sport Sciences, University of Tsukuba, Tsukuba, Japan.

Nobuo Takeshima, Ph.D., Associate Professor, College of General Education, Nagoya City University, Nagoya, Japan; and Visiting Professor, Center for Exercise Science, Department of Health and Human Performance, University of Florida, Gainesville, Florida.

Kiyoji Tanaka, Ph.D., Associate Professor, Institute of Health and Sports Sciences, University of Tsukuba, Tsukuba, Japan.

Reijo Tilvis, M.D., Professor of Geriatrics, University of Helsinki, Helsinki, Finland.

Stephen H. Tolins, M.D., F.A.C.S., Clinical Professor of Surgery, New York Medical College, Valhalla, New York; and Emeritus Associate Professor of Surgery, Albert Einstein College of Medicine, New York, New York.

Jaakko Valvanne, M.D., Ph.D., Geriatrician, Chief Medical Officer, Primary Care, North-Eastern Health Centre, Helsinki, Finland.

Marieke J.G. van Heuvelen, M.Sc., Department of Human Movement Sciences, University of Groningen, The Netherlands.

Takemasa Watanabe, M.D., Lecturer, Department of Health and Psychological Medicine, Aichi Medical University, Nagakute, Japan.

Yutaka Watanabe, M.D., Vice-Director, Division of Cardiology, Higashi Toride Hospital, Ibaraki-ken, Japan.

James M. Waterhouse, B.A., D.Phil., Principal Lecturer, School of Biological Sciences, Liverpool John Moores University, Liverpool, United Kingdom.

Shoichi Yamazaki, Ph.D., Associate Professor, Laboratory of Sports and Health Science, School of Science and Engineering, Ishinomaki Senshu University, Miyagi, Japan.

Yurij T. Yaroshenko, Candidate of Medical Sciences, Leading Research Worker, Department of Clinical Physiology and Pathology of Internal Organs, Institute of Gerontology, Kiev, Ukraine.

Yutaka Yoshitake, Ph.D., Head, Laboratory of Health Promotion Technology, Division of Health Promotion, National Institute of Health and Nutrition, Tokyo, Japan.

Archie Young, B.Sc., M.B., Ch.B., M.D., F.R.C.P., Professor of Geriatric Medicine, Royal Free Hospital School of Medicine, London, United Kingdom.

Preface

Physical Activity, Aging and Sports-Volume III: Toward Healthy Aging-International Perspectives-Part 1. Physiological and Biomedical Aspects is the third volume in the series. Designed to bring together basic concepts and practice to increase knowledge and improve communication in the multidisciplinary areas of exercise, medicine, cardiology, physiology, physical education, rehabilitation, sports and health, the series, thus far, has had a response far exceeding our expectations.

International researchers, clinicians and practitioners have all contributed to this and the two preceding volumes, Volume I: Scientific and Medical Research and Volume II: Practice, Program and Policy. The editors are pleased that the series is developing a comprehensive body of knowledge in the related areas of aging and exercise and sports. Thus, Volume III and Volume IV, scheduled for publication in 1994, are adding another dimension, i.e., the concept of prevention of illness and maintenance of well-being. In order to prevent illness and enjoy a healthy old age, it is important to know and understand the part that exercise and sports play in maintaining and improving health in the later years. This book, based on selected and edited articles from the Third International Conference on Physical Activity and Sports for Healthy Aging held in Jyväskylä, Finland in June 1992, has a number of research articles that we hope will stimulate further investigation and lead to improved practice.

Volume III includes research and theory on functional aging, physiology, cardiovascular performance, osteoporosis, muscles, kinesiology, nutrition, mobility, Master athletes, circadian rhythms, rehabilitation, nutrition and Tai Chi.

Volume IV will continue with articles on behavior, psychology, cognition, personality, motivation, genetic and environmental effects on exercise, life situation determinants, active lifestyles, benefits of exercise, physical activity programs, women and physical activity, successful aging, sports, Senior Olympics and more.

It is anticipated that, as the numbers of older men and women increase throughout the world, more and more knowledge will be needed to understand the aging process in order to keep people mobile and self-sufficient. The research that develops the parameters for better health in old age will also benefit human development throughout the life span so that each child and adult will be able to attain his and her highest capability for performance and health maintenance. Greater knowledge and improved health practices on the part of individuals and families may be the only way to reduce the spiraling costs of health care throughout the world.

These volumes have been developed, first, through papers and presentations on research and practice, followed by the interchange of ideas and knowledge among men and women from all over the world through national and international conferences. Exchange of ideas and discussion of their work with their peers from many disciplines led to the articles contributed by the authors in this book. The papers have been reviewed by leading scientists and practitioners from many countries. The Center for the Study of Aging of Albany, New York is proud through these volumes to bring some of the current knowledge in medicine, exercise physiology, kinesiology, physical education and related fields to a broader audience. We hope the series will benefit us all by promoting more basic research and helping to make practitioners aware of the opportunities to improve the health and quality of life of older people.

The Editors

Sara Harris
Albany, NY, USA

Harri Suominen, Ph.D.
Jyväskylä, Finland

Pertti Era, Ph.D.
Copenhagen, Denmark

Willard S. Harris, M.D.
Tampa, FL, USA

Spring, 1994

Albany, New York

Acknowledgments

The editors wish to thank Eino Heikkinen, M.D., for his interest and support for this book, the members of the Editorial Review Board, the participants in the Third International Conference on Physical Activity, Aging and Sports, and all the contributors. We also thank the many authors whose articles were not selected for this volume for their interest. Special thanks to Jerome L. Fleg, M.D., and Marc Rogers, Ph.D., for their assistance with some of the technical questions in their respective fields.

We acknowledge with gratitude a grant from the Finnish Ministry of Education which has helped with the publication of this book.

The staff of the Department of Health Sciences and the Gerontology Research Center at the University of Jyväskylä, Jyväskylä, Finland was extremely helpful. Special thanks to Pirjo Koikkalainen for her assistance in making this book a reality.

We want to thank the officers and directors of the Center for the Study of Aging for their continuing support of this project: Director of Publications, Jerome Kaplan, Ph.D.; Colonel James L. Anderson, President; Jonathan Harris, M.D.; Edward L. Hirsch; James W. Dougherty, M .D.; Helen Wallace Fitzgerald; and Alfred C. Werner, Ed.D.

Shirley Nunan, administrative assistant and copy editor extraordinary, has done an admirable job. Her continuing interest, enthusiasm and dedication are appreciated. Pauline Lyall of the Center for the Study of Aging staff did an excellent job of typing the manuscripts; Stephanie Richardson, our typographer, has provided outstanding assistance.

PHYSICAL ACTIVITY, AGING AND SPORTS

VOLUME III:
Toward Healthy Aging - International Perspectives
Part 1. Physiological and Biomedical Aspects

Contents

Section 1

Physiology of Exercise and Aging

Aging Changes in Cardiovascular Fitness: Current Research Approaches

Jerome L. Fleg, M.D.

INTRODUCTION

Over the past half century, numerous studies have documented a major decline in maximal aerobic capacity ($\dot{V}O_2$max) with age, usually approximating 10 percent per decade after maturation. The cross-sectional design of most such studies and the well-known declines in physical activity and changes in body composition which accompany the aging process leave doubt regarding the decline in $\dot{V}O_2$max attributable to age *per se*. Several research approaches to offset the shortcomings of these earlier studies have been developed. When $\dot{V}O_2$max is normalized for 24-hour urinary creatinine excretion rather than for total body weight, to adjust for the decrease in muscle mass which occurs with age, the decline in $\dot{V}O_2$max attributable to age is decreased from 55 percent to 11 percent in cross-sectional analysis of nonathletic adults 22 to 87 years old. Longitudinal studies in such populations suggest a decline in $\dot{V}O_2$max of 0.40-0.50 ml•kg•min/yr in men and 0.20-0.35 ml•kg•min/yr in women.

Cross-sectional comparison of older and younger endurance athletes with similar competitive achievements in young adulthood minimizes the confounding effects of differing genetic potential and age-associated declines in physical activity. These studies, as well as longitudinal studies of older athletes who continue to exercise, suggest a decline in $\dot{V}O_2$max of only about five percent per decade, compared with the 10 percent per decade decline observed in sedentary individuals. Furthermore it appears that older athletes who remain highly competitive experience much smaller decrements in $\dot{V}O_2$max than those who reduce their training intensity, despite similar decreases in lean body mass. Recent studies indicate that sedentary individuals in their seventh and eighth decades can achieve relative improvements in $\dot{V}O_2$max with aerobic training similar to those of younger subjects. Taken together, these varied research approaches suggest that the decline in $\dot{V}O_2$max with age is influenced profoundly by age-associated changes in physical activity patterns and body composition. A growing literature suggests that regular and vigorous aerobic exercise can markedly attenuate the decline in $\dot{V}O_2$max attributable to the aging process.

To even the most casual observer of athletic competition, it is evident that maximal performance generally peaks in the 20s and declines gradually thereafter. In the laboratory setting, maximal oxygen consumption, or $\dot{V}O_2$max, is the most universally accepted measurement of cardiorespiratory "fitness." $\dot{V}O_2$max represents the maximal ability of the organism to utilize oxygen during exercise and is determined by the product of maximal cardiac output and maximal capacity of the exercising muscles to extract oxygen from the circulating blood. Numerous cross-sectional and longitudinal studies in sedentary individuals and athletes have documented an age-associated decline in $\dot{V}O_2$max beginning in early adulthood.

Determination of the true decline in $\dot{V}O_2$max due to aging *per se* is a formidable task. Several lifestyle changes which frequently accompany the aging process may have a major influence on $\dot{V}O_2$max. For example, in most industrialized societies, vigorous physical activity declines with age, as illustrated in volunteers from the Baltimore Longitudinal Study of Aging (BLSA), shown in Figure 1 (McGandy et al., 1966). Another such confounding lifestyle variable is the increase in body weight which often occurs over time (Norris and Lundy, 1963). Since $\dot{V}O_2$max is traditionally expressed per kg of body weight, any change in the latter will affect $\dot{V}O_2$max independent of a true change in conditioning status.

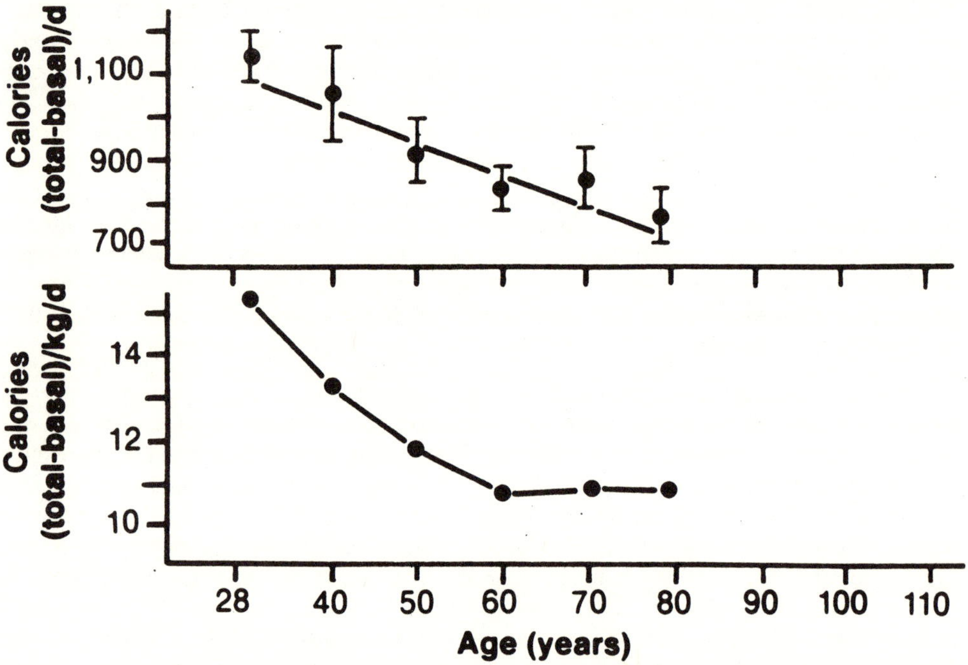

Figure 1. Decline in caloric expenditure with age in volunteers from the Baltimore Longitudinal Study of Aging (BLSA). From McGandy et al., 1966.

The development of cardiovascular or pulmonary disease is another confounding variable in the assessment of age-related changes in $\dot{V}O_2$max. Although those individuals with overt coronary artery disease or congestive heart failure are readily identified and can be excluded from study, the detection and exclusion of subjects with asymptomatic heart disease are much more difficult. For example, overt coronary artery disease was present in only 20 to 30 percent of BLSA volunteers in the seventh and eighth decades (Figure 2) (Gerstenblith et al., 1980). However, additional screening with exercise electrocardiography or thallium scanning would identify an additional 25 to 30 percent of older individuals who should probably also be excluded from studies of normative aging, consistent with the 50 to 70 percent autopsy prevalence of coronary artery disease in the elderly (Elveback and Lie, 1984). Thus, the degree to which lifestyle variables and cardiopulmonary disease are accounted for will significantly affect the results of such studies.

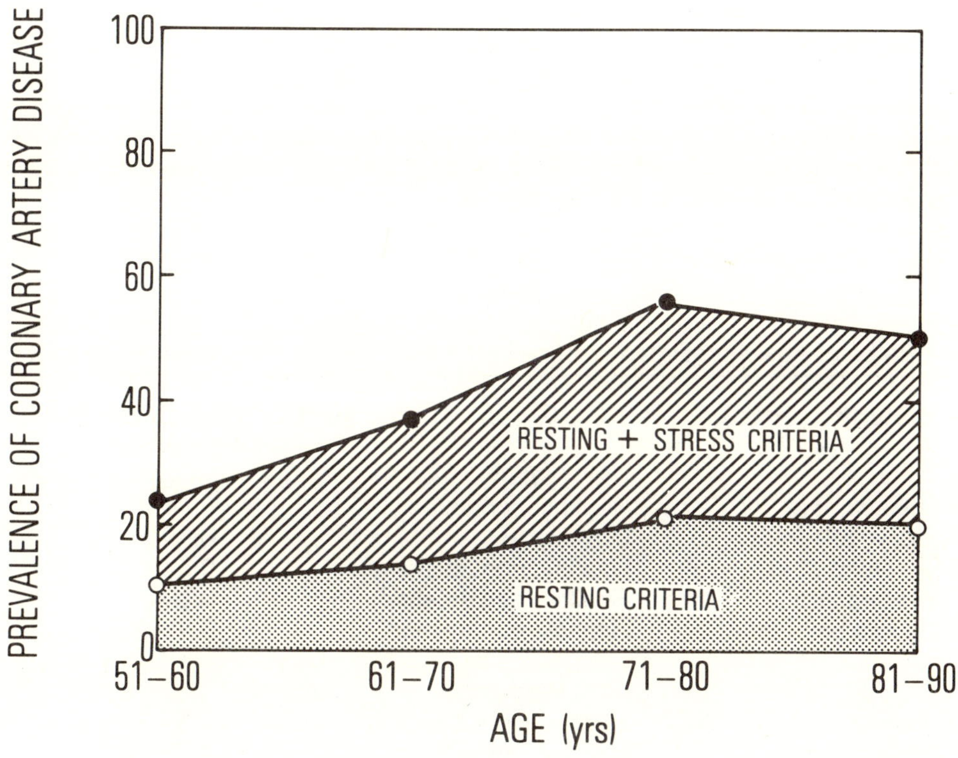

Figure 2. Prevalence of overt and suspected coronary artery disease as a function of age in BLSA volunteers. The lower shaded area represents individuals with evidence of coronary disease by history, physical examination or resting ECG. The upper shaded region indicates asymptomatic individuals with an abnormal exercise ECG and/or exercise thallium scan. Drawn from Gerstenblith et al., 1980.

In this review, five approaches to the delineation of age-associated changes in cardio-respiratory fitness, as represented by $\dot{V}O_2max$, will be taken. These approaches are as follows:

1. Cross-sectional studies of untrained subjects.
2. Cross-sectional studies of athletes and age-matched controls.
3. Longitudinal studies of untrained subjects.
4. Longitudinal studies of athletes.
5. Intervention studies, i.e., training or detraining.

CROSS-SECTIONAL STUDIES OF UNTRAINED SUBJECTS

Many cross-sectional studies over the past half century have documented an age-related decline in $\dot{V}O_2max$ of five to 10 percent per decade between ages 25 and 75 years (Vogel et al., 1986; Robinson, 1938; Åstrand, 1960; Drinkwater et al., 1975; Fleg and Lakatta, 1988; Convertino et al., 1986; Binkhorst et al., 1965; Profant et al., 1972). This decline in $\dot{V}O_2max$ with age parallels the decline in work capacity and is therefore not secondary to increased metabolic efficiency in older subjects. In most such studies, the decline in $\dot{V}O_2max$ with age has averaged 0.40-0.50 ml•kg•min per year in men and 0.20-0.35-ml•kg•min per year in women (Table 1). In general, rates of $\dot{V}O_2max$ decline have been similar in active versus sedentary populations.

TABLE 1

Rates of Age-Associated Decline in $\dot{V}O_2max$ in Cross-Sectional Studies

Study	Group	Rate of $\dot{V}O_2max$ Decline (ml•kg•min•yr)
	Men	
*Robinson et al.	Healthy, nonathletic	0.46
*Vogel et al.	U.S. Army	0.50
*Convertino et al.	Healthy, nonathletic	0.34
*Binkhorst et al.	Healthy, nonathletic	0.39
*Fleg and Lakatta	Healthy, nonathletic	0.39
	Women	
*Åstrand	Healthy, nonathletic	0.35
*Convertino et al.	Healthy, nonathletic	0.33
*Drinkwater et al.	Sedentary	0.30
	Above Average $\dot{V}O_2max$	0.17
*Profant et al.	Sedentary	0.30
	Moderately Active	0.19
*Fleg and Lakatta	Healthy, nonathletic	0.25

Adapted with modifications from Buskirk ER and Hodgson JL. Age and aerobic power: the rate of change in men and women. Federation Proc 1987;46:1824-9.

*see list of References

In a cross-sectional study of carefully screened healthy nonathletic BLSA volunteers aged 22 to 87 years, $\dot{V}O_2max$ during treadmill exercise declined predictably with age in both sexes (Fleg and Lakatta, 1988). Between the ages of 30 and 70 years, $\dot{V}O_2max$ per kg body weight decreased 38 percent in men and 30 percent in women. To explore the role of age-associated changes in body composition on these results, we normalized $\dot{V}O_2max$ in each subject for total muscle mass, as represented by 24-hour urinary creatinine excretion. The rationale for such a normalization is that over 90 percent of oxygen consumed at maximal effort is utilized by the exercising muscles. In both sexes, 24-hour urinary creatinine per kg body weight declined with age, confirming an age-related decline in muscle mass. When $\dot{V}O_2max$ was expressed per mg of creatinine excretion rather than per kg of body weight (Figure 3), the decrease in $\dot{V}O_2max$ explicable by age was reduced from 60 percent to 14 percent in men and from 50 percent to eight percent in women. These results suggest that the age-associated decrease in muscle mass plays a major role in the decline of $\dot{V}O_2max$ with age.

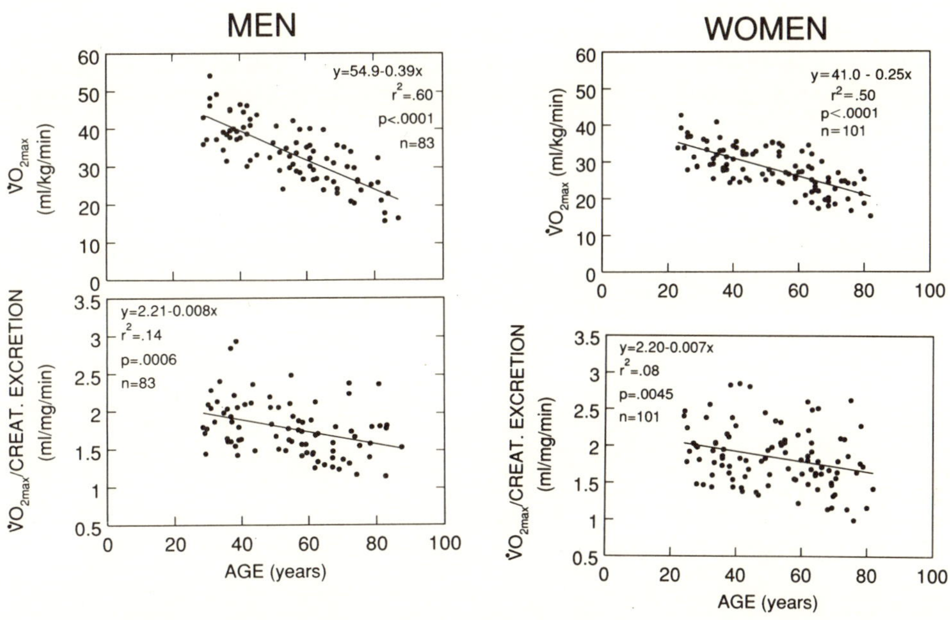

Figure 3. Age-associated decrease in $\dot{V}O_2max$ in carefully screened healthy volunteers.

TOP PANELS. When expressed as the traditional ml/kg/min, $\dot{V}O_2max$ declines strikingly with age.

LOWER PANELS. When $\dot{V}O_2max$ is normalized for 24-hour urinary creatinine excretion, an index of total body muscle mass, the decrease of $\dot{V}O_2max$ with age is markedly attenuated. Adapted from Fleg and Lakatta, 1988.

CROSS-SECTIONAL COMPARISONS OF ATHLETES AND AGE-MATCHED SEDENTARY INDIVIDUALS

Given the significant decline in physical activity with aging, much of the age-associated reduction in $\dot{V}O_2max$ may be mediated by "deconditioning" rather than by age *per se*. One approach used to circumvent the effect of such deconditioning is to examine $\dot{V}O_2max$ responses in highly conditioned endurance athletes over a broad age range. Because endurance athletes are also relatively homogeneous with regard to dietary habits, body build and avoidance of tobacco, excessive alcohol and other deleterious habits, these individuals provide an ideal population for isolating the effect of aging *per se* on aerobic capacity. In one such study, endurance-trained men aged 50 to 72 years were matched to young athletes 19 to 27 years who had similar current habits (Heath et al., 1981). To minimize genetic differences in aerobic capacity, the two groups were also matched for peak running performance times as young adults. In these carefully selected athletes, $\dot{V}O_2max$ averaged 15 percent less in older than younger men. If one assumes that the older athletes had $\dot{V}O_2max$ levels similar to their younger counterparts at identical ages, the extrapolated decline of $\dot{V}O_2max$ in these older athletes approaches five percent per decade, approximately half the rate of sedentary populations; these findings suggest that regular intense physical exercise may attenuate age changes in $\dot{V}O_2max$ (Figure 4). More recently, longitudinal studies in athletes have shown similar results, which will be discussed subsequently.

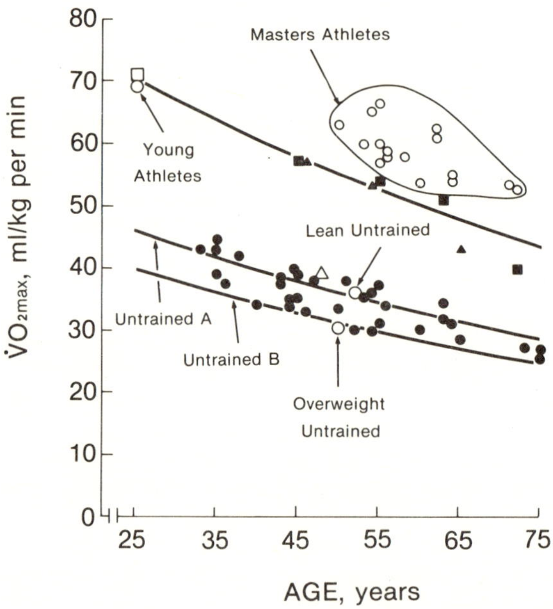

Figure 4. Cross-sectional comparison of $\dot{V}O_2max$ levels in older and younger endurance athletes and untrained subjects from several prior studies. Extrapolation of an age regression in the athletes suggests a decline in $\dot{V}O_2max$ of about five percent per decade, about half the rate of decline in sedentary cohorts. Adapted from Heath et al., 1981.

In younger athletes, $\dot{V}O_2$max is augmented by training-induced increases in both cardiac output and arteriovenous oxygen difference. When the older athletes described above were compared with age-matched sedentary control subjects, the 51 percent higher $\dot{V}O_2$max per kg in the athletes was accomplished by a 19 percent higher cardiac output and a 25 percent higher arteriovenous oxygen difference, estimated by CO_2 rebreathing technique (Hagberg et al., 1985). Direct cardiac imaging during upright cycle exercise in athletes 60 to 79 years old ($\dot{V}O_2$max 51 ± 4 ml•kg•min) and age-matched sedentary controls ($\dot{V}O_2$max 31 ± 4 ml•kg•min) revealed that approximately two-thirds of the difference in $\dot{V}O_2$max was explained by an augmented arteriovenous oxygen difference in the athletes (Fleg, et al., 1988). Thus, cross-sectional studies suggest that peripheral factors are at least as important as central factors (i.e., cardiac output determinants) in achieving high levels of $\dot{V}O_2$max in older endurance trained individuals.

LONGITUDINAL CHANGES OF UNTRAINED SUBJECTS

To infer that age-associated declines in $\dot{V}O_2$max observed in cross-sectional studies represent true longitudinal rates of change is hazardous. Cross-sectional studies tend to minimize aging changes because every age increment represents a progressively more highly selected subset. In other words, not all 20-year-olds will survive to become 70- or 80-year-olds. Longitudinal studies, in which the measurement of interest is made in the same individuals over time, represent the gold standard in assessing the aging process. As expected, these studies are far fewer in number than the more easily-performed cross-sectional type. Unfortunately, several of these longitudinal studies of $\dot{V}O_2$max are confounded by changes in weight or physical activity habits between measurements.

In men initially 40 to 59 years old, $\dot{V}O_2$max declined by an average of 0.40 ml•kg•min per year over 13 years of follow-up (McKeen et al., 1985). Within the overall group, however, substantial variation was observed. Men classified initially as controls experienced a decline averaging only 0.29 ml•kg•min per year compared to a decline of 0.46 ml•kg•min per year in men initially participating in an 18-month exercise program. These rates of decline are confounded by the fact that the controls became more active whereas the exercise group became less active over the 13 years of observation. The average yearly $\dot{V}O_2$max decline of an additional volitionally active control group, who remained more active than the other two groups by self-report, was 0.42 ml•kg•min. More recently, 14 sedentary middle-aged men experienced a decline in $\dot{V}O_2$max from 2.73 to 2.45 1/min over a follow-up averaging 7.9 years (Rogers et al., 1990); this represents a decline of 12 percent per decade or 0.42 ml•kg•min per year—identical to the volitionally active men reported above. A very similar yearly decline of 0.44 ml•kg•min was reported by Åstrand et al. (1973) in 35 active female physical education teachers over a 21-year observation period.

LONGITUDINAL STUDIES IN ATHLETIC INDIVIDUALS

If a major factor in the age-associated decline in $\dot{V}O_2$max is the decrease in physical activity which accompanies aging, then individuals who maintain a high level of activity over time should demonstrate an attenuated rate of $\dot{V}O_2$max decline. At least three longitudinal studies suggest that this hypothesis is correct.

Kasch et al. (1988) measured $\dot{V}O_2$max changes during 20 years of observation in 15 highly motivated men who maintained participation in a supervised exercise program from age 45 to 65 years. The men exercised 3.0 to 3.6 times per week at 77-84 percent of heart rate reserve for about one hour per session throughout the two decades. $\dot{V}O_2$max decreased 12.4 percent (from 44.4 to 38.9 ml•kg•min) over this 20-year period for a mean decline of only 0.27 ml•kg•min per year. The men, however, lost an average of 3.4 kg body weight over the observation period. Thus, if $\dot{V}O_2$max is expressed in liters/min instead of ml•kg•min, the decline of $\dot{V}O_2$max would be 16.3 percent instead of 12.4 percent, or about eight percent per decade. This value lies between the 10 percent per decade decline often quoted for sedentary populations and the five percent decline estimated by Heath et al. (1981) from cross-sectional data of endurance athletes.

More recently Rogers et al. (1990) have measured $\dot{V}O_2$max serially over a 7.5-year mean follow-up in 15 well-trained male Master athletes initially averaging 54.5 years old. The men maintained an exercise frequency of 5.7 days/week over this period although both the mean number of miles run per week (40 ± 5) and the running speed (7:55 ± 0:18 min/mile) were somewhat less than the respective initial values of 50 ± 6 miles and 7:30 ± 0:15 min/mile. During follow-up, $\dot{V}O_2$max declined modestly from 3.68 to 3.54 l/min or from 54.0 to 51.8 ml•kg•min, a decline of 5.5 percent per decade; this rate of decline was half that of the age-matched sedentary control group, mentioned earlier. Body weight remained essentially unchanged in both groups.

Perhaps the best data for examining the role of long-term exercise training in attenuating the age-associated decline in $\dot{V}O_2$max comes from Pollock et al. (1987); these investigators evaluated 24 runners over a 10-year period from an initial mean age of 50 to 82 years. Although all of the men maintained their running mileage over the decade, half of the men maintained their original running speed, while the other half reduced their pace by 1.5 min/mile. Body weight remained nearly constant in both groups although each demonstrated a modest loss of lean body mass. While the group which reduced training intensity experienced a 13 percent reduction in $\dot{V}O_2$max (from 52.5 to 45.9 ml•kg•min), the group which maintained training intensity experienced only a two percent loss of $\dot{V}O_2$max (from 54.2 to 53.3 ml/kg min) over the decade (Figure 5). These compelling data suggest that the decline in maximal aerobic capacity with advancing age can be attenuated markedly by maintaining both a high intensity and quantity of physical activity. However, the possible contributions of genetic factors to these processes cannot be disregarded.

INTERVENTION STUDIES: TRAINING AND DETRAINING

The cross-sectional and longitudinal studies of Master athletes discussed above provide strong evidence that intense aerobic exercise can retard the age-associated decline of $\dot{V}O_2$max in these individuals. For the vast majority of older persons who are relatively sedentary and are not genetically endowed athletes, a more relevant question is whether they too can benefit from regular aerobic exercise training, as evidenced by an increase in $\dot{V}O_2$max. Although early studies suggested that individuals past age 60 did not increase their $\dot{V}O_2$max in response to training (Benestad, 1965; Adams and DeVries, 1973), several recent studies unequivocally support the trainability of older subjects (Figure 6) (DeVries, 1970; Badenhop et al., 1983; Buccola and and Stone, 1975; Sidney and Shephard, 1978; Suominen et al., 1977; Thomas et al., 1985; Tzankoff et al., 1972; Stamford, 1972). These studies demonstrate increases of $\dot{V}O_2$max of five to 24 percent over training periods of eight to 52 weeks. In general, the lower the initial fitness level, the greater the response to training. Further evidence of a training response in the elderly is a well-documented

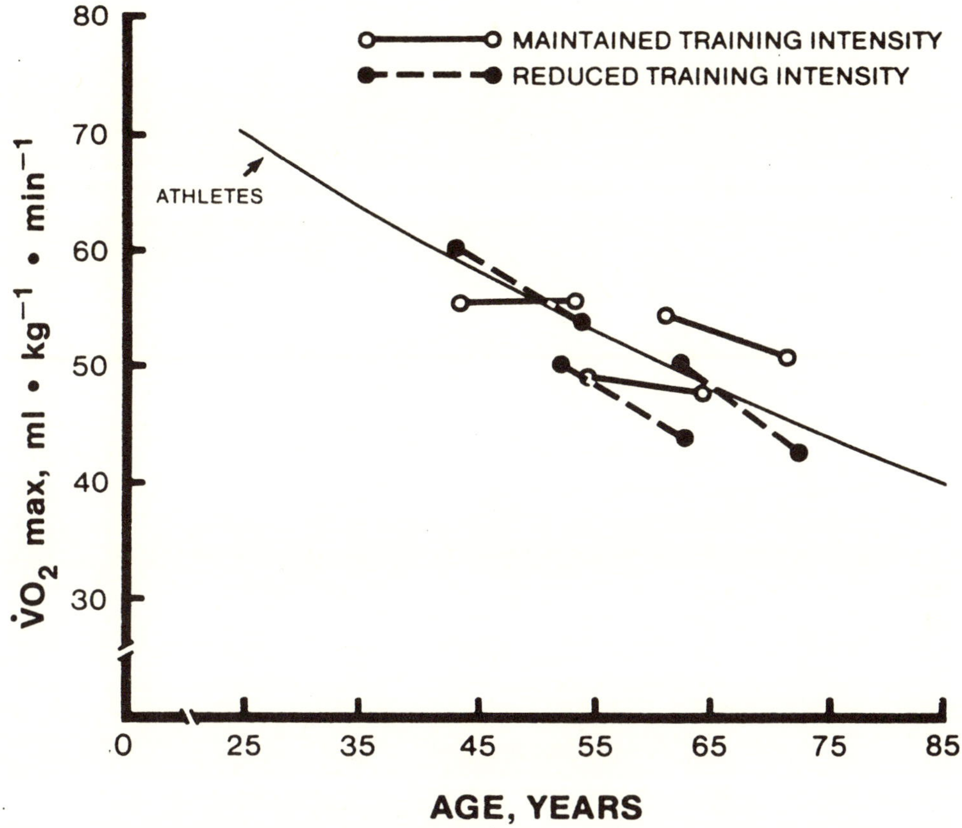

Figure 5. Longitudinal changes in $\dot{V}O_2$max in endurance trained men who maintained or reduced their training intensity over a 10-year follow-up. Solid line represents cross-sectional curve from Heath et al., 1981. From Pollock et al., 1987.

reduction in heart rate response to fixed external exercise loads (Kasch et al., 1988; Buccola and Stone, 1975; Sidney and Shephard, 1978).

In contrast to the threshold of 60 to 70 percent of heart rate reserve (i.e., maximal-resting heart rate), several studies suggest that older individuals may benefit from much lower exercise intensities. Badenhop, et al. (1983) elicited improvements in $\dot{V}O_2$max to nine weeks of exercise at 30-45 percent of heart rate reserve in 14 subjects > 60 years old. A six-month walking program at 40 percent of heart rate reserve augmented $\dot{V}O_2$max by 12 percent in 11 healthy men and women aged 65 ± 3 years (Seals et al., 1984a). An additional six months of training at higher exercise intensity (80 to 85 percent of heart rate reserve) increased $\dot{V}O_2$max by an additional 18 percent. The increase in $\dot{V}O_2$max was accomplished primarily by a widening of the maximal arteriovenous oxygen difference, with little change in the indirectly calculated maximal cardiac output. Of note, reductions of body fat and improvement in insulin sensitivity and serum-lipid levels (Seals et al., 1984b) were observed only after the high intensity regimen.

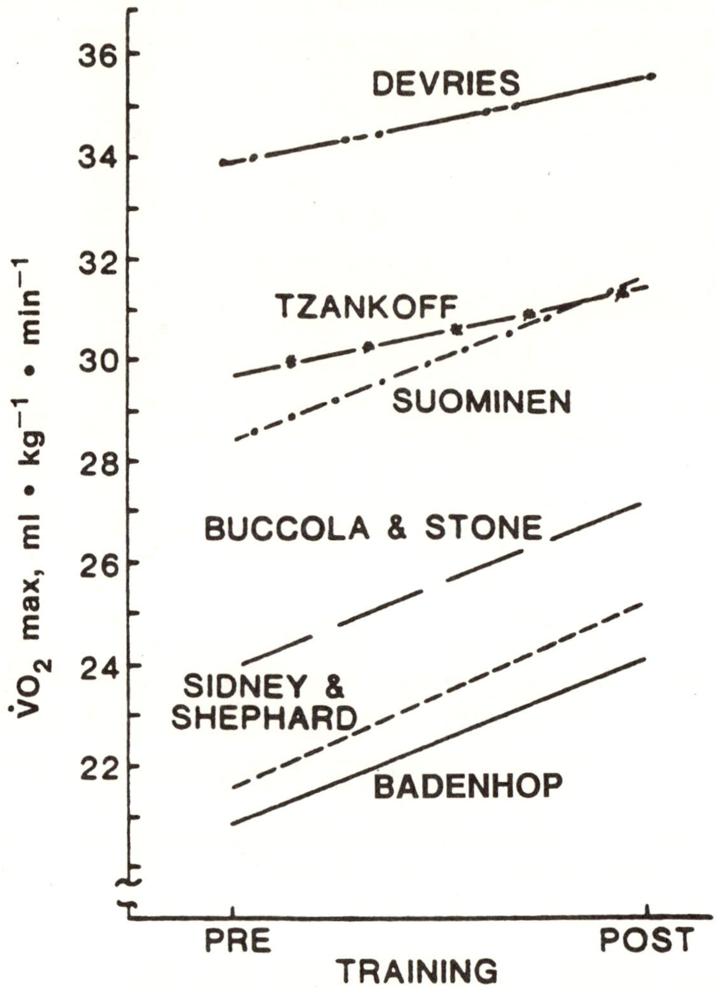

Figure 6. Effects of aerobic training on $\dot{V}O_2$max in several studies of adults > 60 years old. Adapted from Badenhop et al., 1983.

A recent study (Hagberg et al., 1989) has documented that a training response of $\dot{V}O_2$max can be elicited at least through the eighth decade. In 16 subjects 70 to 79 years old, $\dot{V}O_2$max increased by 16 percent after 13 weeks of brisk walking at 50 to 70 percent of $\dot{V}O_2$max and by 22 percent after another 13 weeks of training at 75 to 85 percent of $\dot{V}O_2$max. It is also encouraging that such endurance training programs in healthy older individuals are well tolerated with relatively few orthopedic complications. A major challenge will be to apply such training to the more typical, or even the frail, elderly—groups who stand to benefit greatly because of their more limited baseline exercise capacity.

Additional evidence that the aerobic capacity of older individuals can be modified comes from detraining highly conditioned subjects. Over a 12-week period without exercise, $\dot{V}O_2$max declined from 50.5 to 43.2 ml•kg•min in six male endurance athletes aged 61 ± 8 years (Schulman et al., 1992). After detraining, their $\dot{V}O_2$max expressed per kg of fat-free body mass was similar to those of previously sedentary individuals who had just completed a training program of similar duration. The decline in $\dot{V}O_2$max in the athletes was accompanied by an 18 percent reduction of stroke volume and cardiac output during maximal upright cycle ergometry. Thus, the markedly enhanced aerobic capacity of endurance trained older athletes, although probably in part of genetic origin, is substantially modifiable by changes in physical activity.

CONCLUSION

In the foregoing paragraphs we have briefly explored several lines of evidence that the age-associated decline in maximal aerobic capacity is profoundly influenced by aging changes in physical activity patterns as well as body composition. Thus, much of what we attribute to the aging process may reflect the increasing sedentary lifestyle, loss of muscle mass and increase in adiposity which accompany aging. Although even highly trained senior athletes experience a decline in $\dot{V}O_2$max with age, their rate of decline is only about half the 10 percent per decade observed in sedentary populations. Perhaps more relevant, studies now show that sedentary men and women through the eighth decade can achieve training-induced relative improvements in aerobic capacity similar to younger individuals. The long-term potential for regular exercise to prevent and even reverse much of the age-associated decline in cardiovascular function, thereby reducing disability and enhancing the quality of life, holds great promise for our aging society.

ACKNOWLEDGMENT

The author appreciates the expert secretarial assistance of Paula Wernick and Sharon Thomas.

REFERENCES

Adams GM, DeVries HA. Physiological effects of an exercise training regimen upon women aged 50 to 79. J Gerontol 1973;28:50-5.

Åstrand I. Aerobic work capacity in men and women with special reference to age. Acta Physiol Scand 1960;169(Suppl):1-92.

Åstrand I, Åstrand P-O, Hallback I, Kilbom Å. Reduction in maximal O_2 uptake with age. J Appl Physiol 1973;35:649-54.

Badenhop DT, Cleary PA, Schaal PA, Fox EL, Bartels RL. Physiological adjustments to higher or lower-intensity exercise in elders. Med Sci Sports Exercise 1983;15:496-502.

Benestad AM. Trainability of old men. Acta Med Scand 1965;178:321-7.

Binkhorst RA, Pool J, Van Leeuwen P, Bouhuys A. Maximum oxygen uptake in healthy nonathletic men. Int Z Agnew Physiol Einsehl Arbeitsphysiol 1965;22:10-8.

Buccola VA, Stone WL. Effects of jogging and cycling programs on physiological and personality variables in aged men. Res Q 1975;46:134-9.

Convertino VA, Goldwater DJ, Sandler H. Bedrest-induced peak $\dot{V}O_2$ reduction: association with age, gender and aerobic capacity. Aviat Space Environ Med 1986;57:17-22.

DeVries HA. Physiological effects of an exercise training regimen upon men aged 52-88. J Gerontol 1970;25:325-36.

Drinkwater BL, Horvath SF, Wells CL. Aerobic power in females, ages 10 to 68. J Gerontol 1975;30:385-94.

Elveback L, Lie JT. Continued high prevalence of coronary artery disease at autopsy in Olmstead County, Minnesota 1950 to 1970. Circulation 1984;70: 345-9.

Fleg JL, Lakatta EG. Role of muscle loss in the age-associated reduction in $\dot{V}O_2$max. J Appl Physiol 1988;65:1147-51.

Fleg JL, Schulman S, Gerstenblith G et al. Central versus peripheral adaptations in highly trained seniors (abstr). Physiologist 1988;31:A158.

Gerstenblith G, Fleg JL, VanTosh A et al. Stress testing redefines the prevalence of coronary artery disease in epidemiological studies (abstr). Circulation 1980;62:III-308.

Hagberg JM, Allen WK, Seals DR, Hurley BF, Ehsani AA, Holloszy JO. A hemodynamic comparison of young and older endurance athletes during exercise. J Appl Physiol 1985;58:2041-6.

Hagberg JM, Graves JE, Limacher M et al. Cardiovascular responses of 70-to-79-year-old men and women to exercise training. J Appl Physiol 1989; 66:2589-94.

Heath GW, Hagberg JM, Ehsani AA, Holloszy JO. A physiological comparison of young and older endurance athletes. J Appl Physiol 1981;51:634-40.

Kasch FW, Wallace JP, VanCamp SP, Verity L. A longitudinal study of cardiovascular stability in active men aged 45 to 65 years. Physician Sports Med 1988;16:117-26.

McGandy RB, Barrows CH, Jr., Spanias A, Meredith A, Stone JL, Norris AH. Nutrient intakes and energy expenditure in men of different ages. J Gerontol 1966;21:581-7.

McKeen PC, Rosenberger JL, Slater JS, Nicholas WC, Buskirk ER. A 13-year follow-up of a coronary heart disease risk factor screening and exercise program for 40-to-59-year-old men: exercise habit maintenance and physiologic status. J Cardiac Rehabil 1985;5:510-23.

Norris AH, Lundy T. Trends in selected indices of body composition in men between the age of 30+ and 80 years. Ann NY Acad Sci 1963;110:623-39.

Pollock ML, Foster C, Knapp D, Rod JL, Schmidt DH. Effect of age and training on aerobic capacity and body composition of Master athletes. J Appl Physiol 1987;62:725-31.

Profant GR, Early RG, Nilson KL, Kusumi F, Hofer VG, Bruce RA. Responses to maximal exercise in healthy middle-aged women. J Appl Physiol 1972;33:595-9.

Robinson S. Experimental studies of physical fitness in relation to age. Arbeitsphysiologie 1938;10:251-323.

Rogers MA, Hagberg JM, Martin WH III, Ehsani AA, Holloszy JO. Decline in $\dot{V}O_2$max with aging in Master athletes and sedentary men. J Appl Physiol 1990; 68:2195-9.

Schulman SP, Goldberg A, Becker LC, Lakatta L, Coombs V, Gerstenblith G. Cardiac response to deconditioning in older athletes (abstr). J Am Coll Cardiol 1992;19:386A.

Seals DR, Hagberg JM, Hurley BF, Ehsani AA, Holloszy JO. Endurance training in older men and women. I. Cardiovascular response to exercise. J Appl Physiol 1984;57:1024-9.

Seals DR, Hagberg JM, Hurley BF, Ehsani AA, Holloszy JO. Effect of endurance training on glucose tolerance and plasma lipid levels in older men and women. J Am Med Assoc 1984;252:645-9.

Sidney KH, Shephard RJ. Frequency and intensity of exercise training for elderly subjects. Med Sci Sports 1978;10:125-31.

Stamford BA. Physiological effects of training upon institutionalized geriatric men. J Gerontol 1972;27:451-5.

Suominen HE, Heikkinen E, Liesen H, Michel D, Hollmann E. Effect of eight weeks endurance training on skeletal muscle metabolism in 56-70-year-old sedentary men. Eur J Appl Physiol 1977;37:173-180.

Thomas SG, Cunningham DA, Rechnitzer PA, Donner AP, Howard JH. Determinants of the training response in elderly men. Med Sci Sports Exer 1985;17:667-72.

Tzankoff SP, Robinson S, Pyke FS, Brown CA. Physiological adjustments to work in older men as affected by physical training. J Appl Physiol 1972;33:346-50.

Vogel JA, Patton JF, Mello RP, Daniels WL. An analysis of aerobic capacity in a large United States population. J Appl Physiol 1986;60:494-500.

Effects of Chronic, Intense Endurance Exercise Training on Longitudinal Changes in Maximal Oxygen Uptake in Older Men

Marc A. Rogers, Ph.D.

INTRODUCTION

Aging is associated with a decline in the functional capacity of the cardiovascular system that results in a decreased maximal oxygen uptake capacity ($\dot{V}O_2max$) (Åstrand et al., 1973; Hagberg, 1987; Buskirk and Hodgson, 1987; Pollock et al., 1987; Rogers et al., 1990). Heath et al. (1981) assembled cross-sectional data from 13 published studies in 563 healthy men aged 25 to 75 years and calculated that sedentary men experience a decline in $\dot{V}O_2max$ of about nine percent per decade while Master athletes who continue to engage in regular vigorous endurance training lose only about five percent of their cardiovascular capacity per decade (Figure 1). In the case of Master athletes, this decrease in $\dot{V}O_2max$ contributes to the decline in maximal performance capacity in competitive events, while in sedentary individuals the reduced functional capacity may be manifested by a greater difficulty in carrying out the activities of daily living (ADL). While cross-sectional and early longitudinal studies have suggested that the decrease in $\dot{V}O_2max$ is ~0.45 $ml{\bullet}kg^{-1}\,min^{-1}{\bullet}yr^{-1}$ in sedentary individuals (Hagberg, 1987), there are a number of factors that can potentially affect the rate of decline in the functional capacity of the cardiovascular system with aging. As shown in Table 1, five factors exist that can complicate the study of the aging cardiovascular system and thus need to be taken into consideration when quantifying the reduction of $\dot{V}O_2max$ with increasing age. Diseases such as coronary artery disease and hypertension have a negative effect on cardiac function as do nutritional deficiencies of protein intake and vitamins and minerals. An increase in percent body fat with age results in a decrease in $\dot{V}O_2max$ when expressed in $ml{\bullet}kg^{-1}{\bullet}min^{-1}$, and physical inactivity also reduces oxygen transport capacity. The aging process itself may be manifested by a decrease in the number of cells and a reduction in the efficiency of cellular function, damage to cells and a reduced capacity for cellular repair.

LONGITUDINAL STUDIES

The initial longitudinal study performed to evaluate the effects of aging on the cardiovascular system of young healthy individuals was done in 1949 in a group of 66 physical education students who had a $\dot{V}O_2max$ test and were restudied 20 years later (Åstrand et al., 1973). Men and women who remained habitually active in their leisure and work pursuits experienced a 20 percent decline in $\dot{V}O_2max$, along with a 12 to 15 $beats{\bullet}min^{-1}$ reduction in maximal heart rate. However, it is likely that some increases in physical activity in the months prior to the re-evaluation may have masked the effect of 20 years of aging on $\dot{V}O_2max$ since the subjects knew they were to be retested (Åstrand et al., 1973). In any case, this was the first study to show an approximate reduction in $\dot{V}O_2max$ on the order of 10 percent per decade. It should be mentioned that the subjects in this study were not following an endurance training program, but were nonetheless physically active.

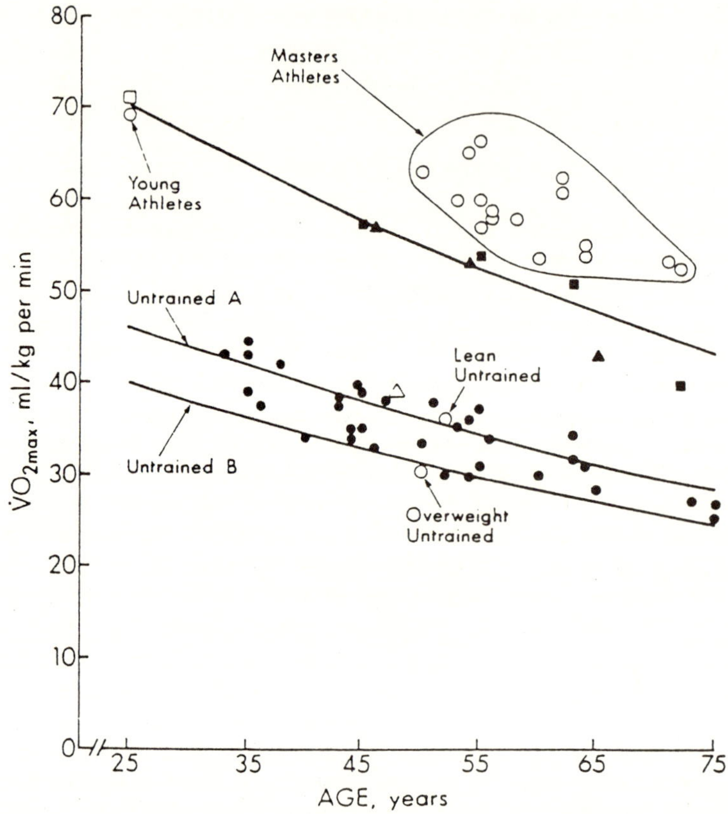

Figure 1. Decline in $\dot{V}O_2max$ with age of healthy, sedentary and endurance-trained men.

0 = Heath et al, 1981

□ = Dill et al, 1967

△ = Robinson et al, 1976

△ = Grimby and Saltin, 1966

● = groups of untrained men from 9 studies

(Reprinted with permission of The American Physiological Society from Heath et al. A physiological comparison of young and older endurance athletes. J Appl Physiol 1981;51:634-640)

TABLE 1

Factors Affecting the Functional Capacity of the Cardiovascular System with Aging

* Disease
* Nutritional Status
* Change in Body Weight
* Physical Inactivity
* Aging Process, *Per Se*

Dill et al. (1967) were the first to test a group of former Olympic caliber distance runners in a 25-year follow-up study. They found that the runners' $\dot{V}O_2max$ had declined at a rate of 1.1 $ml \cdot kg^{-1} \cdot min \cdot yr^{-1}$, a rate of decline much greater than is typical of healthy, sedentary individuals (Buskirk and Hodgson, 1987). The most probable explanation for this accelerated rate of decline was that these champion endurance athletes had attained a very high $\dot{V}O_2max$ as a result of many years of intense training, reaching the "biological ceiling" for cardiovascular capacity in humans. Once their competitive careers were over, however, most of these athletes had completely stopped endurance training and became sedentary. Therefore, the rapid decline cannot be solely attributed to the effects of aging but rather to a combination of aging and the effects of physical inactivity. In support of this hypothesis, one individual in this elite group continued to train over the interim of 20 years and evidenced a much slower rate of decline in $\dot{V}O_2max$, on the order of 0.40 $ml \cdot kg^{-1} \cdot min^{-1} \cdot yr^{-1}$, a rate which was approximately 25 percent slower than the subject with the next slowest rate of change (Dill et al., 1967; Robinson et al., 1976).

EFFECT OF CONSTANT ENDURANCE EXERCISE TRAINING ON $\dot{V}O_2$MAX

In addition to these early studies, Dehn and Bruce (1972) and Kasch and Wallace (1976, 1985) have attempted to determine if continued physical activity can have an effect on the rate of decline in $\dot{V}O_2max$ with aging. Men between the ages of 40 and 72 years were studied before and after 30 months of jogging an average of three miles per week and were found to have a significantly slower rate of decline in $\dot{V}O_2max$, corrected for changes in body weight, than men engaged in recreational activities (Dehn and Bruce, 1972). A subsequent 10-year follow-up study in middle-aged men has shown that training can prevent the decline in $\dot{V}O_2max$, expressed in $l \cdot min^{-1}$ or in $ml \cdot kg^{-1} \cdot min^{-1}$ (Kasch and Wallace, 1976). Even though the subjects in this study were running approximately 15 miles per week at an intensity of greater than 60 percent of $\dot{V}O_2max$, they were probably not receiving a constant training stimulus over the 10 years, since about half of the subjects increased their $\dot{V}O_2max$ by more than 10 percent. This suggests that an *increased* training stimulus probably accounted for the maintenance of $\dot{V}O_2max$ in these subjects over time. The subsequent 18-year follow-up (Kasch and Wallace, 1985) showed a 10 percent decline in $\dot{V}O_2max$ over the intervening eight years when expressed in $l \cdot min^{-1}$, but no change in terms of $\dot{V}O_2max$ in $ml \cdot kg^{-1} \cdot min$-[1] due to the fact that the men had lost 10 pounds. Thus, not only the constancy of the training stimulus but also changes in body weight must be taken into account when ascertaining the effect of aging on the decline in $\dot{V}O_2$max. In this context, 20-year-old and 50-year-old endurance athletes have been matched on the volume of endurance training and their respective performance times to determine the effect of aging, *per se*, on the decline in $\dot{V}O_2$max (Heath et al., 1981). $\dot{V}O_2$max and maximal heart rate were 15 percent lower in the Master athletes, while O_2 pulse during maximal exercise ($\dot{V}O_2$max/maximal heart rate, an index of stroke volume) was similar. These results provide evidence that supports the idea that the decline in $\dot{V}O_2$max is ~5 percent per decade in older endurance-trained individuals and, secondly, that the decline in $\dot{V}O_2$max can be attributed primarily to a reduction in maximal heart rate (Heath et al., 1981).

LONGITUDINAL MASTER ATHLETE STUDIES

A definitive answer to the question regarding the magnitude of the age-related reduction in $\dot{V}O_2$max can be provided only via well-controlled, longitudinal endurance training studies carried out over an extended period of time. With this in mind, Pollock et al. (1987) evaluated the effects of age and training on the $\dot{V}O_2$max and body composition of twenty-four 50-to-80-year-old Master athlete runners over a 10-year period. The athletes in this study were considered to be elite in that they had finished first, second or third in regional or national Masters competition. Table 2 shows the cardiovascular data for the group of 24, initially and at the 10-year follow-up. Even though all the athletes continued their endurance exercise training, they experienced a significant reduction in $\dot{V}O_2$max, maximal O_2 pulse, maximal heart rate and endurance time on the treadmill test. Of further interest was the finding that percent body fat increased (~2 percent) and fat-free weight decreased significantly by about 2 kg (data not shown). Based on activity questionnaires and interviews, it was determined at the follow-up testing that many of the subjects had not maintained a constant training stimulus throughout the intervening years, so therefore the subjects were placed into a competitive group (COMP) or post-competitive (Post-COMP) group. The COMP group consisted of individuals who were "actively training for high-level competition" and who had a daily training intensity that was within 30 seconds per mile of the intensity at the initial testing. The Post-COMP group had ceased to participate in competition and their training intensity had decreased by ~90 seconds per mile. The post-hoc analysis of the data shown in Table 2 indicates that the COMP subjects who maintained a relatively constant training stimulus were able to maintain their $\dot{V}O_2$max and O_2 pulse max over the 10 years of the study, and did not experience a decrease in endurance time on the treadmill, while the subjects who decreased their training experienced a 12 percent decline in $\dot{V}O_2$max as well as significant reductions in maximal O_2 pulse, maximal heart rate and treadmill test time. While it is apparent that regular, vigorous endurance exercise training had the capacity to maintain $\dot{V}O_2$max in the COMP distance runners, they nevertheless had a 7 beats•min^{-1} reduction in maximal heart rate, thus suggesting that stroke volume or oxygen extraction in active skeletal muscle must have been increased from the initial to the follow-up testing. In any case, while this study was the first to show that endurance exercise training can prevent the decline in cardiovascular capacity over 10 years of aging, this exercise effect would probably not last indefinitely.

In 1990, Rogers and co-workers published a study where they remeasured $\dot{V}O_2$max in groups of 60-year-old, healthy, sedentary control and Master athlete subjects who had participated in various exercise and aging studies in the Applied Physiolgy Section at Washington University School of Medicine in St. Louis (Rogers et al., 1990). The Master athletes had been training for an average of 10 years prior to the initial testing and were then retested eight years later while they continued to train and compete in distance running races. All testing of the Master athlete subjects took place at the point of their competitive season when they judged themselves to be in peak fitness. At the follow-up evaluation it was determined from training questionnaires that the Master athletes had reduced the training stimulus (training duration by 10 minutes per day, intensity by ~25 seconds per mile and weekly mileage by ~10 miles) and had a 2:00 performance decrement in their best 10-kilometer (6.2-mile) race times. The control group in this study consisted of healthy, *lean*, individuals of the same age who maintained their body weight and percent body fat over the course of the study but did no regular aerobic training.

TABLE 2

Decline in Cardiovascular Capacity with Aging in Master Athlete Distance Runners

	Total (N=24)	**Comp (N=11)**	**Post-Comp (N=13)**
$\dot{V}O_2max$ (ml • kg^{-1} • min^{-1}			
Initial	53.3 ± 7.5	54.2 ± 7.0	52.5 ± 8.1
10 Yr	49.3 ± 7.1†	53.3 ± 5.4	45.9 ± 6.7†
%Δ	7.5	-	12.6
O_2 Pulsemax (ml • beat^{-1})			
Initial	21.6 ± 3.9	20.7 ± 2.6	22.4 ± 4.6
10 Yr	20.4 ± 3.3*	20.8 ± 2.1	20.0 ± 4.2†
HRmax			
Initial	173 ± 12	177 ± 11	170 ± 13
10 Yr	166 ± 12†	170 ± 11*	163 ± 11†
TM Time (min)			
Initial	9.1 ± 2.6	10.6 ± 3.0	7.9 ± 1.6
10 Yr	8.0 ± 3.0†	9.8 ± 3.2	6.6 ± 2.0†

Values are means ± SE
Significantly different from initial: *$p<0.05$; † $p<0.01$

Comp = competitive runner; Post-comp = non-competitive
HRmax = maximal heart rate
O_2 Pulsemax = maximal oxygen pulse
$\dot{V}O_2max$ = maximal oxygen consumption

(Pollock et al., 1987)

As shown in Table 3, the Master athletes' $\dot{V}O_2max$ declined by five percent, while the age-matched sedentary subjects experienced a twofold greater reduction over the course of the study. Maximal oxygen pulse decreased significantly by 0.02 ml•beat^{-1} in both groups while treadmill time decreased by ~2:00 in the control group with no change in the actively training Master athletes (data not shown). Interestingly, while the sedentary subjects showed a 10 beat•min^{-1} reduction in maximal heart rate per decade that is typically observed in aging studies, the Master athletes' maximal heart rate was maintained at 171 beats•min^{-1} throughout the eight years. This is the first published indication that regular, vigorous endurance exercise training can slow the age-associated reduction in maximal heart rate (Rogers et al., 1990). It may be that in some well-trained older endurance athletes the decline in $\dot{V}O_2max$ is due to a reduction in stroke volume or oxygen extraction, an observation not supported by the findings of Pollock et al. (1987).

TABLE 3

Decline in $\dot{V}O_2max$, O_2Pulsemax and HRmax with Aging in Sedentary Subjects and Master Athletes

	Master Athletes (N=15)	Controls (N=14)
$\dot{V}O_2max$ (l•min^{-1})		
Initial	3.68 ± 0.13	2.73 ± 0.14
8 Yr	3.54 ± 0.14*	2.45 ± 0.12†
$\dot{V}O_2max$ (ml•kg^{-1}•min^{-1})		
Initial	54.0 ± 1.7	33.9 ± 1.7
8 Yr	51.8 ± 1.8*	30.6 ± 1.6†
% Δ	4.7	9.7
O_2Pulse_{max} (ml•beat^{-1})		
Initial	0.32 ± 0.01	0.20 ± 0.01
8 Yr	0.30 ± 0.01*	0.18 ± 0.01*
HRmax		
Initial	171 ± 3	171 ± 3
8 Yr	171 ± 3	163 ± 4†

Values are means ± SE
Significantly different from initial: *$p<0.05$; † $p<0.01$
HR_{max} = maximal heart rate
O_2 $Pulse_{max}$ = maximal oxygen pulse
$\dot{V}O_2max$ = maximal oxygen consumption

Modified from Rogers et al, 1990.

RATES OF DECLINE IN $\dot{V}O_2$MAX WITH AGING

The loss of cardiovascular capacity ($\dot{V}O_2$max) with aging can be expressed not only in terms of an absolute value ($\dot{V}O_2$max in $l \cdot min^{-1}$), a relative amount per unit of body weight ($ml \cdot kg^{-1} \cdot min^{-1}$) and a percent decrease in $\dot{V}O_2$max per decade but also in terms of a rate, *e.g.*, $\dot{V}O_2$max in $ml \cdot kg^{-1} \cdot min^{-1}\ yr^{-1}$. Summary Table 4 shows the results of four, relatively well-controlled eight to 15-year longitudinal studies in healthy trained men who were initially in their late 20's (Marti et al., 1991; Marti and Howald, 1990) or mid 50's (Pollock et al., 1987; Rogers et al., 1990) and the corresponding rates of decline in $\dot{V}O_2$max. In most cases, the sedentary control subjects showed the greatest rates of decline in $\dot{V}O_2$max, ranging from 0.44 to 1.11 $ml \cdot kg^{-1} \cdot min^{-1}\ yr^{-1}$, while those endurance-trained individuals who maintained the relative quantity and quality of their training program with a constant stimulus evidenced the slowest rate of decline in $\dot{V}O_2$max. A comparison of the rate of decline in $\dot{V}O_2$max of Marti et al.'s (1991) 20-year-old runners (0.33 $ml \cdot kg^{-1} \cdot min \cdot 1 yr^{-1}$) with the 55-year-old runners of Rogers and coworkers (1990) (0.32 $ml \cdot kg^{-1} \cdot min^{-1} yr^{-1}$) surprisingly shows that aging itself may not affect the rate of decline of the maximal capacity of the cardiovascular system, all other things being equal. The fact that young and older distance runners who maintain their training may have equivalent rates of decline in $\dot{V}O_2$max suggests that reductions in cardiovascular capacity may be due to changes in physical

TABLE 4

Rate of Decline of $\dot{V}O_2$max with Aging in Well-trained Subjects

Study	Group	Duration (yr)	Rate ($ml \cdot kg^{-1} \cdot min^{-1} \cdot yr^{-1}$)
Marti et al. (1991)	Runners/Orienteers (current)	15	0.33
	Runners/Orienteers (former)	15	1.07
	Controls	15	0.57
Marti and Howald (1990)	Runners/Bobsledders (Highly Active)	15	0
	Runners/Bobsledders (Active)	15	0.54
	Controls	15	1.11
Rogers et al. (1990)	Master Athlete Runners	8	0.32
	Controls	8	0.44
Pollock et al. (1987)	Master Athlete Runners (Comp)	10	0.09
	Master Athlete Runners (Post-Comp)	10	0.66

Comp, current = presently involved in competition
Duration = length of followup
Post-Comp, former = formerly involved in competition but still training
0 = no change

activity rather then the effects of aging, *per se*. This notion is supported by the fact that the young subjects in Marti's studies maintained a more intense training stimulus in terms of duration and intensity(Marti et al., 1991; Marti and Howald, 1990).

CONCLUSION

Early cross-sectional and longitudinal studies that were undertaken to document the effects of aging on the cardiovascular system failed to take into account a number of factors that independently and perhaps synergistically could result in a decreased functional capacity, factors such as the presence of disease, nutritional status, changes in body weight and physical inactivity. Considerable recent evidence now indicates that physical activity in the form of regular, vigorous endurance exercise training can temporarily prevent the decline in $\dot{V}O_2$max with aging (Pollock et al.,1987) or decrease the rate of decline in actively training individuals when compared to healthy, yet sedentary, age-matched controls. The cross-sectional data from Heath et al. (1981) in a large sample of healthy individuals plus the longitudinal data from Rogers et al. (1990) in Master athletes indicate that deterioration of the cardiovascular system as the result of the aging process *per se* in men who maintain a relatively constant exercise training stimulus appears to result in a decline in $\dot{V}O_2$max of only ~5 percent per decade in comparison to the 10 percent reduction typically seen in healthy, sedentary men. This seems to indicate that roughly 50 percent of the decline in $\dot{V}O_2$max with aging is the result of physical inactivity and therefore is potentially preventable.

ACKNOWLEDGEMENTS

The author's research was originally supported in part by National Institute on Aging Program Project Grant #AG-05562. Special appreciation is extended to the Master athlete distance runners (LP, RJ, OH, ES, PS, CH, JG, ED, RS, JAB, HC, LG, DS, TR, LE, NC, TKC) for their time, dedication and interest in our exercise and aging research. This manuscript is dedicated to the memory of the Reverend Ray Sears who was a distance runner for the last 65 of his 80 years.

REFERENCES

Åstrand I, Åstrand P-O, Hallback I, Kilbom Å. Reduction in maximal O_2 uptake with age. J Appl Physiol 1973;35:649-54.

Buskirk ER, Hodgson JL. Age and aerobic power: the rate of change in men and women. Federation Proc 1987;46:1824-9.

Dehn MM, Bruce RA. Longitudinal variations in maximal oxygen uptake with age and activity. J Appl Physiol 1972;33:805-7.

Dill DB, Robinson S, Ross JC. A longitudinal study of 16 champion runners. J Sports Med Phys Fitness 1967;7:4-27.

Grimby G, Saltin, B. Physiological analysis of physically well trained middle-aged and old athletes. Acta Med Scand 1966;179:513-26.

Hagberg, JM. Effect of training on the decline of $\dot{V}O_2$max with aging. Federation Proc 1987;46:1830-3.

Heath GW, Hagberg JM, Ehsani AA, Holloszy JO. A physiological comparison of young and older endurance athletes. J Appl Physiol 1981;51:634-40.

Kasch FW, Wallace, JP. Physiological variables during 10 years of endurance exercise. Med Sci Sports 1976;8:5-8.

Kasch FW, Wallace, JP, Van Camp, SP. Effects of 18 years of endurance exercise on the physical work capacity of older men. J Cardiac Rehabil 1985;5:308-12.

Marti B, Howald, H. Long-term effects of physical training on aerobic capacity: controlled study of former elite athletes. J Appl Physiol 1990; 69:1451-9.

Marti B, Knobloch M, Riesen W, Howald H. Fifteen-year changes in exercise, aerobic power, abdominal fat and serum lipids in runners and controls. Med Sci Sports Exerc 1991;23:115-22.

Pollock ML, Foster C, Knapp P, Rod JL, Schmidt DH. Effect of age and training on aerobic capacity and body composition of Master athletes. J Appl Physiol 1987;62:725-31.

Robinson S, Dill DB, Robinson RD, Tzankoff SP, Wagner JA. Physiological aging of champion runners. J Appl Physiol 1976;41:46-51.

Rogers MA, Hagberg JM, Martin III WH, Ehsani AA, Holloszy JO. Decline in $\dot{V}O_2$max with aging in Master athletes and sedentary men. J Appl Physiol 1990; 68:2195-9.

Age-Related Decline of Aerobic Capacity in Aged Runners

Mitsuru Higuchi, Ph.D., Yutaka Yoshitake, Ph.D., Keiko Ishii, R.D.
Michiko Koda, M.S., Toshiki Ohta, M.D., Shuhei Kobayashi, M.D.

INTRODUCTION

Maximal oxygen uptake has been widely accepted as a good index of the functional capacity of the cardiorespiratory system. The maximal oxygen uptake in adults decreases with age (Åstrand et al., 1973), some of which decline seems to be the inevitable deterioration of the adaptive mechanisms of the heart and circulation.

Heath et al. (1981) have summarized data from nine mostly cross-sectional studies and noted that a nine percent per decade average decline in maximal oxygen uptake expressed in terms of ml/kg body weight/min occurred from the age of 25 years. Furthermore, they hypothesized, on the basis of a comparison of young and Master athletes, that if physical activity level and body composition remain relatively constant the deterioration attributable to the aging process *per se* results in a decline in maximal oxygen uptake of approximately five percent per decade. However, only limited data are available to evaluate the decline of maximal oxygen uptake in Master athletes who have been regularly training for vigorous endurance exercise.

Recently, follow-up studies on aerobic capacity in Master athletes have been published by Pollock et al. (1987) and Rogers et al. (1990). The decline in rates of maximal oxygen uptake in Master athletes, aged 62 years on the average at the follow-up, were 0.40 and 0.32 ml/kg/min/year in the studies of Pollock et al. (1987) and Rogers et al. (1990), respectively.

However, no data are available to evaluate maximal oxygen uptake decline associated with advancing age after 60 or 70 years in Master athletes. In the present study, we therefore remeasured maximal oxygen uptake in a group of Master athletes aged over 60 years after an average follow-up period of 6.5 years to obtain further information regarding the influence of regularly performed endurance exercise on the decline of maximal oxygen uptake with aging.

SUBJECTS

Subjects were seventeen Master athletes, who were 60 to 78 years old when they participated in our previous cross-sectional study (Fuchi et al., 1989). The Master athletes had been training regularly for an average of 13 years before they were first tested (T_1) in our laboratory (range three to 40 years) and were competing in local 5-km, 10-km, or marathon races. The seventeen endurance-trained men (aged 67 to 83 years) were retested after a 6.5-year follow-up (T_2). All subjects continued their endurance running training. The physical characteristics, training conditions, and race speeds of the Master athletes are shown in Table 1. The subjects were not taking any medications known to affect endurance exercise performance. The study was approved by the Human Studies Committee at National Institute of Health and Nutrition, and all subjects provided written informed consent.

TABLE 1

Physical Characteristics, Training Conditions, and Race Speeds for Master Athletes

Variables	Initial	Follow-up
Age, years	65.6 ± 5.1	72.0 ± 4.7*
Height, cm	162 ± 4	162 ± 4
Weight, kg	54 ± 3.8	54.1 ± 4.5
Fat-free weight, kg	47.8 ± 2.9	47.3 ± 3.5
Estimated body fat, %	11.5 ± 1.8	13.0 ± 2.7*
Consecutive years of training, years	13.0 ± 8.8	19.1 ± 8.3*
Training distance, km/week	46.8 ±19.9	38.6 ± 20.7
Race time		
5 km, min (11)	21.8 ± 1.8	24.2 ± 2.1*
10 km, min (12)	43.8 ± 3.6	48.3 ± 4.7*

mean ±SD n=17, Numbers in parentheses are sample size if different from 17.
*p<0.01 vs. initial testing.

METHOD

Exercise Testing and Measurement of Maximal Oxygen Uptake

All subjects underwent a history and physical examination, a resting electrocardiogram, and a maximal exercise test according to the protocol of Saltin and Åstrand (1967) on a motor-driven treadmill to determine their maximal oxygen uptake. All exercise tests were terminated as the result of subject fatigue. The criteria for obtaining maximal oxygen uptake were: (1) a plateau of maximal oxygen uptake against workload, or (2) respiratory exchange ratio >1.

Treadmill speed was varied depending on the race-time of each subject (generally 10 m/min less at the follow-up test than at the initial test). The inclination of the treadmill was increased by 2.6 percent every three minutes. The expired gases were collected in Douglas bags during the last two to three minutes of each period. The volume of the expired gases was measured with a dry gas meter. The oxygen and carbon dioxide content of the collected gases was analyzed using a paramagnetic and infrared gas-analyzer (Minato Medical Science Gas Analyzer, MG-360) calibrated with gases analyzed by the Scholander technique. Heart rates were recorded electrocardiographically.

Body Composition

Skinfold thickness measurements were made with a caliper at two sites (subscapular and triceps). Body density was estimated from the skinfold thickness measurements using the equation developed for a Japanese population (Nagamine and Suzuki, 1964). Relative body fat (percent) was estimated from this value (Brozek et al., 1963).

The Master athletes' initial and follow-up tests were both conducted during a competitive session.

STATISTICS

Paired t-tests were used to determine significant differences in the dependent variables over time. Data are presented as means ± standard deviation (SD).

RESULTS

Physical Characteristics

Although the body weights of the Master athletes did not change significantly between the initial and follow-up evaluations, percent body fat, estimated from skinfolds, was increased significantly from initial to follow-up testing (Table 1).

Training Data

Weekly training distance declined slightly, although the change was not statistically significant, from initial to follow-up testing. Their average running speed of 5-km or 10-km in the recent year was slower by nine to 10 percent at the follow-up than it was at the initial evaluation (Table 1).

All subjects performed respiratory exchange ratio >1 at both the initial and follow-up testing, and nine of 11 subjects terminated the exercise test at a plateau of maximal oxygen intake against workload at the initial and follow-up testing, respectively. The data for maximal oxygen uptake, whether expressed in terms of liters/min, ml/kg body weight/min, or ml/kg fat-free weight/min show a significant decline by 10 to 12 percent from the initial to follow-up evaluations. Maximal heart rate did not decrease (170 vs. 167 beats/min). Oxygen pulse at maximal heart rate was remarkably reduced by 10 percent. Maximal pulmonary minute ventilation decreased significantly from 89 to 79 liters/min from the initial to the follow-up testing (Table 2).

TABLE 2

Maximal Oxygen Uptake and Related Variables of Master Athletes

Variables	Initial	Follow-up
Maximal oxygen uptake		
l/min	2.64 ± 0.31	2.32 ± 0.24*
ml/kg /min	48.5 ± 4.5	42.9 ± 4.3*
ml/kg fat-free weight/min	55.1 ± 4.8	49.4 ± 4.6*
Maximal heart rate, beats/min	170 ± 10	167 ± 9
Maximal oxygen pulse, ml/kg/beat	0.29 ± 0.03	0.26 ± 0.03*
Maximal ventilation, l/min	89.3 ± 15.0	79.4 ± 12.4*

mean ± SD. n=17 *p<0.01 vs. initial.

DISCUSSION

We previously studied cross-sectionally the age-related decline of maximal oxygen uptake and related variables by matching body composition and weekly running mileage in fifty-five male long-distance Master runners who could run at a 10-km race speed within approximately 80 percent of the speed of Japanese Master athletes recorded in each age group. In these runners, 10-km-run velocity decreased significantly with advancing age at a rate of six percent per decade, 1.7 m/min/year (Fuchi et al., 1989). The maximal oxygen uptake also decreased significantly with increase in age at a rate of approximately seven percent per decade (0.44 ml/kg/min/year).

In the present longitudinal study, the average rate of decline in 10-km race speed was 3.2 m/min/year, which was steeper than that obtained by the previous cross-sectional study. The decline of maximal oxygen uptake averaged 0.87 ml/kg/min/year, which was higher than the value obtained by the cross-sectional study. The decline rate of the maximal oxygen uptake for our Master athletes was also remarkably higher than those obtained by both Pollock et al. (1987) and Rogers et al. (1990). In this regard, the Master athletes in the studies of both Pollock et al. (1987) and Rogers et al. (1990) were younger (62.3 ± 9.1 and

62.0 ± 2.3 years at follow-up, respectively) than our Master athletes (72.0 ± 4.7 years at follow-up). Furthermore, in the Master athletes who participated in the studies of Pollock et al. (1987), the eleven subjects were still highly competitive and continued to train at the same running mileage (approximately 35 miles per week) and intensity. The other 13 Master athletes became noncompetitive and slightly reduced their running mileage, from 26 to 22 miles per week, and reduced training intensity. The results in the study of Pollock et al. (1987) showed that the competitive group maintained its maximal oxygen uptake: the rate of decline in maximal oxygen uptake was only 0.09 ml/kg/min/ year; while the non-competitive group showed a significant decline of maximal oxygen uptake from initial test to 10-year follow-up: the rate of decline in maximal oxygen uptake was 0.64 ml/kg/min/year. Rogers et al. (1990) also demonstrated that the Master athletes who maintained higher intensity and weekly mileage in their training had a slower rate of decline in maximal oxygen uptake (0.32 ml/kg/min/year) with aging.

In the present study, although the Master athletes did not substantially reduce their running mileage, they mentioned that they could not maintain higher levels of training intensity because of fatigue. As indicated by Pollock et al. (1987), it appears that older athletes, particularly aged over 70 years, have the most difficulty in maintaining their performance times, which could be associated with their training conditions. Taking these studies into consideration, the rate of decline in maximal oxygen uptake for our Master athletes is reasonable.

It has been widely accepted that the increase in body weight and decrease in the habitual level of physical activity that typically occur with aging contribute to the decline of maximal oxygen uptake when expressed in terms of ml/kg body weight/min. In the present study, although the Master athletes did not change their body weights from the first testing to the follow-up testing, they increased the estimated percent of body fat content, which was associated with a slight reduction of lean body weight as shown in Table 1. As shown in Table 2, the Master athletes decreased their maximal oxygen uptake by 11.5 percent and 10.5 percent when expressed in terms of ml/kg body weight/min and ml/kg fat-free weight/min, respectively, from the initial testing to the follow-up testing.

Fleg and Lakatta (1988) have shown in a cross-sectional study that a large portion of the age-associated decline in maximal oxygen uptake in nonendurance-trained individuals, 22 to 87 years of age, is explained by the loss of muscle mass, which was observed with advancing age. Rogers et al. (1990), however, have indicated significant decrease of maximal oxygen uptake in terms of ml/kg body weight/min in sedentary men (9.7 percent) and Master athletes (4.1 percent) without changes of fat-free weight from the initial to the follow-up testing. Pollock et al. (1987) observed that Master athletes decreased their maximal oxygen uptake by 7.5 percent and 4.6 percent when expressed in terms of ml/kg body weight/min and ml/kg fat-free weight/min, respectively, from the initial to the follow-up testing. In this context, we considered that in aging Master athletes the decrease of maximal oxygen uptake might be induced by some other factors in addition to the loss of muscle mass with aging.

In the present study, although there was no statistical difference in heart rate at the point of maximal oxygen uptake between the initial and follow-up tests, a significant decrease was observed in oxygen pulse at maximal heart rate. Fuchi et al. (1989) indicated that the age-related decline of maximal oxygen uptake in Master athletes was mainly explained by the central factors (represented by the decline of maximal heart rate and maximal cardiac output), rather than by a peripheral factor (represented by maximal arterio-venous oxygen difference). Therefore it could be considered that stroke volume was mainly reduced in the Master athletes from the initial to follow-up tests. Coggan et al. (1990) indicated that Master athletes have higher levels of mitochondrial enzyme activities and greater muscle capillarization compared with the matched young athletes despite having a lower maximal oxygen uptake. These findings suggest that the decline of maximal oxygen uptake in Master athletes could be explained by the cardio-respiratory system rather than skeletal muscle function.

As shown in Figure 1, we observed a higher rate of age-related decline in maximal oxygen uptake than did either Pollock et al. (1987) or Rogers et al. (1990). Pollock et al. (1987) tried to assess whether or not there was a sharp reduction in maximal oxygen uptake after age 70. From their results they concluded that Master athletes above 70 years of age do not show the sharp reduction of maximal oxygen uptake with aging and, also, that their previous cross-sectional study (Pollock et al., 1974), using a small sample for subjects 70 years and older, can be misleading. However, Pollock et al. (1987), also described that the cell sizes among groups in the literature were too small to attempt any conclusions at that time. Therefore, further studies are needed to determine whether sharp reductions of maximal oxygen uptake occur after the age of 70 years in Master athletes.

CONCLUSION

These results suggest that the decline in maximal oxygen uptake capacity with age may be greater in runners aged above 60 years of age who reduce training mileage and intensity than in runners aged less than 60 years and that it could be very difficult to prevent the age-related decrease of maximal oxygen uptake in older Master runners who can not maintain their training intensities.

ACKNOWLEDGEMENTS

We would like to acknowledge Dr. Marc Rogers, the Department of Kinesiology, University of Maryland, for his constructive comments.

This study was supported by the Research Grant on Aging and Health, and by the Research Grant on Cardiovascular Diseases, Ministry of Health and Welfare, Japan.

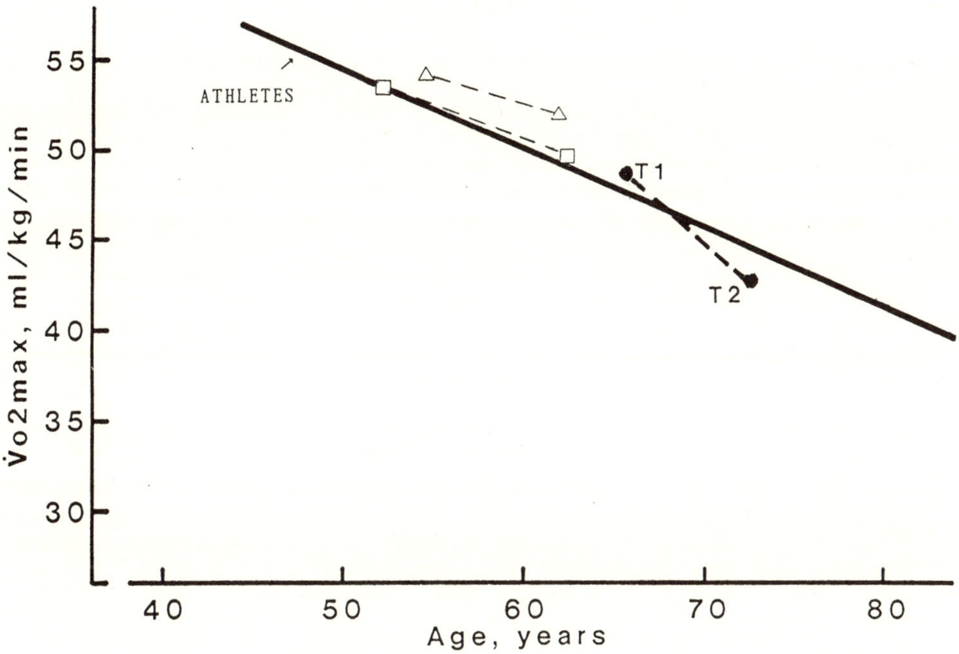

Figure 1. Maximal oxygen uptake ($\dot{V}O_2max$)of endurance Master runners. Linear regression line for endurance runners is obtained by the cross-sectional study of Fuchi et al. (1989).

Longitudinal studies:

Present Study: ● - - ●

Pollock et al. (1987): □ - - □

Rogers et al. (1990): △ - - △

T_1=initial and T_2=follow-up data in the present study

Decline rate of $\dot{V}O_2max$

0.32 ml/lg/min/year: cross sectional study of Fuchi et al. (1989)

0.44 ml/kg/min/year: present study.

0.87 ml/kg/min/year: Pollock et al. (1987).

0.40 ml/kg/min/year: Rogers et al. (1990).

REFERENCES

Åstrand I., Åstrand P-O, Hallback I, Kilbom Å. Reduction in maximal oxygen uptake with age. J Appl Physiol 1973;35:649-54.

Brozek J, Grand J, Anderson JT, Keys A. Densitometric analysis of body composition: revision of some quantitative assumptions. Ann NY Acad Sci 1963;110:113-40.

Coggan AR, Spina RJ, Rogers MA et al. Histochemical and enzymatic characteristics of skeletal muscle in Master athletes. J Appl Physiol 1990;68:1896-901.

Fleg JL, Lakatta EG. Role of muscle loss in the age-associated reduction in $\dot{V}O_2$ max. J Appl Physiol 1988;65:1147-51.

Fuchi T, Iwaoka K, Higuchi M, Kobayashi S. Cardiovascular changes associated with decreased aerobic capacity and aging in long-distance runners. Eur J Appl Physiol 1989;58:884-9.

Heath GW, Hagberg JM, Ehsani AA, Holloszy JO. A physiological comparison of young and older endurance athletes. J Appl Physiol 1981;51:634-40.

Nagamine S, Suzuki S. Anthropometry and body composition of Japanese young men and women. Hum Biol 1964;36:8-15.

Pollock ML, Foster C, Knapp D, Rod JL, Schmidt DH. Effect of age and training on aerobic capacity and body composition of Master athletes. J Appl Physiol 1987;62:725-31.

Pollock ML, Miller Jr HS, Wilmore J. Physiological characteristics of champion American track athletes 40 to 75 years of age. J Gerontol 1974;29: 645-9.

Rogers MA, Hagberg JM, Martin III WH, Ehsani AA, Holloszy JO. Decline in $\dot{V}O_2$max with aging in Master athletes and sedentary men. J Appl Physiol 1990;68:2195-9.

Saltin B, Åstrand P-O. Oxygen uptake in athletes. J Appl Physiol 1967;23:353-8.

Longitudinal Assessment of Aerobic Work Capacity in the Elderly

Nobuo Takeshima, Ph.D., Kiyoji Tanaka, Ph.D, Takemasa Watanabe, M.D.
Fumio Kobayashi, M.D., Takashi Kato, M.D.

INTRODUCTION

The magnitude of the exercise effect is related to the initial level of cardiorespiratory fitness, training stimulus (intensity, frequency, and duration of exercise sessions), and duration of the training program. It is thought that physical exercise has a favorable effect on aerobic work capacity of older individuals. Hagberg et al. (1989) demonstrated that elderly men and women over 70 years old significantly improved cardiorespiratory fitness as a result of endurance exercise conditioning at moderate to high intensity. Recently, lactate threshold has been used as an index of aerobic work capacity and of training intensity in normal individuals as well as in patients with coronary heart disease, hypertension, and obesity (Davis et al., 1979; Meyer and Weideman, 1985; Urata et al., 1987; Henritze et al., 1985; Tanaka et al., 1986, 1989). However, studies on the increase of lactate threshold (Blumenthal et al., 1989; Belman and Gaesser, 1991) or ventilatory threshold (Thomas et al., 1985) with aerobic exercise in the elderly are inconsistent. It remains to be established whether improvement in aerobic work capacity or other attributes (e.g., serum lipids) requires a training intensity at or above the intensity corresponding to the lactate threshold.

The role of exercise frequency in determining exercise effects on the elderly has received little attention. In addition, most previous studies on the effect of exercise in the elderly used a training duration of less than 48 weeks (Badenhop et al., 1983; Seals et al., 1984; Yerg et al., 1985; Thomas et al., 1985). The present study was conducted to quantify the exercise training effects of a one-day-per-week program in comparison with a three-day-per-week program, and the long-term effect of a one-day-per-week program in the elderly was also evaluated.

SUBJECTS

Fourteen subjects were divided into two groups: a high-frequency group, who trained three times a week (n=8, 69.4 ± 4.4 years) and a low-frequency group, who trained once a week (n=6, 69.7 ± 3.6 years). None of the subjects had previously engaged in any regular exercise training program. The health status of the participants was determined from the following screening procedures: medical history, physical examination, hematological evaluation, urinalysis, chest x-ray, blood pressure, resting electrocardiogram (ECG), and graded exercise testing with ECG monitoring. None of the subjects had a personal history of heart attack, stroke, diabetes mellitus or hypertension. No significant differences between groups in pre-treatment baseline values were found in age, body mass index, oxygen uptake corresponding to lactate threshold, maximal oxygen uptake, heart rate corresponding to lactate threshold, and maximal heart rate.

METHODS

In the first phase of the project, subjects trained three days per week or one day per week, respectively, for 12 weeks. Following the 12-week exercise program, all subjects continued daily exercise once a week for three-and-a-half years.

Exercise Testing

A Monark cycle ergometer was used for the exercise testing. Following two-minute warm-up cycling at 0 watt, the power output was increased 15 watts every minute until voluntary exhaustion. The pedal rate was kept at 60 revolutions per minute. All measurements of expired gases were determined by standard techniques of open-circuit spirometry, using Mijnhardt Oxycon System. Gas analyzers for O_2 and CO_2 were calibrated immediately prior to and after each testing session with standard gases of known concentrations. Oxygen uptake, minute ventilation, and heart rate corresponding to lactate threshold and their maximal values were measured during exercise. Heart rate was continuously monitored via a 12-lead electrocardiogram (ML8000, Fukuda Electronics Co.). All subjects took the 12-minute walk distance test. The walk distance as a general endurance performance index was determined by self-selected pace walking (Takeshima et al., 1992).

Lactate Threshold

For detection of lactate threshold, a series of venous blood samples (1 ml each) were drawn every minute during exercise in the upright position from an antecubital vein of the right arm. Blood lactate determination was performed by the enzymatic-electrode method with a Cobas analyzer (Baxter Co.). Lactate threshold was conceptually defined as the point at which the rate of lactate production and diffusion exceeded the rate of its removal, and was detected as the point in exercise of increasing intensity at which lactate increased in a non-linear fashion. For discerning the point at which the increase of lactate became non-linear, the log-log transformation method was used (Beaver et al., 1985).

Assessment of Other Variables

Systolic and diastolic blood pressures, serum lipids and lipoproteins, hematological variables, and physical fitness variables were also measured. An atherogenic index (AI) was calculated as low-density lipoprotein cholesterol/high-density lipoprotein cholesterol. The details of blood analysis have been described elsewhere (Tanaka et al., 1989).

Exercise Conditioning

Each exercise session consisted of 10 to 15 minutes of warm-up and flexibility exercise, 30 minutes of cycling on a stationary ergometer, 30 minutes of recreational activities (walking, aerobic dancing, or mini-tennis), and five to ten minutes of cool-down activities. Training intensity corresponded to the watts or heart rate associated with the lactate threshold determined by the exercise test. After the 12-week exercise program, all subjects of both groups continued to participate in exercise conditioning programs once a week.

Statistics

The pre- and post-test data were analyzed by the paired t-test. To determine whether there were significant differences between high- and low-frequency groups, unpaired t-test was utilized. Cochran-Cox and Welch tests were used when the variance of each variable was significantly different between two groups. Statistical significance was set at $p<0.05$.

RESULTS

No significant group differences were obtained in pre-treatment baseline values for age, body mass index, oxygen uptake corresponding to lactate threshold, maximal oxygen uptake, heart rate corresponding to lactate threshold, and maximal heart rate (Tables 1 and 2). The effects of the 12-week exercise program were found to be significant for oxygen uptake corresponding to lactate threshold (16.8 ± 3.2 →19.3 ± 3.7 ml/kg/min), maximal oxygen uptake (28.9 ± 6.5 →32.5 ± 6.6 ml/kg/min), and 12-minute walk distance (1406 ± 210 → 1460 ± 208 m) in the high-frequency group, while no significant changes were observed in the low-frequency group (Table 2).

TABLE 1

Characteristics of the Subjects

Group	High-frequency	Low-frequency
Age (yr)	69.4 ± 4.4	69.7 ± 3.6
Height (cm)	158.8 ± 6.6	157.6 ± 4.3
Weight (kg)	56.9 ± 8.3	56.9 ± 9.0
Body mass index	22.6 ± 2.8	22.8 ± 2.4
Systolic blood pressure (mm Hg)	128.8 ± 13.2	128.5 ± 9.1
Diastolic blood pressure (mm Hg)	75.8 ± 12.6	81.7 ± 8.8

At 3.5 years follow-up of the program, however, in the high frequency group all the three variables that had increased significantly regressed to the pre-treatment baseline values, and the atherogenic index significantly increased from 2.40 ± 1.36 to 2.94 ± 1.06 (Table 3).

DISCUSSION

The American College of Sports Medicine (ACSM) has recommended that training intensity during conditioning sessions should not be prescribed to exceed 85 percent nor should it be lower than 50 percent of maximal oxygen uptake. For asymptomatic adults the average conditioning intensity is usually between 60 percent and 70 percent of maximal oxygen uptake (ACSM, 1986). Moreover, the ACSM (1986) suggests that, for sedentary persons regardless of whether they are asymptomatic or symptomatic, exercise frequency should be a minimum of three days per week and exercise duration should be at least 20 to 30 minutes per day. Although several factors can influence aerobic work capacity response to exercise training, it is generally agreed that exercise intensity is the key factor. In fact, the magnitude of improvement in the elderly has been linked to exercise intensity in many studies (Badenhop et al., 1983; Niinimaa et al., 1978; Seals et al., 1984; Sidney et al., 1978). These studies have shown that higher exercise intensities elicit greater increases in aerobic work capacity than lower exercise intensities.

TABLE 2

Physiological Effects of Exercise Conditioning on Aerobic Capacity in Each Group

Group	Pre	Post	After 3.5 Years
<u>High-Frequency</u>			
Oxygen uptake corresponding to lactate threshold (ml/kg/min)	16.8 ± 3.2	19.3 ± 3.7*	14.8 ± 1.6#
Heart rate corresponding to lactate threshold (beats/min)	105.9 ± 11.9	109.6 ± 14.0	106.5 ± 5.8
Maximal oxygen uptake (ml/kg/min)	28.9 ± 6.5	32.5 ± 6.6*	26.1 ± 4.4#
Maximal heart rate (beats/min)	154.1 ± 17.3	156.8 ± 15.3	155.4 ± 14.7
12-min walk distance (m)	1405.6 ± 209.5	1460.0 ± 207.5*	1197.8 ± 128.7#
<u>Low-Frequency</u>			
Oxygen uptake corresponding to lactate threshold (ml/kg/min)	14.2 ± 2.6	14.2 ± 2.1	13.2 ± 1.7
Heart rate corresponding to lactate threshold (beats/min)	102.8 ± 6.6	99.2 ± 12.5	105.5 ± 8.5
Maximal oxygen uptake (ml/kg/min)	22.8 ± 2.5	23.3 ± 2.2	22.3 ± 3.0
Maximal heart rate (beats/min)	153.7 ± 9.4	150.8 ± 11.5	148.2 ± 14.1
12-min walk distance (m)	1280.8 ± 80.2	1351.7 ± 111.8	1137.8 ± 105.2

* Significantly different from pre-value
# Significantly different from post-value

TABLE 3

Effects of Exercise Conditioning on Serum Lipids in Each Group

Group	Pre	Post	After 3.5 Years
High-Frequency			
Triglycerides (mg/dl)	116.6 ± 58.3	104.4 ± 50.9	118.3 ± 50.5
Total Cholesterol (mg/dl)	221.0 ± 38.3	205.6 ± 38.9*	222.6 ± 36.1
High-density lipoprotein cholesterol (mg/dl)	62.6 ± 18.2	58.0 ± 14.9	53.2 ± 16.8#
Atherogenic Index	2.40 ± 1.36	2.40 ± 1.39	2.94 ± 1.06#
Low-Frequency			
Triglycerides (mg/dl)	122.0 ± 56.3	108.5 ± 57.9	135.7 ± 75.0#
Total Cholesterol (mg/dl)	236.0 ± 43.3	212.0 ± 34.2*	231.0 ± 18.6
High-density lipoprotein cholesterol (mg/dl)	57.2 ± 14.1	56.5 ± 13.3	50.9 ± 11.3
Atherogenic Index	2.84 ± 0.90	2.45 ± 0.63	3.17 ± 0.94#

* Significantly different from pre-value
\# Significantly different from post-value

However, Katch et al. (1978) have indicated that even if subjects are exercising at the same relative percent of oxygen uptake or of maximal heart rate, the metabolic stress is not constant across subjects. The intensity of lactate threshold varies widely, from 50 percent or below to 70 percent or above maximal oxygen uptake, in normal elderly men and women (Takeshima et al., 1990). Yoshitake (1986) has shown a significant relationship among the noradrenaline, systolic blood pressure, rate-pressure product and blood lactate observed during submaximal exercise in middle-aged and elderly women. Especially the systolic blood pressure and rate-pressure product steeply increased at levels above the lactate threshold. Thus, the lactate threshold level may be a better intensity threshold to use to determine the exercise intensity for endurance training for elderly persons than the percent of maximal oxygen uptake.

Previous studies have utilized the lactate threshold level hypothesis as an optimal exercise intensity in patients with coronary heart disease (Tanaka et al., 1992), hypertension (Seals and Hagberg, 1984; Urata et al., 1987), and obesity (Tanaka et al., 1986, 1989). In the present study, the 12-week exercise program at the lactate threshold intensity were found to have beneficial effects on oxygen uptake corresponding to lactate threshold, maximal oxygen uptake, 12-minute walk distance and total cholesterol. It is very important that, in sedentary older men and women regardless of whether they are asymptomatic or symptomatic, exercise training contributes not only to increasing physical fitness but also to health related factors such as lipid and lipoprotein profiles. Failure to observe significant exercise-induced changes in lipids and/or lipoprotein variables except for total cholesterol may have been due to a lack of adequate exercise or of control over the subjects' condition (i.e., dietary habits). Further studies are needed to clarify effects of exercise training on serum lipid and lipoproteins.

The role of exercise frequency in determining the effects of exercise training on older people has received little attention. Studies generally show that a frequency of three days per week produces significant training effects (Denis et al., 1984; Gaesser et al., 1984; Massicotte et al., 1979; Pollock et al., 1975; Thomas et al., 1985; Wilmore et al., 1980). The results obtained in the present study also indicate that a 12-week exercise program contributed significantly to increased aerobic work capacity in the high-frequency group, while no significant differences were observed in the low-frequency group. Exercise frequency of one day per week does not appear to be an adequate stimulus to maintain increased aerobic work capacity.

Although all the subjects in the high-frequency group continued to do the same aerobic exercise once a week for an additional three-and-a-half years after the 12-week exercise program, it was not an adequate stimulus to maintain their initial training effect. Wood et al. (1984) suggest that the amount of exercise (i.e., 1200 to 1500 kcal per week of moderate-intensity exercise for 12 weeks or more) is more important than intensity to obtain significant increases in high-density lipoprotein cholesterol of healthy ambulatory men and women. In our program, in which elderly subjects exercised one day a week for 3.5 years, no increase in aerobic work capacity was obtained.

CONCLUSION

It can be concluded that a one-day-a-week exercise program at the intensity of lactate threshold and duration of 30 to 60 minutes will not increase aerobic work capacity in the elderly after either 12 weeks or three-and-a-half years. Three-days-a-week exercise programs elicited significant physiologic benefits (oxygen uptake corresponding to lactate threshold and maximal oxygen uptake) after 12 weeks, but when frequency of training was reduced to one day per week the training effect was lost. Elderly persons who finish a regular exercise program should continue some kind of habitual exercise at least three days per week.

REFERENCES

American College of Sports Medicine. Guidelines for Exercise Testing and Prescription, 3rd Edition. Philadelphia: Lea & Febiger, 1986.

Badenhop DT, Cleary PA, Schaal SF, Fox EL, Bartels RL. Physiological adjustments to higher- or lower-intensity exercise in elders. Med Sci Sports Exerc 1983;15:496-502.

Beaver WL, Wasserman K, Whipp BJ. Improved detection of lactate threshold during exercise using a log-log transformation. J Appl Physiol 1985;59:1936-40.

Belman MJ, Gaesser GA. Exercise training below and above the lactate threshold in the elderly. Med Sci Sports Exerc 1991;23:562-8.

Blumenthal JA, Emery CF, Madden DJ et al. Cardiovascular and behavioral effects of aerobic exercise training in healthy older men and women. J Gerontol 1989;44:M147-57.

Davis JA, Frank MH, Whipp BJ, Wasserman K. Anaerobic threshold alterations caused by endurance training in middle-aged men. J Appl Physiol 1979;46:1039-46.

Denis C, Dormois D, Lascour JR. Endurance training, $\dot{V}O_2$max, and OBLA: a longitudinal study of two different age groups. Int J Sports Med 1984;5:167-73.

Gaesser GA, Rich RG. Effects of high- and low-intensity exercise training on aerobic capacity and blood lipids. Med Sci Sports Exerc 1984;16:269-74.

Hagberg JM, Graves JE, Limacher M et al. Cardiovascular responses of 70-to-79-year-old men and women to exercise training. J Appl Physiol 1989;66:2589-94.

Henritze J, Weltman A, Schurrer R, Barlow K. Effects of training at and above the lactate threshold on the lactate threshold and maximal oxygen uptake. Eur J Appl Physiol 1985;54:84-8.

Katch V, Weltman A, Sady S et al. Validity of the relative percent concept for equating training intensity. Eur J Appl Physiol 1978;39:219-27.

Massicotte D, Avon G, Corriveau G. Comparative effects of aerobic training on men and women. J Sports Med 1979;19:23-32.

Meyer K, Weideman H. Die Bedeutung vonfixer anarobier Schwelle, Trainingslaktat und Trainingshertzfrequentz fur ein Fahradergometertraining mit Hertzinfarkpatienten. Z Kardiol 1985;74: 466-74.

Niinimaa V, Shephard RJ. Training and oxygen conductance in the elderly. I. The respiratory system. J Gerontol 1978;33:354-61.

Pollock ML, Dimmick J, Miller HS, Kendrick Z, Linnerud AC. Effects of mode of training on cardiovascular function and body composition of adult men. Med Sci Sports 1975;7:139-45.

Seals DR, Hagberg JM. The effects of exercise training on human hypertension: a review. Med Sci Sport Exerc 1984;16:207-15.

Seals DR, Hagberg JM, Hurley BF, Ehsani AA, Holloszy JO. Endurance training in older men and women. I. Cardiovascular response to exercise. J Appl Physiol 1984;57:1024-29.

Sidney KH, Shephard RJ. Frequency and intensity of exercise training for elderly subjects. Med Sci Sports Exerc 1978;10:125-31.

Takeshima N, Kobayashi F, Watanabe T, Sumi K, Tanaka K, Kato T. Responses to a submaximal-maximal stress test in the elderly. In: Kaneko, M, ed. Fitness for the Aged, Disabled, and Industrial Worker. Illinois: Human Kinetic Books, 1990:107-12.

Takeshima N, Tanaka K, Kobayashi F, Sumi K, Watanabe T, Kato T. Validity of the maximal aerobic capacity estimated from submaximal cycling exercise and field performance tests in the elderly. Jpn J Phys Fitness Sports Med 1992;41:295-303.

Tanaka K, Yoshimura T, Okuda T et al. Physiological alterations on obese women: the effects of caloric restriction plus physical training at an intensity corresponding to or above anaerobic threshold. Bull Phys Fitness Inst 1986;62(Suppl):26-40

Tanaka K, Kim H, Wakita M, Nakadomo F, Hazama T, Maeda K. Effects of anaerobic conditioning plus caloric restriction in obese middle-aged women. Jpn J Appl Physiol 1989;19:495-504.

Tanaka K, Watanabe Y, Hiyama T, Takeda M, Yoshimura T. Changes in vital age of CHD patients following a supervised aerobic conditioning program. J Jpn Atheroscler Soc 1992;20:661-7.

Thomas SG, Cunningham DA, Thompson J, Rechnitzer PA. Exercise training and ventilation threshold in elderly. J Appl Physiol 1985;59:1472-6.

Thomas SG, Cunningham DA, Rechnitzer PA, Donner P, Howard JH. Determinants of the training response in elderly men. Med Sci Sports Exerc 1985;17:667-72.

Urata H, Tanabe Y, Kiyonaga A et al. Anti-hypertensive and volume-depleting effects of mild exercise on essential hypertension. Hypertension 1987;9:245-52.

Wilmore JH, Davis JA, O'Brien RS, Vodak PA, Walder GR, Amsterdam EA. Physiological alternations consequent to 20-week conditioning programs of bicycling, tennis and jogging. Med Sci Sports Exerc 1980;12:1-8.

Wood PD, Williams P, Haskell WL. Physical activity and high density lipoproteins. In: Miller NE, Miller GJ, eds. Clinical and Metabolic Aspects of High-Density Lipoproteins. London: Elsevier Science Publishers, 1984:133-65.

Yerg JE, Seals DR, Hagberg JM, Holloszy JO. Effects of endurance exercise training on ventilatory function in older individuals. J Appl Physiol 1985;58:791-4.

Yoshitake Y. Changes of cardiovascular, sympathoadrenal and metabolic response during exercise corresponding to lactate threshold of middle-aged and elderly women. J Hyg 1986;40:867-71.

Physical and Physiological Characteristics in Middle-Aged and Aged Swimmers

Michiko Koda, M.S., M. Miyashita, Ph.D., M. Mutoh, M.D.
Mitsuri Higuchi, Ph.D., Yutaka Yoshitake, Ph.D., Toshiki Ohta, M.D.

INTRODUCTION

Swimming is considered to be a beneficial popular exercise, as are walking and jogging, for middle-aged and older individuals. The guidelines for exercise prescription by the American College of Sports Medicine (1990) suggest that various endurance game activities can maintain cardiorespiratory fitness and body composition and endurance in the healthy adult. Fuchi et al. (1986), Higuchi et al. (1987) and Fuchi et al. (1989) have shown that middle-aged and older long-distance runners had a higher maximal oxygen uptake than that of age-matched untrained individuals, and that runners had a lower percent of body fat than untrained.

However, little information is available to evaluate the effects of regular swimming exercise on body composition and aerobic capacity in middle-aged and older people. Therefore, the purpose of the study was to evaluate the physical and physiological characteristics of Master swimmers by comparing these characteristics with those of age-matched runners and untrained subjects.

SUBJECTS

Sixteen male and 42 female swimmers over 40 years of age volunteered to participate in this study. They regularly (twice or three times per week) performed the swimming workouts. The mean distance in the swimming workouts was 7500 m/wk for males and 3000 m/wk for females, respectively. The swimmers were compared with age-matched runners (male: n=44, female: n=65) and untrained subjects (male: n=35, female: n=80). All participants gave their informed consent to participate in the study.

METHODS

Height, body weight, and subscapular and triceps skinfold thicknesses were measured. The skinfold measurements were made on the right side of the body with a caliper. The total skinfold fat was defined as the sum of the two skinfolds measured.

Maximal oxygen uptake was obtained during treadmill exercise using a walking protocol (Bruce and Horsten, 1969) for swimmers and for untrained individuals and a running protocol for runners (Saltin and Åstrand, 1967). The expired gases were collected in Douglas bags during the last two to three minutes of each period. The criteria for obtaining maximal oxygen uptake were: 1) a plateau of maximal oxygen uptake against workload, and 2) respiratory exchange ratio (>1.0).

Statistics

Student's t-tests were used to determine significant differences between the groups. The level of statistical significance was set at $p<0.05$.

RESULTS

Data on physical and physiological measures are presented in Tables 1-1 and 1-2 for male and in Tables 2-1and 2-2 for female swimmers. Swimmers were taller than runners and untrained individuals of both sexes. As shown in Table 1, the male swimmers had higher body mass index (kg/m^2) and higher body weights than did runners; both these measurements were similar to those of untrained men. However, the sum of skinfold thicknesses in swimmers was lower than that of untrained men. In the females, body mass index and sum of skinfold thicknesses in swimmers were lower than those in untrained women, whereas swimmers had a similar body mass index but higher skinfold thicknesses when compared to the runners.

Both male and female swimmers had higher maximal oxygen uptake expressed as ml/kg body weight/min than untrained individuals had but lower than runners had.

DISCUSSION

In males, although the sum of skinfold thicknesses of swimmers was lower than that of untrained subjects, body mass index was not significantly different between swimmers and untrained subjects. This finding suggests that male middle-aged and aged swimmers had less body fat than untrained men. On the other hand, sum of skinfold thicknesses and body mass index of swimmers was higher than those of runners in both sexes. This could be partly explained by higher levels of subcutaneous fat deposits in swimmers that might be induced by an adaptive response to exercise in water. However, follow-up studies are needed to confirm this possibility. Although there was no significant difference in body mass index between swimmers and untrained, whose body mass index was below the borderline of overweight, body fat content estimated from skinfold thickness measurements were less in swimmers than in untrained counterparts. This suggests that regular swimming exercise is useful to modify an increase in body fat content.

Kobayashi et al. (1980) have shown that in 60- to 69-year-old male subjects maximal oxygen uptake of the runners was 2.56 1/min (50 ml/kg/min), and that of untrained men was 1.74 l/min (29 ml/kg/min). The aerobic capacities in runners and untrained subjects obtained in the present study were similar to the data in Kobayashi's study. The maximal oxygen uptake capacity expressed as ml/kg body weight/min in swimmers was higher than in untrained individuals, but was lower than in runners. In water, however, body weight by no means has the same loading factor as in running (Holmer, 1974). In water, therefore, it is possible that the swimmers had levels of maximal oxygen uptake capacity (in terms of liters/min) similar to the runners. This result indicates that regular swimming exercise could increase aerobic power.

TABLE 1-1

Physical Characteristics in Male Subjects

	Age group	n	Age (yr)	Height (cm)	Weight (kg)	BMI (kg/m^2)
Swimmers	40	4	47.5 + 2.1	167.2 4.5	63.8 * 3.7	22.9 2.2
	50	6	53.1 3.1	169.8 * 3.6	66.8 * 4.3	23.2 * 1.4
	60	6	65.8 * 2.2	165.8 * 3.7	58.3 6.9	21.2 2.1
Runners	40	10	47.2 # 1.5	162.3 4.6	55.9 # 4.9	21.2 1.4
	50	14	53.9 2.4	163.2 4.4	55.8 # 4.2	20.9 # 1.1
	60	20	62.8 2.5	160.5 4.1	53.5 # 4.2	20.8 # 1.3
Untrained	40	9	43.4 2.5	167.0 7.2	62.1 7.5	22.3 2.0
	50	9	53.4 2.5	164.3 5.3	62.5 7.7	23.1 2.1
	60	17	64.2 2.6	161.6 6.0	59.1 7.8	22.6 2.4

mean
±SD

* Significantly different swimmers vs. runners $p<0.05$
+ Significantly different swimmers vs. untrained $p<0.05$
# Significantly different runners vs. untrained $p<0.05$

TABLE 1-2

Physical and Physiological Characteristics in Male Subjects

	Age group	Sum of skinfold (m^2)	$\dot{V}O2max$ (l/min)	$\dot{V}O2max$ (ml/kg/min)	Training volume (km/wk)
Swimmers	40	20.7 11.7	3.2 + 0.3	49.5 *+ 3.8	6.0 2.8
	50	23.7 * 6.0	3.0 + 0.4	44.7 *+ 5.4	5.9 2.3
	60	19.8 6.3	2.4 + 0.4	40.3 *+ 3.6	10.0 5.7
Runners	40	15.1 # 2.5	3.2 # 0.4	57.8 # 5.4	56 32
	50	17.4 # 5.2	2.9 # 0.3	52.2 # 4.9	51 24
	60	16.5 # 3.9	2.7 # 0.3	49.9 # 4.0	55 21
Untrained	40	25.6 5.5	2.5 0.2	41.0 5.2	
	50	30.3 7.5	2.0 0.5	32.4 6.2	
	60	24.9 7.4	1.8 0.3	29.9 3.0	

mean
±SD

* Significantly different swimmers vs. runners $p<0.05$
+ Significantly different swimmers vs. untrained $p<0.05$
# Significantly different runners vs. untrained $p<0.05$

TABLE 2-1

Physical Characteristics in Female Subjects

	Age group	n	Age (yr)	Height (cm)	Weight (kg)	BMI (kg/m²)
Swimmers	40	23	45.7 2.7	157.0 5.5	52.0 5.3	21.1 1.6
	50	44	53.5 3.2	154.1 4.7	48.1 + 6.2	20.2 + 2.3
	60	8	63.9 3.2	154.3 5.7	55.6 * 4.3	23.4 1.4
Runners	40	18	44.4 2.9	154.9 4.1	51.8 7.2	21.5 2.4
	50	31	53.3 2.4	153.9 4.8	50.2 5.4	21.2 # 1.8
	60	16	64.3 3.0	150.1 4.8	48.1 # 5.5	21.4 # 2.7
Untrained	40	22	45.3 2.2	154.2 4.8	53.1 6.0	22.4 2.7
	50	28	54.1 3.1	152.5 4.8	52.6 5.3	22.6 2.3
	60	30	64.0 2.3	150.7 5.4	53.7 8.2	23.6 3.1

mean
±SD

* Significantly different swimmers vs. runners $p<0.05$
\+ Significantly different swimmers vs. untrained $p<0.05$
\# Significantly different runners vs. untrained $p<0.05$

TABLE 2-2

Physical and Physiological Characteristics in Female Subjects

	Age group	Sum of skinfold (mm)	$\dot{V}O2max$ (l/min)	$\dot{V}O2max$ (ml/kg/min)	Training volume (km/wk)
Swimmers	40	32.7 +	1.9 *+	37.4 *+	4.5
		7.6	0.3	4.2	3.5
	50	30.2 +	2.0 +	41.5 +	3.3
		8.2	0.3	5.8	1.4
	60	38.8 *	1.7 +	29.6 *+	2.4
		5.8	0.3	3.5	1.5
Runners	40	27.7 #	2.4 #	46.9 #	53
		10.7	0.3	7.5	17
	50	31.7 #	2.0 #	40.7 #	43
		9.3	0.3	5.4	24
	60	27.9 #	1.8 #	36.6 #	38
		6.8	0.2	5.1	15
Untrained	40	40.4	1.6	30.8	
		12.3	0.2	5.2	
	50	39.6	1.6	30.4	
		10.2	0.2	2.8	
	60	39.6	1.4	26.6	
		10.5	0.2	2.9	

mean
±SD

* Significantly different swimmers vs. runners $p<0.05$
\+ Significantly different swimmers vs. untrained $p<0.05$
\# Significantly different runners vs. untrained $p<0.05$

In females, the maximal oxygen uptake capacity of 50-year-old swimmers was similar to that of runners, but was higher than that of the untrained in the respective age groups. This finding suggests that the intensity and the period of aerobic training in female 50-year-old swimmers might have been at the same level as those of the age-matched runners.

CONCLUSION

In conclusion, the beneficial effects of regular swimming exercise on health status in middle-aged and aged people are: 1) to restrain increase in body fat content with age, and 2) to reduce the decline of maximal oxygen uptake that is typically associated with the aging process.

ACKNOWLEDGEMENTS

We would like to acknowledge Dr. Marc Rogers, the Department of Kinesiology, the University of Maryland, who provided helpful comments on this paper.

This study was supported by the Research Grant on Aging and Health, and by the Research Grant on Cardiovascular Diseases, Ministry of Health and Welfare, Japan.

REFERENCES

American College of Sports Medicine. Position Stand. The recommended quantity and quality of exercise for developing and maintaining cardiorespiratory and muscular fitness in healthy adults. Med Sci Sports Exerc 1990;22:265-74.

Bruce RA, Horsten TR. Exercise stress testing in evaluation of patients with ischemic heart disease. Prog Cardiovasc Dis 1969;11:371-90.

Fuchi T, Higuchi M, Yamakawa K, Ozawa M, Kobayashi S. Aerobic capacity of middle-aged and older endurance athletes. Japanese J Sport Sci 1986;5:341-6.

Fuchi T, Iwaoka K, Higuchi M, Kobayashi S. Cardiovascular changes associated with decreased aerobic capacity and aging in long-distance runners. Eur J Appl Physiol 1989;58:884-9.

Higuchi M, Iwaoka K, Fuchi T, Kobayashi S. A physiological profile of excellent Masters long distance runners. Japan J Sport Sci 1987;6:400-6.

Holmer I. Physiology of swimming man. Acta Physiol Scand 1974; suppl 407:1-55.

Kobayashi K, Kitamura K, Matsui H. Aerobic power of non-athletic and athletic men, ages 20 to 72 years. Japan J Phys Educ 1980;24:313-23.

Saltin B, and Åstrand P-O. Oxygen uptake in athletes. J Appl. Physiol 1967; 23:353-8.

Assessment of Ventilatory Threshold in Older Women: Comparison Among Three Methods

Giuseppe De Vito, M.D.
Concetta Pulejo, A.P.
Laura Capranica, M.Sc.
Francesco Figura, M.D.

INTRODUCTION

The main purposes of exercise testing for older people are to evaluate the fitness of the subjects and to define the risk associated with varying workloads. Using this information, it is also possible to establish the appropriate intensities for exercise prescription. At present, there is no consensus regarding the most effective methods of assessing cardiorespiratory fitness in elderly populations and the selection of an appropriate test protocol which permits obtaining accurate data in this population.

Maximal oxygen consumption measurements, correlated to cardiovascular function, are commonly used in different populations to evaluate physical fitness (Dehn and Bruce, 1972; Buskirk and Hodgson, 1987; Rivera et al., 1989; Frontera et al., 1990). Although peak results are readily determined, they are strictly dependent on subject motivation and difficult to obtain in elderly populations. In fact, only a proportion of older subjects can reach a plateau of oxygen consumption during a maximal exercise test (Sidney and Shephard, 1977).

Furthermore, the selection of ergometric tests for exercise test protocols in the elderly is still being debated. In fact, cycle ergometers may not be suitable for older populations because of lack of recent experience of cycling, stiffer joints and reduced muscular efficiency associated with cycling (Shephard, 1987). On the other hand, although walking on a treadmill involves an activity familiar to everyone, some subjects, at particular speeds and grades, become less efficient mechanically (Bruce, 1985).

As an alternative to maximal tests, submaximal tests have been proposed. In fact, the advantages of this kind of test are both a reduction in risk and ease of administration. Controversy also exists regarding the most appropriate methodology for assessment of submaximal exercise procedures and parameters. From early studies in the 1960's, several investigators proposed the anaerobic threshold (AT) as a good indicator of physical fitness. Furthermore, Farrell (1979) showed that, among various indices proposed to predict the endurance performance, the intensity of exercise corresponding to the anaerobic threshold yielded the highest correlation with the subject's endurance. Regarding the non-invasive detection of AT, this parameter has been used as an effective gauge of physical fitness in patients as well as in healthy normal subjects (Beaver et al., 1986). This kind of threshold, based on pulmonary ventilation measurements, has been called the ventilatory threshold ($\dot{V}$eT). The $\dot{V}$eT in the elderly can represent a good indicator of work capability, at least until the seventh decade of life (Foster et al., 1986). In fact, while $\dot{V}O_2$max decreases with age, the $\dot{V}$eT declines more slowly. This may be explained because the $\dot{V}$eT can be maintained with normal levels of daily activities, such as walking, while the former needs higher training stimuli (Wasserman et al., 1973; Thomas et al., 1985; Posner et al., 1987).

At present, the most common procedures to assess the ventilatory threshold are: a) the simplified v-slope method ($\dot{V}$eTvs); b) the pulmonary ventilation method $\dot{V}$eT$\dot{V}$E); c) the equivalents method ($\dot{V}$eTeq). In the present study, these three methods were compared to determine which one is the most effective in ventilatory threshold identification in an older female group.

METHODS

Subjects

Physical characteristics and body mass index (BMI) of twenty-three mildly active healthy women ranging in age from 54 to 69 years are reported in Table 1.

TABLE 1

Characteristics of Subjects

N = 23	Age (yr)	Body Mass (kg)	Stature (cm)	BMI (kg/m^2
Mean	61	65	160	25.3
SD	4.9	7.3	6.4	3
Min	54	55.5	149	20.2
Max	69	87	174	33.2

BMI=Body mass index.

To exclude subjects with physical impairment, every subject underwent a medical examination which included: pulmonary function tests, resting and exercise electrocardiogram, and arterial blood pressure measurement. Subjects with any of the following conditions were excluded from the study: significant cardiovascular or pulmonary disease, blood pressure >165/90/mmHg, or uncontrolled metabolic disease. Prior to the test each subject was informed about the nature of the experimental protocol and possible risks associated with it and asked to sign a consent form.

Exercise Protocol

Exercise testing was conducted no sooner than two hours after a light meal. The test protocol was developed specifically for this study. Each subject performed incremental work rate test on a treadmill at a constant speed of four km/h. The test started with a three-minute warm-up at 0 percent slope; thus a 2.5 percent increase in the slope of the treadmill was established at one-minute intervals. The test was conducted until volitional exhaustion. Indeed, 18 subjects out of 23 (78 percent) protracted the test as far as the conditions of $\dot{V}O_2$max attainment were documented (RQ>1.1, HR equal or near to maximal and plateau in $\dot{V}O_2$ uptake).

Equipment and Measurements

Heart rate (HR) was continuously recorded during the test by means of standard electrocardiography. Pulmonary ventilation ($\dot{V}$E), oxygen uptake ($\dot{V}O_2$) and carbon dioxide output ($\dot{V}CO_2$) were measured every 30 seconds by a computerized open-circuit pneumotach (Jaeger, EOS Sprint model). Power output, corresponding both to $\dot{V}$eT and to $\dot{V}O_2$max, was calculated according to Mathews and Fox (1976).

Assessment of Ventilatory Threshold

For each subject the ventilatory threshold ($\dot{V}O_2$ml•kg^{-1}•min^{-1}) was detected using the three following graphic methods, and consequently plotting the physiological values measured during the test:

a) the v-slope method ($\dot{V}$eTvs), which detects the break point in the relationship of the CO_2 output versus O_2 uptake plot, corresponding to the excess of the CO_2 output generated from the buffering of hydrogen ions (Sue et al., 1988).

b) the pulmonary ventilation method ($\dot{V}$eT$\dot{V}$E), which detects the non-linear increase in pulmonary ventilation that occurs at certain levels of O_2 consumption or workload (Wasserman and McIlroy, 1964);

c) the ventilatory equivalents method ($\dot{V}$eTeq), which detects a systematic increase of ventilatory equivalent for O_2 ($\dot{V}$E/$\dot{V}O_2$) without a concomitant increase in ventilatory equivalent for CO_2 ($\dot{V}$E/$\dot{V}CO_2$) (Davis, 1985).

Three skilled researchers were asked to detect $\dot{V}$eT on each plot. In case of disagreement, the data were averaged. To be considered valid the threshold had to be clearly identified by at least two researchers.

Statistical Analysis

The correlation matrix was calculated between the $\dot{V}O_2$max, $\dot{V}$eTvs, $\dot{V}$eT$\dot{V}$E, $\dot{V}$eTeq, BMI and age variables. F and t-student's analyses were used to assess the linearity of regression line (Sachs, 1984). A 0.05 level of confidence was chosen for all statistical comparisons.

RESULTS

Descriptive statistics of the assessed physiological parameters at $\dot{V}$eT and $\dot{V}O_2$max occurrence are listed in Table 2. Regarding $\dot{V}$eT methods, no statistically significant differences were found between the parameters.

TABLE 2

Values (means ± SD) of Some Physiological Quantities Measured at V̇eT and V̇O_2max Occurrence. The Percentage of Threshold Identification for Each Method is also Reported.

	V̇eTvs	V̇eTV̇E	V̇eTeq	V̇O_2max
V̇O_2(l•min^{-1})	1.05 ± 0.2	1.04 ± 0.1	1.05 ± 0.2	1.38 ± 0.24
V̇O_2(ml•kg•min^{-1})	16.4 ± 2.2	16.0 ± 2	16.4 ± 2	21.2 ± .2.2
V̇E (l•min-^{1})	27.5 ± 5.3	27.7 ± 4.4	26.9 ± 5	40.7 ± 11
HR (b•min^{-1})	130.4 ± 10	132.5 ± 11	132.5 ± 9	151 ± 8
Power (watt)	65 ± 30	61 ± 28	64 ± 32	98 ± 24
% of V̇eT Identification	78.4	61	82.6	78.4

At V̇eT occurrence in the three methods, the mean values of oxygen uptake, pulmonary ventilation, heart rate and power output ranged from 16 to 16.4 ml•kg^{-1}•min^{-1}, 27 to 27.7 l•min^{-1}, 131 to 133 beats•min^{-1}, and 64 to 71 watt, respectively. The same table shows the mean values of maximal oxygen uptake (21.2 ± 2, ml•kg^{-1}•min-^{1}). The highest percentage of success for V̇eT identification was 83 percent for the V̇eTeq, and the lowest was 61 percent for the V̇eTV̇E method.

Table 3 shows the correlation coefficients between all the considered variables. All methods resulted in significant correlation to one another and to V̇O_2max ($p<0.01$). No significant correlations were found between BMI and the other variables. Age showed a significant relation only to V̇eTV̇E ($p<0.05$).

DISCUSSION

Ventilatory threshold has been used to predict the work rate below which physical work can be performed for prolonged periods of time. In the elderly, this non-invasive submaximal exercise parameter is particularly suitable to assess cardiovascular fitness and to define the appropriate workloads for training programs (Marchetti et al., 1991). Wasserman and Whipp (1973) emphasized the importance of the protocol to obtain valid data in V̇eT measurements. In this study, the chosen one-minute increment interval seemed convenient, and no subject showed any discomfort. On the other hand, it must be stressed that with elderly people it is necessary to prolong the familiarization session with the measurement apparatus. In fact, hyperventilation, which can impair the data, was frequently observed during the resting phase prior to the test. This was probably due to the higher level of anxiety often reported in elderly people.

TABLE 3

Simple Correlations Coefficients Among All the Considered Methods $\dot{V}O_2max$, Body Mass Index (BMI) and Age

	$\dot{V}O_2max$	$\dot{V}eTvs$	$\dot{V}eT_{\dot{V}E}$	$\dot{V}eTeq$	BMI
$\dot{V}O_2max$					
$\dot{V}eTvs$	0.65*				
$\dot{V}eT_{\dot{V}E}$	0.83**	0.80**			
$\dot{V}eTeq$	0.69*	0.76**	0.68*		
BMI	0.49	0.12	0.15	0.14	
Age	0.22	0.32	0.58*	0.32	0.37

*$p<0.05$; **$p<0.01$

Results showed the equivalents method to be the easiest to graphically detect $\dot{V}eT$. A reasonable explanation for this result has not yet been found. Caiozzo et al. (1982) reported that this "dual" criterion provides a more specific determination of $\dot{V}eT$ in that it is clearly delineated from other causes of non-linear increases in ventilation such as neurogenic factors or exercise-induced hypoxemia. The high correlation observed between methods, when compared to one another and to $\dot{V}O_2max$, indicates that all of them could be used to determine the $\dot{V}eT$. These results do not agree with those reported by Wasserman et al. (1973) and McLellan et al. (1981), who found a negative correlation between $\dot{V}eT$ and $\dot{V}O_2max$.

CONCLUSION

The data suggest that, as with younger populations, ventilatory threshold can be reliably measured if strict criteria are met, at least until the seventh decade of life. The equivalents method resulted in the most effective $\dot{V}eT$ identification.

ACKNOWLEDGEMENT

This research was supported by a grant of the Ministry of the University and of the Scientific and Technological Research of Italy.

REFERENCES

Beaver WL, Wasserman K, Whipp B. A new method for detecting anaerobic threshold by gas exchange. J Appl Physiol 1986;60:2020-7.

Bruce RA. Functional aerobic capacity, exercise and aging. In: Andres R, Bierman EL, Hazzard WR, eds. Principles of Geriatric Medicine. New York: McGraw Hill, 1985:87-103.

Buskirk ER, Hodgson JL. Age and aerobic power: the rate of change in men and women. Federation Proc 1987;46:1824-9.

Caiozzo VJ, Davis JA, Ellis JF et al. A comparison of gas exchange indices used to detect the anaerobic threshold. J Appl Physiol 1982;53:1184-9.

Davis JA. Anaerobic threshold: review of the concept and directions for future research. Med Sci Sports Exerc 1985;17:6-18.

Dehn M, Bruce RA. Longitudinal variations in maximal oxygen intake with age and activity. J Appl Physiol 1972;33:805-7.

Farrell PA, Wilmore JH, Coyle EF, Billing JE, Costill DL. Plasma lactate accumulation and distance running performance. Med Sci Sports Exerc 1979;11:338-44.

Foster VL, Hume GJE, Dickinson AL, Chatfield SJ, Byrnes WC. The reproducibility of $\dot{V}O_2max$, ventilatory, and lactate thresholds in elderly women. Med Sci Sports Exerc 1986;18:425-30.

Frontera WR, Meredith CN, O'Reilly KP, Evans WJ. Strength training and determinants of $\dot{V}O_2max$ in older men. J Appl Physiol 1990;68:329-33.

Marchetti M, DeVito G, Venturoli PG. La soglia anaerobica nell'anziano. Med Sport 1991;44:1-7.

Mathews DK, Fox EL. The Physiological Basis of Physical Education and Athletics, 2nd Ed. Philadelphia: W.B. Saunders Company, 1976:64-6.

McLellan T, Skinner J. The use of the aerobic threshold as a basis of training. Can J Appl Sports Sci 1981;6:197-201.

Posner JD, Gorman KM, Klein HS, Cline CJ. Ventilatory threshold: measurement and variation with age. J Appl Physiol 1987;63:1519-25.

Rivera AM, Pels AE, Sady SP, Sady MA, Cullinane EM, Thompson PD. Physiological factors associated with the lower maximal oxygen consumption of master runners. J Appl Physiol 1989;66:949-54.

Sachs L. Applied Statistics, 2nd Ed. New York: Springer-Verlag, 1984.

Shephard RJ. Physical Activity and Aging, 2nd Ed. London: Croom Helm, 1987:92.

Sidney HK, Shephard RJ. Maximum and submaximum exercise tests in men and women in the seventh, eighth, and ninth decades of life. J Appl Physiol 1977;43:280-7.

Sue DY, Wasserman K, Moricca B, Casaburi R. Metabolic acidosis during exercise in patients with chronic obstructive pulmonary disease: use of the v-slope method for anaerobic threshold determination. Chest 1988;94:931-8.

Thomas SG, Cunningham DA, Thompson J, Rechnitzer PA. Exercise training and "ventilation threshold" in elderly. J Appl Physiol 1985;59:1472-6.

Wasserman K, McIlroy MB. Detecting the threshold of anaerobic metabolism in cardiac patients during exercise. Am J Cardiol 1964;14:844-52.

Wasserman K, Whipp BJ, Koyal SN, Beaver WL. Anaerobic threshold and respiratory gas exchange during exercise. J Appl Physiol 1973;35:236-43.

Functional Reserves of the Cardiovascular System in Elderly Trained Men

Oleg V. Korkushko, M.D.
Yurij T. Yaroshenko

INTRODUCTION

Aging is an inevitable and dynamic process that leads to the weakening of the organism's viability and adaptive capacities, thus increasing the probability of death. These processes, however, are accompanied by the development of adaptive mechanisms aimed at maintenance of the organism's homeostasis. A set of such adaptive mechanisms is referred to as a vitauct. The study into regularities of this process and its mastering opens the pathway for the control over life span (Frolkis and Muradian, 1991).

An optimal motor regimen is one of the possible influences upon the processes of vitauct. Moderate physical exercise was shown to increase the life span of rats (Goodrick, 1980; Holloszy and Smith, 1987), while hypokinesia and maximal physical loads resulted in a significant (2.8-fold) decrease of experimental animal life span (Muravov, 1976).

Physical training has an extensive and versatile effect upon the elderly organism. Nevertheless, the significance of an active motor regimen is frequently underestimated in medical practice. As a result, the volume of motor activity is unjustifiably limited in old age.

There are publications both in favor of practicing physical exercise in older age (Shephard, 1986; Gorman and Pozner, 1988) and against. Physical exercise at age 65 to 85 was reported not to make any changes in the physiological and psychological status in 50 percent of cases, while in 15 percent the status changed for the worse (Blumenthal et al., 1982). Although Edington et al. (1972) reported a certain "threshold of age" after which physical training produces negative rather than positive effects, Lakatta and Spurgeon (1987) failed to confirm the existence of the above threshold for physical exercises.

The mechanisms by which the process of adaptation to long-term exercise training is formed in the elderly remain uncertain. The possibilities for bringing the above mechanisms into play are also uncertain.

The purpose of the present investigation was to reveal the functional capacities of the cardiorespiratory system in elderly subjects who are apparently healthy and who practice endurance training. Our approach was to assess the ability to develop training effects in older persons who had never practiced exercise training on a regular basis but who started doing it regularly at the age of 60 and over.

METHODS

Subjects

Two groups of apparently healthy male subjects aged 60 to 89 years with varying levels of motor activity were selected. Group 1 consisted of 60 persons (20 for each age decade), who had not been engaged in either intensive physical work or programmed exercise training. Group 2 was made up of 50 persons (20 aged 60 to 69, 20 aged 70 to 79, and 10 aged 80 to 89), who had been active in exercise training as members of health groups and joggers' clubs. All of Group 2, mostly intellectuals, began training at the age of 60 and over. None of them had previously been active in sports; their lifestyle included a moderate motor regimen. Length of training of those aged 60 to 69 was three to eight years (average 5.7 years), in those aged 70 to 79 years was five to 18 years (average 12.0 years), and in subjects aged 80 to 89 was 10 to 28 years (average 17.2 years).

The analysis of their training cycle revealed the total energy expenditure for exercise training to be 600 to 800 kcal/day. Training included daily gymnastic exercises (45 to 60 minutes) and jogging sessions (four to six times a week). The jogging distance was 20 to 42 km/week (average 28.2 ± 0.89 km). Heart rate during training reached 75 percent of the maximum for the given age, the intensity not exceeding the limit of aerobic zone of energy provision. Most of the study subjects had been examined on a regular inpatient basis at the Clinical Department of the Ukrainian Institute of Gerontology, Kiev. No evidence of cardiovascular, respiratory, endocrine and neural pathology was found clinically and/or instrumentally.

Experimental Procedures

Load Test . The level of physical working capacity and its cardiorespiratory provision were evaluated through the continuous and gradual increase in workload (initial load 25w with a 25w increase every five minutes) on a bicycle ergonometer, while the subjects were sitting up, until reaching a submaximal heart rate, viz., 85 percent of maximum for the given age (Hossack and Bruce, 1982), provided that no clinical and electrocardiographic symptoms of overloading occurred (Anderson, 1971).

Electrocardiographic Control . Electrocardiograms were taken at initial stage and during restitution using 12-standard-lead electrocardiograph 6-NEK-4 (GDR). During investigation, the electrocardiogram was recorded each minute in MC5 lead using teleelectrocardiograph "Sirecust" (Siemens, FRG).

Central Hemodynamics and Gas Exchange. The arterial blood pressure was measured using auscultatory method at initial stage, at minutes two and four of each incremental load, and during restitution. The cardiac output was measured by means of impedance plethysmography (Kubicek et al., 1966) at initial stage, at 25w, and at submaximal load (Rheoplethysmograph 4RG-2M, USSR). The ventilation and gas exchange were determined by means of an automated gas analyzer "Oxycon-4" (Mijnhardt, Netherlands).

Intracardiac Hemodynamics and Myocardial Contractility. The intracardiac hemodynamics and left ventricular systolic and diastolic functions were studied in the group of 60- to 69-year-old subjects by means of echocardiography (Ekosector, Smith Kline Instrument, UK). Measurements were made at initial stage and 30 minutes after administration of beta-adrenergic-receptor stimulating agent isoprenalin (0.15 mg/kg body weight, sublingually). Indices of intracardiac hemodynamics and left ventricular systolic and diastolic function were estimated using graphoanalytical computer "Numonics," USA.

Spectral Analysis of Cardiac Rhythm. The state of autonomic control of heart function was studied by spectral analysis of cardiac rhythm (PC SM-4, USSR), using the method described in detail earlier (Korkushko et al., 1991). The level of the parasympathetic regulation was evaluated based on the power of high-frequency component of cardiac rhythm spectrum within the range 0.2-0.4 Hz and its percent contribution to total spectral power (Pomeranz et al., 1985). The state of the sympathetic link of the autonomic regulation was assessed from the power of low-frequency component of the spectrum within the range 0.01-0.05 Hz and its percent contribution to total spectral power (Weise et al., 1987), as well as from the index of tension and amplitude of variation pulsometry mode (Baevsky et al., 1984). R-R intervals were registered in supine and sitting positions at initial stage and at minutes three to five of each incremental load after reaching the steady state.

RESULTS

Central and Intracardiac Hemodynamics and Myocardial Contractility at Rest

In the subjects engaged in regular long-term exercise training (Group 2, as described under "Subjects" in the "Methods" section), there was a tendency for a rearrangement of hemodynamics towards a more economical function even at rest. Thus, the cardiac index was similar to that of untrained subjects but was maintained at the expense of high values of the stroke index, with the heart rate having significantly lower values. Other hemodynamic indices at rest did not differ significantly between the groups of trained and untrained (Group 1) subjects, which were defined in the "Methods" section.

The analysis of resting intracardiac hemodynamics revealed no significant exercise-related differences. Thus, the end-diastolic and end-systolic indices were almost the same in both groups (Table 1).

The values of left ventricular mass, the left ventricular mass index, and the index of end-diastolic volume/left ventricular mass were similar in both groups as well. No differences between the two groups were found at diastole in the thickness of either the left-ventricular posterior wall or the interventricular septum. In contrast, the trained subjects at systole had a thicker posterior wall of the left ventricle and a thicker interventricular septum than did the untrained subjects and also displayed higher values of the ejection fraction and of the normalized volumic rate of blood flow within the first third of the ejection phase.

In subjects who practiced exercise training on a regular basis there were also significant changes in the indices of left ventricular diastolic filling, such as a higher peak of relaxation rate and a larger filling fraction within the rapid filling phase (Table 1).

Physical Working Capacity and its Hemodynamic Provision

The level of body functional reserves can be objectively assessed during workload tests. In those subjects who were on regular exercise training, the standard 25w load study clearly revealed an economizing effect of training, seen in a decrease of heart rate and an increase of stroke index. A decrease was also noted in the increment in the arterial blood pressure in response to standard workload. The level of peripheral vascular resistance was lower in comparison with untrained subjects (Table 2).

TABLE 1

Indices of Intracardiac Hemodynamics and Left Ventricular Systolic and Diastolic Functions in Apparently Healthy Elderly Untrained and Trained Men (M ± SE)

	Untrained	**Trained**
Heart rate, beats/min	66.3 ± 2.0	55.3 ± 1.5***
End-diastolic index, ml/m²	67.9 ± 1.9	71.5 ± 2.6
End-systolic index, ml/m²	27.1 ± 1.1	26.2 ± 1.2
Stroke index, ml/m²	41.6 ± 1.5	45.7 ± 1.5
Cardiac index, l/min/m²	2.62 ± 0.09	2.60 ± 0.13
Thickness of left ventricular posterior wall at systole, cm	1.56 ± 0.02	1.62 ± 0.02*
Thickness of left ventricular posterior wall, cm	1.01 ± 0.01	1.01 ± 0.01
Thickness of interventricular septum at systole, cm	1.17 ± 0.05	1.34 ± 0.03**
Thickness of interventricular septum at diastole, cm	1.07 ± 0.05	1.10 ± 0.04
Left ventricular mass, g	246.6 ± 7.1	248.6 ± 7.8
Left ventricular mass/ body area, g/m²	128.6 ± 4.3	136.6 ± 4.3
End-diastolic volume/left ventricular mass, ml/g	0.53 ± 0.01	0.53 ± 0.01
Ejection fraction, %	61.1 ± 0.70	63.6 ± 0.39 ***
Degree of shortening of small axis of left ventricle	32.4 ± 0.4	34.9 ± 0.46***
Normalized rate of circular shortening of myocardial fibers, c^{-1}	1.05 ± 0.02	1.11 ± 0.03
Normalized volumic rate of blood flow within the Ist third of ejection phase, c^{-1}	2.10 ± 0.03	2.35 ± 0.05 ***
Peak of relaxation rate, mm/c	104.3 ± 2.0	118.6 ± 1.4 ***
Fraction of fast filling, %	50.4 ± 0.4	55,4 ± 0.3 ***
Fraction of slow filling, %	24.0 ± .0.2	20.9 ± 0.5 ***
Fraction of systole of atrium, %	25.6 ± 0.3	23.9 ± 0.3 ***

Note: Significant differences of indices or measurements between Groups.

* $p < 0.05$ **$p < 0.01$ *** $p < 0.001$

TABLE 2

Changes of Hemodynamics in Response to Standard Load (25 W) in ApparentlyHealthy Elderly Untrained (1) and Trained (2) Men (M ± SE)

Age, yr	**60 - 69**		**70 - 79**		**80 - 89**	
Groups	**1 n = 20**	**2 n=20**	**1 n=20**	**2 n=20**	**1 n=10**	**2 n=10**
Heart rate, beats/min	90.1 ± 1.95	76.2 ± 2.07***	95.3 ± 2.88	78.4 ± 2.72***	92.2 ± 3.12	74.0 ± 1.94***
Stroke index, ml/m²	57.1 ± 2.57	68.0 ± 3.78*	51.2 ± 2.10	62.1 ± 2.99**	54.7 ± 2.30	63.2 ± 2.51*
Cardiac index, 1/min/m²	5.1 ± 0.20	5.1 ± 0.22	4.9 ± 0.20	4.8 ± 0.17	5.0 ± 0.17	4.7 ± 0.28
Total peripheral resistance, dynes -sec -cm^{-5}	921 ± 30.4	835 ± 27.1*	1046 ± 50.8	979 ± 37.9	1010 ± 29.9	881 ± 41.7*
Systolic blood pressure, mm Hg	150.5 ± 2.87	137.5 ± 3.89*	160.5 ± 3.12	143.0 ± 3.90**	164.0 ± 5.33	138.0 ± 2.28***
Diastolic blood pressure, mm Hg	88.5 ± 2.55	79.5 ± 1.31**	88.5 ± 1.59	84.0 ± 2.61	81.0 ± 2.90	67.0 ± 78***

Note: Significant differences of indices or measurements between Groups 1 and 2.

* $p < 0.05$ ** $p < 0.01$ *** $p < 0.001$

The trained vs. untrained subjects were able to cope with a greater volume of load (Table 3). Thus, at age 60 to 69 the value of submaximal workload was 29.5 percent higher than that of their untrained counterparts and approximated the volume of load performed by apparently healthy men aged 40 to 49 (Korkushko and Yaroshenko, 1986). A similar picture was observed within the subsequent two age decades. In particular, the relative increment of submaximal workload in trained men of the ninth decade even increased (to 36.7 percent) compared to the control.

An increase in the workload power was accompanied by an increase in oxygen consumption at submaximal load level in all age groups. Oxygen transport to periphery increased at the expense of the increase of submaximal systolic index, the maximal heart rate being statistically insignificant between the study groups. Maximal rate of blood flow increased by means of the increased stroke index.

Intracardiac Hemodynamics and Myocardial Contractility: Effect of Pharmacological Stimulation of Beta-Adrenergic Receptors

In view of the difficulty of studying intracardiac hemodynamics and myocardial contractility under conditions of workload by means of echocardiography, a pharmacological load was produced with the beta-adrenostimulator, isoprenalin (isoproterenol). Isoprenalin administration led to an increase of the end-diastolic volume and ejection fraction, and a decrease of the end-systolic volume, the latter being more marked in the trained subjects (Table 4). In trained vs. untrained subjects, the cardiac output at the peak effect of isoprenalin was more increased, an effect due to the more marked increase of both stroke volume and heart rate. A thorough analysis of myocardial contractility showed a significantly higher increment of contractility following isoprenalin administration. In both study groups, with regard to indices of left ventricular diastolic filling, the administration of isoprenalin increased the peak of the rate of relaxation and the fraction of filling during the fast filling phase. This may signify the improvement of myocardial relaxation and of early filling by the stimulation of beta-adrenoreceptors. The above indices were significantly higher in the trained subjects.

Autonomic Regulation of Cardiac Rhythm

The comparison of resting indices of spectral analysis of cardiac rhythm revealed no essential differences as far as exercise training was concerned. However, at all levels of workload the dispersion of respiratory component of the spectrum was significantly higher in the trained subjects, thus indicating a more effective utilization of the functional reserves of the parasympathetic nervous system. Parallel to this, differences were noted in the dynamics of indices characterizing a degree of tension of the sympathetic part of the autonomic nervous system. Thus, at 25 and 50w, the dynamics of mode amplitude and tension index was similar in both groups. But with increasing loads, the mode amplitude was increasing at the same pace in the trained, whereas in the untrained subjects it reaches maximum at 50w, remaining unchanged thereafter (Figure 1).

TABLE 3

Results of Submaximal Exercise Test in Apparently Healthy Elderly Untrained (1) and Trained (2) Men (M ± SE)

Age, yr	**60 - 69**		**70 - 79**		**80 - 89**	
Groups	**1** n = 20	**2** n = 20	**1** n = 20	**2** n = 20	**1** n = 10	**2** n = 10
Workload, W	110.0 ± 3.87	142.5 ± 3.62 ***	88.0 ± 5.24	115.0 ± .48**	72.5 ± 4.25	95.0 ± 47**
Total volume of work, kJ	79.2 ± 3.94	134.4 ± 6.55***	53.0 ± 4.76	88.2 ± 5.51***	36.4 ± 3.66	61.8 ± 4.40**
Oxygen consumption, $ml \bullet min^{-1} \bullet kg^{-1}$	29.8 ± 1.30	37.1 ± 2.31*	26.5 ± 1.57	31.6 ± 1.61*	23.1 ± 0.93	27.7 ± 1.29**
Heart rate, beats/min	134.4 ± 3.34	138.6 ± 1.78	127.4 ± 2.88	125.8 ± 3.36	119.9 ± 3.80	116.6 ± 4.12
Stroke index, ml/m^2	59.8 ± 2.24	73.9 ± .77**	50.8 ± 3.36	63.0 ± 3.96*	52.5 ± 3.28	64.0 ± 4.40*
Cardiac index, $l/min/m^2$	8.0 ± 0.37	10.2 ± 0.43***	6.7 ± 0.39	7.9 ± 0.40*	6.3 ± 0.34	7.5 ± 0.45*
Systolic blood pressure, mm Hg	183.5 ± 5.29	186.0 ± 6.81	189.5 ± 3.63	192.0 ± 7.16	190.5 ± 4.49	177.0 ± 6.57
Diastolic blood pressure, mm Hg	92.0 ± 2.14	88.6 ± 2.14	97.0 ± 1.89	92.0 ± 3.63	90.0 ± 2.64	74.0 ± 3.58**

Note: Significant differences of indices or measurements between Groups 1 and 2.

*$p < 0.05$ **$p < 0.01$ *** $p < 0.001$

TABLE 4

Isoprenalin-Induced Changes in the Indices of Intracardiac Hemodynamics, Myocardial Contractility and Left Ventricular Diastolic Filling in Apparently Healthy Untrained and Trained Men Aged 60-69 (M ± SE)

	Untrained			Trained		
	Before Isoprenalin	After Isoprenalin	Relative changes, %	Before Isoprenalin	After Isoprenalin	Relative changes, %
End-diastolic volume, ml	130.6 ± 4.1	135.6 ± 4.5	3.8 ± 0.9	125.3 ± 5.7	131.2 ± 6.1	4.7 ± 1.0
End-systolic volume, ml	52.1 ± 2.5	50.2 ± 2.8	3.7 ± 2.2	45.8 ± 2.63	39.5 ± 2.4	-15.1 ± 1.6***
Stroke volume, ml	78.4 ± 1.8	86.7 ± 2.2	10.6 ± 1.5	79.5 ± 3.2	91.7 ± 3.9	15.5 ± 1.8*
Cardiac output, l/min	5.2 ± 0.1	6.1 ± 0.2	17.6 ± 3.2	4.4 ± 0.3	6.2 ± 0.4	43.6 ± 7.7**
Ejection fraction, %	60.3 ± 0.6	64.0 ± 0.6	6.2 ± 0.6	63.8 ± 0.5	70.1 ± 0.8	9.9 ± 1.1**
Normalized volumic rate of blood flow within the Ist third of ejection phase, c^{-1}	2.09 ± 0.03	2.59 ± 0.07	23.7 ± 2.1	2.33 ± 0.07	3.12 ± 0.1	34.3 ± 4.5*
Peak of relaxation rate, mm/c	104.3 ± 2.0	117.1 ± 2.4	12.4 ± 1.8	118.0 ± 1.7	143.0 ± 4.1	21.2 ± 3.0*
Fraction of fast filling, %	50.4 ± 0.4	55.4 ± 0.3	9.9 ± 0.5	54.2 ± 0.3	61.3 ± 0.4	13.1 ± 0.7**
Fraction of slow filling, %	24.0 ± 0.2	20.9 ± 0.5	13.1 ± 1.7	23.9 ± 0.5	17.9 ± 0.3	-24.9 + 1.9***
Fraction of systole of atrium, %	25.6 ± 0.3	23.9 ± 0.3	-6.2 ± 0.6	21.9 ± 0.3	20.9 ± 0.5	-4.5 + 1.9

Note: Significant differences of relative changes in indices or measurements between Groups 1 (untrained) and 2 (trained).

* $p < 0.05$ ** $p < 0.01$ *** $p < 0.001$

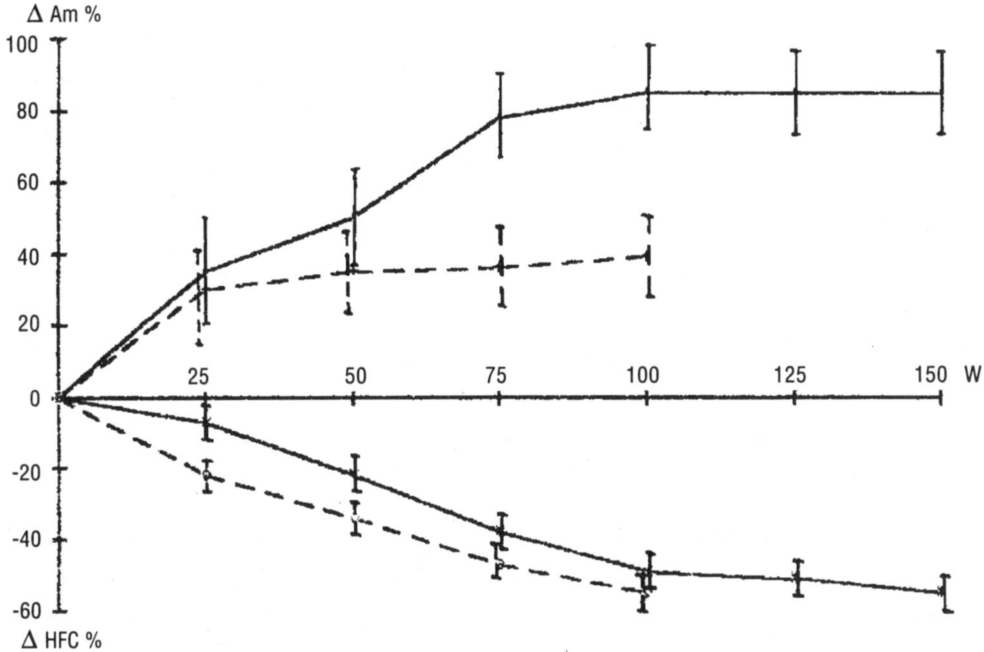

Am - Relative changes of amplitude of variation pulsometry mode during exercise

HFC - Relative changes of high-frequency component of cardiac rhythm spectrum during exercise

Figure 1. Autonomic regulation of cardiac rhythm in the process of stepwise increase of exercise in apparently healthy trained (solid line) and untrained (broken line) men aged 60-69

DISCUSSION

Change of Maximal Capabilities of Cardiorespiratory System During Exercise Training

According to published data, the increase of body reserves due to exercise training in young subjects shows itself primarily in the increase of physical working capacity and maximal oxygen consumption (Blomqvist and Saltin, 1983; Schaible and Scheuer, 1985).

In regard to the improvement of the older organism's performance as a physiological system through exercise training, the question remains to be solved and the literature data are controversial.

Numerous reports provide evidence for an increase of physical working capacity and maximal oxygen consumption in elderly persons owing to exercise training (Adams and de Vries, 1973; Suominen et al., 1977; Bortz, 1982; Seals et al., 1984; Hagberg, 1987; Hagberg et al., 1989).

On the other hand, Benestad (1965), Usutani et al. (1979) and Goertren et al. (1984) reported no essential changes of the parameters characterizing aerobic working capacity in elderly persons during exercise training. The above discrepancies can be accounted for by the different training programs used. In particular, the lack of training effect was linked with a low intensity of training workloads, which failed to cause adaptation of the cardiovascular system. The high level of the organism's aerobic capacities, which we observed in the endurance trainees, indicated that the organism's performance could be improved through exercise training at any age including that of 80 to 89 years.

In young subjects the positive effect of exercise training upon the hemodynamics is thought to be related to the dilation of cardiac cavities, the increase of myocardial mass and the decrease of peripheral vascular resistance (Blomqvist and Saltin, 1983). At the same time, Ehsani (1987) reported lack of direct evidence for the effects of exercise training upon rise of the myocardial contractility in humans.

The question arises whether or not the mechanism mediating the positive effect of training is active in old age. Discussions are still underway in the literature concerning the possible increase of maximal cardiac output in older persons through exercise training. In particular, Niinimaa and Shephard (1978) failed to find any reliable data in favor of such a possibility.

In our study, the maximal value of cardiac index was higher in trained vs. untrained subjects. It was also noted that substantial part of the blood flow was provided for by the rise of the stroke index at stable maximal heart rate.

To assess the range of adaptive capacities of myocardial contractility, we analyzed the changes that occurred in left ventricular systolic and diastolic function following an acute pharmacological load with isoprenalin. Such an approach allowed us to characterize the contribution made by the mechanisms of adrenergic regulation to the maintenance of myocardial contractility with special reference to the level of physical fitness.

In trained elderly males, isoprenalin produced a more significant positive effect upon myocardial contractility and relaxation compared to their untrained elderly counterparts. This indicates that regular exercise training improves the reactive capacity of the cardiovascular system. In this context, interesting data reported by Spurgeon et al. (1983) can be mentioned. They found that physical training had no effect on myocardial contractility of the young rats, whereas the old animals showed a delay in the development of age changes in a number of parameters of myocardial contractility.

The differences in the cardiovascular response to isoprenalin which we found in the elderly men with varying physical activity can be conditioned by the adaptive rearrangement of the autonomic regulation. Indeed, the results of our spectral analysis of cardiac rhythm provide evidence that the reserve capacities of the sympathetic system are greater in the trained elderly subjects than in their untrained counterparts. For instance, at 50w the elderly trained persons displayed almost a twofold reserve for the enhancement of sympathetic influences upon the cardiac rhythm. The above reserve capacities in the untrained subjects were insignificant. Such rearrangement of autonomic regulation of cardiac rhythm in trained elderly subjects promotes lesser tension of the sympathetic regulation at low and moderate load power, resulting in a better preservation of residual capacities at submaximal load power.

Thus, regular exercises, even if they are started at an elderly age, not only promote the maintenance of higher initial indices of the systolic and diastolic function of the heart, but also improve the reactive capacities of the cardiovascular system and its regulatory mechanisms. It is of note that the main mechanism of positive effects of training in the elderly seems to be the improvement in the quality of heart performance.

Economization of Cardiovascular Function During Training in Elderly Persons

The effect of economization of functions, observed during exercise training, promotes the extension of the range of the organism's functional capacities and the increase of performance of the oxygen transport system. This effect is reflected in values taken both at rest and with standard load (Schaible and Scheuer, 1985). Is the economizing effect of motor activity still retained in old age?

Our trained subjects showed, both at rest and with standard load, a clear economizing effect of training, seen in a decrease of the heart rate and an increase of stroke volume, and a decrease of increment of arterial blood pressure in response to workload. With standard workload, the level of peripheral vascular resistance was lower compared to that observed in the untrained subjects. Such a rearrangement of hemodynamics improved heart performance and widened the range of hemodynamic reactivity at workload.

According to our data, the resting values of end-diastolic and end-systolic index did not differ between the study groups. The results obtained by Grutinger (1984) and Stein et al. (1980) in their studies of endurance-trained young people revealed an increase of the end-diastolic volume. Bachl et al. (1983) investigated elderly men (69.4 ± 5.6 years), who practiced training on a bicycle ergometer, and, using echocardiography, found an increase of end-diastolic diameter of the left ventricle and thickness of its posterior wall and septum. At the same time, Merrill (1988) in his investigation involving 16 women (average age 65 years), who took part in a 12-week physical training program on bicycle ergometer, failed to reveal any essential changes in stroke volume, despite the increase in the functional capacities of the cardiovascular system.

Our results can be explained, at least in part, by the fact that with age even without exercise training there occurs an increase in end-diastolic volume, while its further increase in the process of training probably limits the passive-elastic properties of the myocardium of the elderly.

In our studies, the left ventricular mass and the left ventricular mass index were almost the same in both groups. These results are in agreement with the data of Savage et al. (1990), who showed that exercise training led to an increase of left ventricular mass in persons aged 50- but produced no effect on left ventricular mass in those aged 50+. These data also confirm experimental findings pertinent to evaluation of the effect of training on the rate and efficacy of protein and RNA synthesis in the myocardium of young and old rats aged eight and 25 months, respectively (Starnes et al., 1983). The rate of protein and RNA synthesis was shown to decline with age. Physical training program (five times a week for 21 weeks) appeared to have no effect upon these processes.

Thus, elderly subjects were shown to have limited capacities to adapt to physical load due to changes in intracardiac hemodynamics and development of myocardial hypertrophy. We have shown, however, that in old age there are possibilities for the exercise training-dependent improvement of left ventricular filling parameters.

At 25 to 75w, the trained vs. untrained elderly subjects showed more economical use of the reserve capacities of the sympathetic part of the autonomic nervous system. This may indicate that the regular exercise training reduces functional tension within the system of autonomic regulation in conditions of physical strain, widens the range of adaptive capacities, improves the quality of regulation, and promotes the reliability of the organism's function.

Analysis of data in the literature showed that, in addition to the improvement by exercise training of the hemodynamic response to physical load in the elderly persons, some important mechanisms of peripheral adaptation to exercise training still remain in the elderly. Thus, during the process of training, elderly subjects showed a rise in the activity of some enzymes in the muscle tissue (Suominen et al., 1977) and an increase of oxidative activities of the mitochondria, although, in contrast to the young subjects, the number of mitochondria remained unchanged (Orlander and Aniansson, 1980). In rats, exercise training prevented age-related decrease of cytochrome C in the myocardium and activity of aldolase and superoxide dismutase (Starnes et al., 1983).

Analysis of the literature and our own data suggests that the main mechanisms mediating the effect of exercise training are retained in the elderly. Still, in view of the age-related decrease that occurs in the rate and efficacy of synthesis of biochemical substrates and proteins, the importance of myocardial hypertrophy in the development of training effect decreases and the time needed for its attainment lengthens.

CONCLUSION

Intensive exercise endurance training within the range of aerobic energy production, even if it is started at an elderly age, promotes a significant increase of the organism's performance. Extension of the range of an organism's adaptive capacities manifests itself in a rise of maximal adaptive capacities, as well as in a more economical response to standard loads. It is essential to note that exercise training influences most those links of an organism's function in which age-related changes are most significant. The data presented substantiate the notion that active muscle activity should be used widely as a highly effective method to stimulate functions and to extend the range of adaptive capacities.

Regular endurance training promotes the deceleration of age-related changes in oxygen transport and the maintenance of the organism's reserves, thereby serving as a basis for the prevention of premature aging and the attainment of active longevity.

Note: According to the Ukrainian Institute of Gerontology's classification, "Elderly" age is the period from 60 to 74 years; and "Old" age is the period 75 to 89 years.

REFERENCES

Adams GM, de Vries HA. Physiological effects of an exercise training regimen upon women aged 52-79. J Gerontol 1973;28:50-5.

Anderson KL, Shephard RJ, Denolin H, Varnauskas E, Masironi R. Fundamentals of Exercise Testing. Geneva: WHO, 1971:41.

Bachl N, Baumgartl P, Huber G, Fasching I. Leistungsfahigkeit und kardialebelastbardkeit alterer sporttreibender. Z Herz Kreislauf 1983;15:262-73.

Baevsky RM, Kirilov OI, Kletskin SZ. Mathematical Analysis of Cardiac Rhythm Changes During Stress. Moscow: Nauca, 1984:133.

Benestad AM. Trainability of old men. Acta Med Scand 1965;178:321-7.

Blomqvist CG, Saltin B. Cardiovascular adaptations to physical training. Ann Rev Physiol 1983;45:169-89.

Blumenthal JA, Schocken DD, Needels TL, Hindle P. Psychological and physiological effects of physical conditioning of the elderly. J Psychosom Res 1982;36:505-10.

Bortz WM. Disease and aging. JAMA 1982;248:1203-8.

Edington DW, Cosmas AC. Exercise and longevity, evidence for a threshold age. J Gerontol 1972;27:341-3.

Ehsani AA. Cardiovascular adaptations to exercise training in the elderly. Fed Proc 1987;46:1840-3.

Frolkis VV, Muradian KK. Life Span Prolongation. Boca Raton: CRC Press, 1991:6.

Goertren D, Sterfass R, Sopko G, Leon A. The functional capacity and physical activity levels of women over 60 years of age. J Sport Med Phys Fit 1984;24:30-6.

Goodrick CL. Effects of long-term voluntary wheel exercise on male and female Wistar rats. Gerontology 1980;26:22-3.

Gorman KM, Posner JD. Benefits of exercise in old age. Clin Geriat Med 1988; 4:181-92.

Gruttinger WF. The cardiovascular response to chronic physical exertion and exercise training: an echocardiographic review. Am Heart J 1984;108:1014-8.

Hagberg JM. Effect of training on the decline of $\dot{V}O_2max$ with aging. Fed Proc 1987;46:1830-3.

Hagberg JM, Graves JE, Limacher M et al. Cardiovascular responses of 70-to-79-year-old men and women to exercise training. J Appl Physiol 1989; 66:2589-94.

Holloszy JO, Smith EK. Effects of exercise on longevity of rats. Fed Proc 1987;46:1850-3.

Hossack KF, Bruce RA. Maximal cardiac function in sedentary normal men and women: comparison of age-related changes. J Appl Physiol 1982;53:799-804.

Korkushko OV, Shatilo VB, Plachinda YuI, Shatilo TV. Autonomic control of cardiac chronotropic function in man as a function of age: assessment by power spectral analysis of heart rate variability. J Auton Nerv Syst 1991; 32:191-8.

Korkushko OV, Yaroshenko YT. Age-related changes of physical working capacity and its cardiorespiratory support. Vestn AMS USSR 1986;10:42-7.

Kubicek WG, Karnegis JN, Patterson RP, Witsoe DA, Mattson RH. Development and evaluation of an impedance cardiac output system. Aerosp Med 1966;37:1208-12.

Lakatta EG, Spurgeon HA. Effect of exercise on cardiac muscle performance in aged rats. Fed Proc 1987;46:1 844-9.

Merrill JD. Endurance training in older women: maximal and submaximal cardiovascular response. J Appl Gerontol 1988;7:181-92.

Muravov IV. Motor regimen, biological age and life span. In: Gerontology and Geriatrics 1975. Year-Book. Kiev, 1976:88-96.

Niinimaa V, Shephard RJ. Training and 0_2 conductance in the elderly. II. The cardiovascular system. J Gerontol 1978;33:362-7.

Orlander J, Aniansson A. Effects of physical training on skeletal muscle metabolism and ultrastructure in 70-to-75-year-old men. Acta Physiol Scand 1980;109:149-54.

Pomeranz B, Macaulay RJB, Candill MA et al. Assessment of autonomic function in humans by heart rate spectral analysis. Am J Physiol 1985;248:H151-3.

Savage DD, Levy D, Dannenberg AL, Garrison RG, Castelli WP. Association of echocardiographic left ventricular mass with body size, blood pressure and physical activity (the Framingham Study). Am J Cardiol 1990;65:371-6.

Schaible TF, Scheuer J. Cardiac adaptations to chronic exercise. Prog Cardiovasc Dis 1985;27:297-324.

Seals DR, Hagberg JM, Harley BF, Ehsani AA, Holloszy JO. Endurance training in older men and women. I. Cardiovascular response to exercise. J Appl Physiol 1984;57:1024-28.

Shephard RJ. Physical training for the elderly. Clin Sports Med 1986;5:515-30.

Spurgeon HA, Stenbach MF, Lakatta EG. Chronic exercise prevents characteristic age-related changes in cardiac contraction. Am J Physiol 1983; 244:H513-8.

Starnes JW, Edington DW, Beyer RE. Myocardial protein synthesis during aging and endurance exercise in rats. J Gerontol 1983;38:660-5.

Stein RA, Mitchelli D, Diamond J, Horwitz B, Krasnow N. The cardiac response to exercise training echocardiographic analysis at rest and during exercise. Am J Cardiol 1980; 46:219-25.

Suominen H, Heikkinen E, Liesen H, Michel D, Hollmann W. Effects of 8 weeks' endurance training on skeletal muscle metabolism in 56-70-year-old sedentary men. Eur J Appl Physiol 1977;37:173-80.

Usutani S, Nishiyama K, Sugawara K et al. Studies on physical fitness of middle and old aged people. Comparison of health state and physical fitness between recreational exercise group and non-exercise group. Hirosaki Med J 1979;31:147-75.

Weise F, Heydenreich F, Runge U. Contributions of sympathetic and vagal mechanisms to the genesis of heart rate fluctuations during orthostatic load: a spectral analysis. J Auton Nerv Syst 1987;21:127-34.

Effects of Aging and Overload Training on Left Ventricular Diastolic Function in National Competitive Weight Lifters

Michael Sagiv, Ph.D.
David Ben-Sira, Ph.D.
Amira Sagiv, R.N.

INTRODUCTION

Recently, diastolic left ventricular filling has been shown to be affected not only by ventricular property but also by aging (Downes et al., 1989; Kuo et al., 1987) and by loading conditions (Gardin et al., 1987; Stoddard 1989), which may mask or mimic changes in compliance. Previous studies have shown that hearts of subjects engaged in predominantly pressure overload activities such as weight lifting exercise, develop a concentric left ventricular hypertrophy (Braunwald, 1984) which may differ in its function when compared with normal subjects (Menapace et al., 1982). The aging influence on cardiovascular performance during exercise has been widely investigated. Studies have shown that aging of the myocardium produces changes in left ventricular function (Lakatta and Yin, 1982; Templeton et al., 1979, Yin et al., 1980). This can be assessed by Doppler echocardiographic measurement of transmittal flow velocities (Kitabatake et al., 1982; Rokey et al., 1985). The present study has been designed to examine the effects of aging and lifelong chronic overload training on left ventricular filling properties. Isometric exercise rather than isotonic stress was applied because primarily it induces an increase in afterload similar to that seen during weight lifting training and because of its negligible effects on heart rate. Secondly, Doppler studies during isometric stress are easier to perform than during dynamic exercise.

METHODS

Subjects

Forty-eight healthy males volunteered for this study. They were divided into four groups: 14 young men (29 ± 6 years), 10 older men (52.5 ± 1.1 years), 14 young weight lifters engaged in heavy weight lifting at the national level in the last five years (28 ± 6 years) and 10 older former weight lifters (51 ± 3 years) who competed at the national level for at least five years. None of the normal subjects was a member of a competitive team. None suffered from hypertension, diabetes mellitus, hyperlipidemia, ischemic heart disease, or cardiomyopathy. Physical examination and resting 12-lead electrocardiogram were normal in all subjects. In addition, all subjects had a normal graded treadmill exercise test with a mean exercise capacity of 9.1 ± 2 METs in the older groups and 13.2 ± 2 METs in the younger groups. In order to match work capacity of the young subjects, four older normal subjects were excluded from the study due to low work capacity (lower than 8 METs). Informed consent obtained from each volunteer was approved by the Clinical Science Center Committee on Human Subjects.

Procedure and Measurements

The first session was devoted to habituation to the deadlift maneuver. In addition, all subjects were given a verbal reminder that smoking, eating, caffeine, and physical activity were not allowed for 12 hours prior to testing. During the second session, isometric exercise which involved the hands, hips, legs, and lower back muscle groups (deadlift) was measured with a platform-mounted strain gauge bridge. Subjects stood on the platform and grasped a T-bar connected to the strain gauge by an adjustable link chain. The output of the device was coupled to the screen of an IBM PC computer so that subjects could observe the magnitude of the deflection (Figure 1).

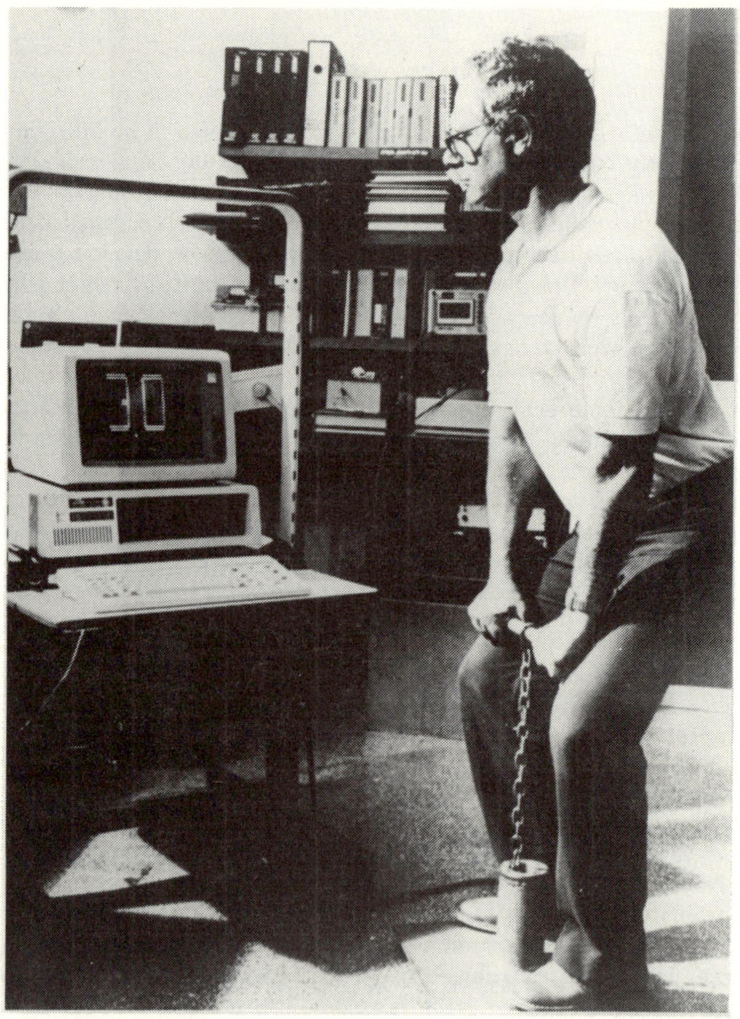

Figure 1. Subject position during isometric deadlift

Studies of isometric deadlift were performed at 30 percent of maximum voluntary contraction for three minutes. The 30 percent level was controlled by visual observation of the recorder output from the deadlift platform. Rhythmic breathing was maintained and Valsalva maneuver discouraged by continual prompting during isometric exercise and visual control with an automated system (Oxycon-4 metabolic cart produced by Mijnhardt, Netherlands).

Oxygen consumption was measured during the third minute with an automated system using the automated metabolic cart system Oxycon-4. Heart rate and electrocardiogram were monitored using bipolar chest lead CM5 and a Burdick C/5 recorder and oscilloscope. Five-second recordings were obtained at the end of each minute of isometric exercise. Blood pressure was monitored using a standard sphygmomanometer cuff and mercury manometer mounted at eye level. Recordings were taken at the last 30 seconds of the third minute of isometric maneuver. Validation of blood pressure auscultation during isometric exercise was evaluated in another study by Sagiv et al. (1985). Mean arterial blood pressure (MABP) was calculated using the equation: MABP = DBP + 1/3 (SBP-DBP), where: DBP = Diastolic Blood Pressure, SBP = Systolic Blood Pressure.

Complete Doppler echocardiographic studies were performed at rest, utilizing an Interspec Apogee TM ultrasound system equipped with 2- and 3-MHz transducers. Using two-dimensionally directed M-mode echocardiographic records, the diameters of the aorta and left atrium were measured from the parasternal long-axial view, and left ventricular end-diastolic and systolic diameters and interventricular septal and left ventricular posterior wall thicknesses were measured from the parasternal short-axial views just below the mitral valve level. Left ventricular ejection fraction was determined according to the Teichholz method (1976). Pulsed Doppler interrogation was performed from the apical four-chamber view with a 5-mm sample volume at the level of the mitral annulus, while less than a 10-degree angle between the Doppler cursor line and long axis of the left ventricle was maintained (Figure 2).

Peak blood velocity through the mitral value during early diastole (E) and presystole (A), the E/A peak velocity ratio, the time-velocity integral of the whole inflow period (T-TVI), the E-TVI, the A-TVI, and the atrial filling fraction (AFF percent) were measured. Correction for heart rate was performed by dividing the filling parameters by the square root of the R-R interval. AFF was calculated by using the following equation: AFF = (A-TVI) / (T-TVI) x 100. The Doppler parameters at left ventricular inflow were measured at rest and at the end of the third minute of isometric stress.

Statistical Methods

Comparisons between and among groups and conditions were made using multi-analysis of variance with repeated measures. The Tukey post hoc procedure was used for specific comparison at the $p<0.05$ level of significance. All values are presented as the mean ± 1 SD.

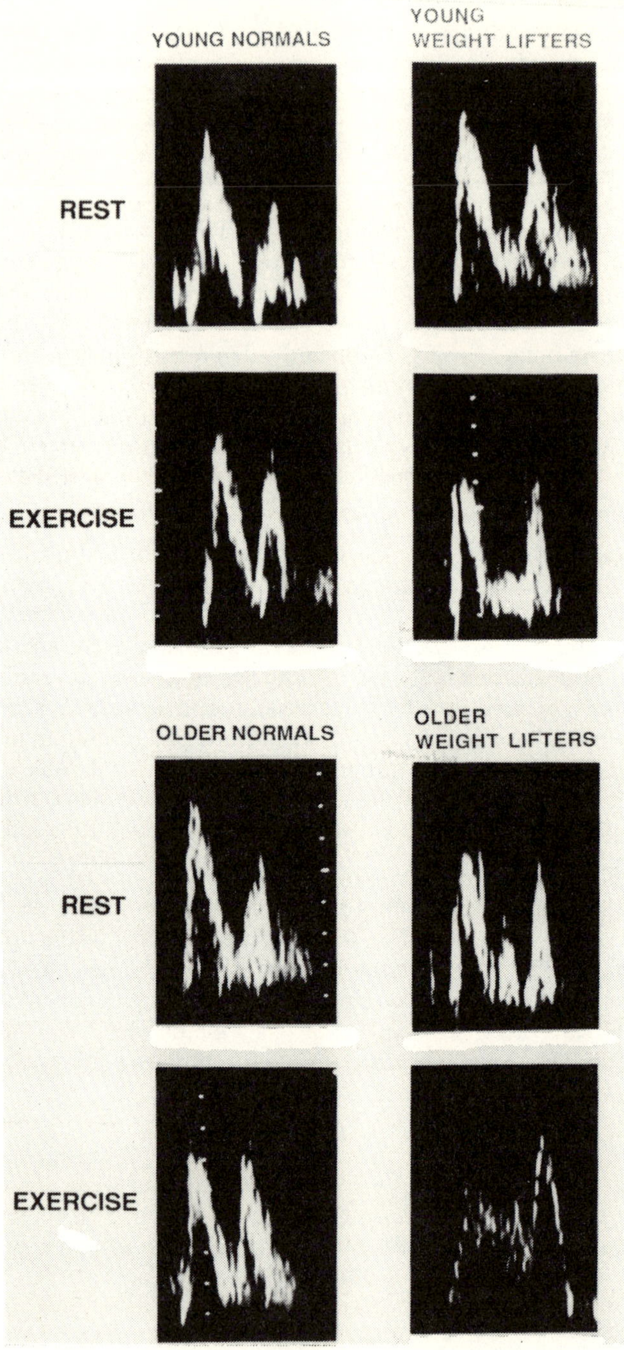

Figure 2. Representative pulsed Doppler echocardiographic recordings of velocity-time profiles obtained in young and older normal subjects and in young and older weight lifters at rest and during deadlift at 30 percent of maximal voluntary contraction.

RESULTS

Each group completed the study without difficulty or abnormal symptoms, dysrhythmias, or ischemic electrocardiographic responses. Mean descriptive data for the four subject groups are presented in Table 1. Means, standard deviations and results for left ventricular diastolic function and hemodynamic responses at rest and during isometric exercise bout are shown in Tables 2 and 3. Isometric tension at 30 percent of maximal voluntary contraction during deadlift maneuver was significantly ($p<0.001$) higher in the two young groups than in the two older groups, with the significantly ($p<0.05$) highest value seen in the young weight lifters.

Left atrial size, left ventricular end systolic and diastolic dimensions, mitral E-point septal separation, aortic dimension and ejection fraction were within the normal range and with similar values in all subjects. The thickness of the interventricular septum and left posterior walls in the young weight lifters were significantly ($p<0.05$) greater than in the other groups. Thus, the young weight lifters had evidence of left ventricular hypertrophy. Doppler studies did not reveal valvular regurgitation in any of the subjects. Auscultation also was negative for valvular regurgitation.

TABLE 1

Mean Descriptive Data in the Four Experimental Groups
(values are mean ± SD)

Variable	Young normals	Young weightlifters	Older normals	Older weightlifters
N of cases	14	14	10	10
Age (yrs)	29 ± 6	28 ± 9	52.5 ± 1.1*	51 ± 3*
Weight (kg)	66 ± 10	65 ± 12	70 ± 3*	63 ± 5
Height (cm)	165 ± 10*	176 ± 9	173 ± 3	163 ± 6*
LA (cm)	3.4 ± 0.3	3.2 ± 0.2	3.5 ± 0.4	3.1 ± 0.3
EDD (cm)	4.4 ± 0.5	4.3 ± 0.2	4.1 ± 0.3	4.1 ± 0.4
ESD (cm)	3.1 ± 0.3	2.8 ± 0.2	3.3 ± 0.3	2.9 ± 0.3
SPW (cm)	1.1 ± 0.1	1.4 ± 0.15*	1.0 ± 0.1	1.1 ± 0.1
PW (cm)	1.0 ± 0.1	1.4 ± 0.11*	1.0 ± 0.1	1.1 ± 0.2

* Significant differences between groups ($p<0.05$)

LA = Left atrium dimension, EDD = Left ventricular end diastolic dimension, ESD = Left ventricular end systolic dimension, SPW = Interventricular septum thickness, PW = Posterior wall thickness

TABLE 2

Hemodynamic Measurements at Rest and During Isometric Exercise in the Four Experimental Groups (values are mean ± SD)

Variable	Condition	Young		Old		Probability		
		Normals	Weightlifters	Normals	Weightlifters	Group	Effort	Group Effort
HR ($B \cdot min^{-1}$)	Rest	74.7 ± 6	71.4 ± 5	74.2 ± 10	71 ± 6	N S		
	Exercise	94.2 ± 8	96.0 ± 9	90.4 ± 10	89.1 ± 6	N S	0.05	N.S
SBP (mm Hg)	Rest	121 ± 12	130 ± 11	122 ± 14	124 ± 12	N S		
	Exercise	188 ± 10	204 ± 10	190 ± 15	192 ± 9	N S	0.05	0.05
DBP (mm Hg)	Rest	74 ± 10	77 ± 9	71 ± 7	70 ± 10	N S		
	Exercise	98 ± 7	102 ± 6	100 ± 9	104 ± 7	N S	N.S	N S
MABP (mm Hg)	Rest	89.7 ± 6	94.7 ± 7	88.0 ± 8	88.1 ± 7	N S		
	Exercise	128 ± 8	136 ± 10	130 ± 8	133.4± 7	0.05	0.05	0.05
$\dot{V}o2$ ($ml \cdot kg^{-1} \cdot min^{-1}$)	Rest	3.2 ± 0.4	3.2 ± 0.6	3.5 ± 0.7	3.7 ± 0.5	N S		
	Exercise	10.1 ± 1.0	11.7 ± 1.8	10.2 ± 1.2	10.3 ± 1.7	N S	0.05	N S

NS = Not Significant; HR = Heart Rate; SBP = Systolic Blood Pressure; DBP = Diastolic Blood Pressure; MABP = Mean Arterial Blood Pressure; $\dot{V}O_2$ = Oxygen Consumption.

TABLE 3

Doppler Measurements at Rest and During Exercise for the Four Experimental Groups
(values are mean ± SD)

Variable	Condition	Young		Old		Probability		
		Normals	Weightlifters	Normals	Weightlifters	Group	Effort	GroupxEffort
E $(cm \cdot sec^{-1})$	Rest	65.0 ± 8	66.0 ± 14	61.8 ± 12	45.0 ± 10*	0.05		
	Exercise	60.8 ± 11	66.9 ± 14	56.0 ± 11	41.1 ± 8	0.05	0.05	0.05
A $(cm \cdot sec^{-1})$	Rest	42.1 ± 10	45.9 ± 6.7	45 ± 10	40 ± 6	N S		
	Exercise	55.2 ± 16	70.0 ± 10*	60 ± 10	52 ± 8	0.05	0.05	0.05
E/A ratio	Rest	1.45 ± 0.6	1.48 ± 0.37	1.37 ± 0.3	1.13 ± 0.22*	0.05		
	Exercise	1.18 ± 0.22*	0.94 ± 0.11	0.94 ± 0.2	0.79 ± 0.11*	0.05	0.05	0.05
ETVI (cm)	Rest	10.3 ± 2.5	10.4 ± 2.6	9.8 ± 1.8	5.5 ± 1.7*	0.05		
	Exercise	9.06 ± 1.3	7.43 ± 1.8*	9.1 ± 1.3	6.6 ± 1.4*	0.05	0.05	0.05
ATVI (cm)	Rest	3.4 ± 0.7	3.73 ± 0.9	3.2 ± 0.8	2.4 ± 0.6*	0.05		
	Exercise	3.85 ± 0.8	5.73 ± 1.5*	4.0 ± 0.6	3.2 ± 1.1	0.05	0.05	0.05
TTVI (cm)	Rest	13.7 ± 2	14.0 ± 3	13.0 ± 1.8	7.9 ± 1.9*	0.05		
	Exercise	12.9 ± 2	13.2 ± 3	13.1 ± 1.9	9.8 ± 2.1*	0.05	N S	N S
AFF (%)	Rest	19.8 ± 5	21.8 ± 3.6	24.6 ± 6	30.1 ± 3.9*	0.05		
	Exercise	29.8 ± 6	38.0 ± 6.4*	30.5 ± 8	33.0 ± 4.3	0.05	0.05	0.05
MVC (kg)	Rest	—	—	—	—	—		
	Exercise	238 ± 20*	329 ± 30*	192 ± 17	197 ± 22	0.05	—	0.05

* This group differs from the others at that condition

E = Mitral peak early diastole, A = Presystolic maximal velocity, ETVI = Mitral early diastolic time velocity, ATVI = Mitral presystolic time velocity, TTVI = Total time velocity integral, AFF = Atrial filling fraction, MVC = Maximal voluntary contraction.

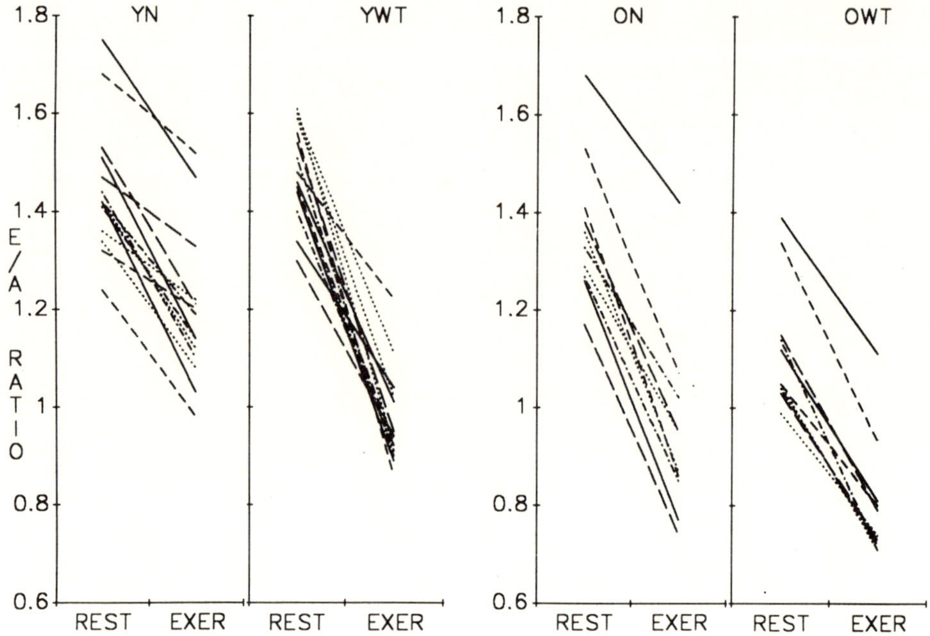

Figure 3. Individual data for mitral early diastole/presystolic maximal velocity ratio (E/A) at rest and during isometric exercise (EXER) in young normals (YN), young weight lifters (YWT), old normals (ON) and old weight lifters (OWT).

Hemodynamic Responses

Heart rate did not differ between the groups at rest and during exercise. Mean heart rate was significantly ($p<0.05$) higher during deadlift than at rest for all the groups. Systolic and diastolic blood pressure at rest were similar in each group. During isometric deadlift, all groups showed significant ($p<0.05$) increases from resting values in blood pressure. Systolic blood pressure during exercise bout was significantly ($p<0.05$) higher in the young weight lifters, while diastolic blood pressure was significantly ($p<0.05$) higher with the highest value in the older weight lifting group compared to the other groups. Oxygen uptake increased significantly ($p<0.05$)from rest to deadlift in all groups. However, oxygen uptake values were significantly ($p<0.005$) higher in the younger weight lifting group than in the other groups during deadlift maneuver.

Left Ventricular Diastolic Filling

The E wave peak velocity was significantly ($p<0.05$) lower in the older weight lifters than in the other three groups, and it remained so during the isometric bout. At rest, the A peak velocity did not differ significantly between groups. During exercise, the A peak velocity of all subjects increased significantly ($p<0.05$) from resting values, with significantly ($p<0.05$) higher values in the young weight lifting subjects. The E/A ratio was thus significantly ($p<0.05$) reduced at rest and during isometric exercise in the older weight lifters compared to the other three groups. All subjects had lower ($p<0.05$) values for E/A ratio during exercise from resting values. No significant differences were found at rest and during exercise between the two young groups and the older normals in regard to TTVI. However, in the older weight lifting subjects, significantly ($p<0.05$) lower values were found at rest and during isometric deadlift compared with the other three groups. At rest and during isometric deadlift, the ETVI and ATVI differed significantly ($p<0.05$) in the older weight lifting subjects from the other subjects having lower values. During exercise bout, the young weight lifting group differed significantly ($p<0.05$) from the other normal subjects having reduced ETVI and increased ATVI from resting values. Atrial filling fraction differed significantly ($p<0.05$) at rest in the older weight lifters. All subjects increased significantly ($p<0.05$) those values from resting values, with the highest increase ($p<0.05$) in the young weight lifting group.

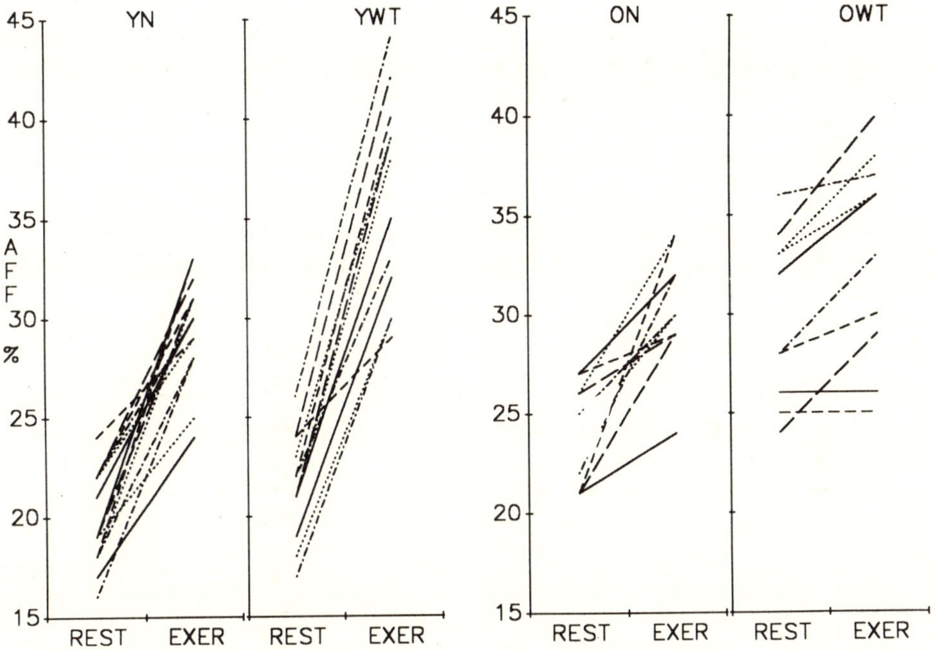

Figure 4. Individual data for atrial filling fraction (AFF) at rest and during isometric exercise (EXER) in young normals (YN), young weight lifters (YWT), old normals (ON) and old weight lifters (OWT).

DISCUSSION

This study indicated that at rest atrial contribution to total diastolic filling increased, in the absence of left ventricular pathology, owing to the aging process alone. During isometric deadlift, the different patterns found at rest among the groups were more prominent. With increased afterload, the young weight lifters showed a significantly higher value of systolic blood pressure compared to the other three groups. This response may be attributed to the higher absolute tension exerted for three minutes by the young weight lifters. However, calculations of the mean arterial blood pressures did not reveal significant differences between groups. This pressor response is in agreement with previous studies (Sagiv et al., 1985; Sagiv et al., 1988a). The similar increases in blood pressure during exercise may be because they were performing contractions at the same percent of maximal voluntary contraction. Heart rate rose significantly from rest to exercise; this increase during isometric deadlift has been previously reported (Sagiv et al., 1985; Sagiv et al., 1988a; Seals et al., 1983). This increase, however, differs significantly from that observed during dynamic exercise (Asmussen, 1981). Although significant differences in heart rate were observed from rest to isometric maneuver, it seems unlikely that the differences in heart rate responses in the present study are a factor that altered diastolic filling properties and time dependent variables (Goldberg, 1988). With rapid heart rates, the time available for cardiac filling is abbreviated to such an extent that it infringes on the phase of rapid ventricular filling. Under the circumstances, left ventricular filling properties may be altered. In contrast, bradycardia prolongs the period of ventricular filling. However, as the major inflow occurs early in diastole, it provides for only a small increase in end-diastolic volume.

The differences from rest to exercise for all subjects may be due to reduction in central blood volume, following large increase in intrathoracic and abdominal pressures, along with increment in afterload during isometric bout. This reduction in central blood volume and increases in afterload in turn may alter venous return and diastolic filling properties, by disturbing the pressure-flow relationship of the venous system and by increasing systemic venous resistance.

The results obtained in the older weight lifters at rest and during exercise demonstrated a significant reduction in diastolic function compared to the normal older men and young ones. Previous studies on elderly subjects have shown results similar to those found here in the older weight lifters of an age-related augmentation in the atrial component of left ventricular filling (Downes et al., 1989; Kuo et al., 1987; Stoddard et al., 1989). It is likely that these differences are related to changes with chronic overload training and age in the passive phase of left ventricular diastolic pressure-volume relationship. This response suggests that the combined chronic overload training and aging might reduce the inotropic state in the older weight lifters.

The failure to augment contractility in the older weight lifters may be the cause of reduced diastolic function (Sagiv et al., 1988a). Under normal conditions during exercise, adrenergic stimulation increases the frequency of contractile responses which, while stronger, are also briefer. Thus, the typical response of the heart to adrenergic stimulation is a sinus tachycardia in which each contraction, although more forceful, relaxes more rapidly and is abbreviated to a prolonged lusitropic stage which in turn facilitates filling at increased heart rates (Katz, 1990). In addition, decreases in end-systolic dimension and an increase in contractile state, as seen in the young subjects (Sagiv et al., 1988a; Sagiv et al.,

1988b), will increase atrioventricular pressure gradient at the time of mitral value opening (Yellin et al., 1980).

The results from the young weight lifters demonstrated normal left ventricular relaxation indices and filling properties at rest. However, during isometric deadlift, abnormal filling properties were noted, namely, reduced E/A ratio and mitral early diastolic time velocity, and an increase in A, mitral presystolic time velocity, and atrial filling fraction. The differences from rest to exercise in the young weight lifters compared to the two normal groups may be due to a larger reduction in central blood volume due to a higher voluntary contraction performed and not to fundamental differences in the properties of the myocardium. In addition, during isometric bout, the mechanism responsible for the decrease in venous return is a reflex increase in sympathetic activity, possibly related to earlier recruitment of type II fibres (Palatini,1988). This sympathetic activity will increase levels of catecholamines, which will promote deactivation at the sarcomere level by augmenting calcium sequestration by the sarcoplasmic reticulum (Morad et al., 1978). This in turn will change the velocity of relaxation, which is directly related to end-systolic load (Gaasch et al., 1980).

CONCLUSION

Although this study has shown significant differences in Doppler indices of diastolic function during isometric exercise, it is likely that, in the young weight lifters and in both normal groups, these differences are related to differences in the stroke volume and arterial pressure responses and not to fundamental differences in the properties of the myocardium. As for the older weight lifting group, this study suggests that at rest they relied more on atrial contribution for left ventricular filling than on the passive phase of ventricular filling. Isometric exercise stress increased the reliance on the atrial support, as was seen in previous studies of elderly subjects.

REFERENCES

Asmussen E. Similarities and dissimilarities between static and dynamic exercise. Circ Res 1981(Suppl. I);48:3-10.

Braunwald E. Heart Disease: A textbook of cardiovascular medicine. Philadelphia: W.B. Saunders, 1984:413-93.

Downes RT, Nomeir AM, Smith MK, Stewart PK, Little CM. Mechanism of altered pattern of left ventricular filling with aging in subjects without cardiac disease. Am J Cardiol 1989;64:523-7.

Gaasch WH, Blaustein AS, Andrias CW, Donahue RP, Avitall B. Myocardial relaxation. II. Hemodynamic determinants of rate of left ventricular isovolumic pressure decline. Am J Physiol 1980;239:H1-6.

Gardin JM, Rohan MK, Davidsen DM et al. Doppler transmitral flow velocity parameters: relationship between age, body surface area, blood pressure and gender in normal subjects. Am J Noninvas Cardiol 1987;1:3-10.

Goldberg ST, Allen HD, Marx GR, Donnerstein RL. Doppler Echocardiography, 2nd ed. Philadelphia: Lea & Febiger, 1988:285.

Katz AM. Interplay between inotropic and lusitropic effects of cyclic adenosine monophosphate in the myocardial cell. Circulation 1990;82(Suppl I): I7-11.

Kitabatake A, Inoue M, Asao M et al. Blood flow reflecting diastolic behaviour of the left ventricle in health and disease. A study by pulsed Doppler technique. JPN Circ J 1982;46:92-102.

Kuo LC, Quinones MA, Rokey R, Sartori M, Abinader EG, Zoghbi WA. Quantification of atrial contribution to left ventricular filling by pulsed Doppler echocardiography and the effect of age in normal and diseased hearts. Am J Cardiol 1987;59:1147-78.

Lakatta EG, Yin PCP. Myocardial aging functional alterations and related cellular mechanisms. Am J Physiol 1982;242:927-41.

Menapace FJ, Hammer WJ, Ritzer TF et al. Left ventricular size in competitive weight lifters: an echocardiographic study. Med Sci Sports Exerc 1982;14:72-5.

Morad M, Weiss J, Cleeman L. The inotropic action of adrenaline on cardiac muscle: does it relax or potentiate tension? Eur J Cardiol 1978;7(Suppl): 53-62.

Palatini P. Blood pressure behaviour during physical activity. Sports Med 1988;5:353-74.

Rokey R, Kuo LC, Zoghbi WA, Limacher MC, Quinones MA. Determination of parameters of left ventricular diastolic filling with pulsed Doppler echocardiography: comparison with cineangiography. Circulation 1985;71:543-50.

Sagiv M, Hanson P, Besozzi M, Nagle F. Left ventricular responses to upright isometric handgrip and deadlift in men with coronary artery disease. Am J Cardiol 1985;55:1298-1302.

Sagiv M, Goldhammer E, Abinader GE, Rudoy J. Aging and the effect of increased after-load on left ventricular contractile state. Med Sci Sports Exerc 1988a;20:281-4.

Sagiv M, Hanson P, Goldhamer E, Ben-Sira D, Ruddy J. Left ventricular and hemodynamic responses during upright isometric exercise in normal young and elderly men. Gerontology 1988b;34:165-70.

Seals DR, Washburn RA, Hanson PG, Nagle F, Painter P. Increased cardiovascular response to static contraction of large muscle groups. J Appl Physiol 1983;54:434-7.

Stoddard MF, Pearson AL, Kern MJ, Atcleeiff J, Mrosek DG, Labovitz AJ. Influence of alteration in preload on the pattern of left ventricular diastolic filling as assessed by Doppler echocardiography in humans. Circulation 1989;79:1226-36.

Templeton GH, Platt MR, Willerson JT, Weisfeldt ML. Influence of aging on left ventricular hemodynamics and stiffness in beagles. Circ Res 1979;44:189-94.

Teichholz LE, Kreulen T, Herman MV, Gorlin R. Problems in echocardiographic volume determination. Echocardiographic angiographic correlations in the presence or absence of asynergy. Am J Cardiol 1976;37:7-11.

Yellin EL, Sonnenblick EH, Frater RWM: Dynamic determinants of left ventricular filling: an overview. In: Bann J, Arntzenius AC, Yellin EL, eds. Cardiac Dynamics. The Hague/Boston/London: Martinus Nijhoff Publishers, 1980: 145-58.

Yin FCP, Spurgeon HA, Weisfeldt ML, Lakatta EG. Mechanical properties of myocardium from hypertrophied rat heart. Circ Res 1980;46:292-300.

Structural and Functional Features in Old Amateur Runners: An Echo-Doppler Study

Gastone Sabbadini, M.D.
Lorenzo Pascazio, M.D.
Giorgio Delbello, M.D.
Guido Curri, M.D.

INTRODUCTION

"Athlete Heart" and other effects of physical exercise have been well studied in adult, highly trained, competitive athletes (Bekaert et al., 1981; Brown et al., 1983; Ehsani et al., 1978; Fegard et al., 1984; Mumford and Prakash, 1981; Snoeckx et al., 1982; Wieling et al., 1981). The majority of these studies were carried out with young subjects (18 to 30 years of age, average 23), primarily males, in diverse athletic activities (running, swimming, bicycling, rowing, weight-lifting). Cardiac responses to exercise have been less well studied in elderly subjects who are not competitive but are sufficiently trained (Heath et al., 1981). Moreover, data on anatomy and functional regulation of the circulatory system in athletes are not easily available in the literature (Pyorala et al., 1967; Sebban et al., 1981). The circulatory system is very complex in its structure and function; for example, the human brain differs significantly from other organs of the body: it accounts for only two percent of body weight, but receives 15 percent of cardiac output and consumes 20 percent of body oxygen supply in the basal state (Stephens and Stilwell, 1969). Today, several aspects of the heart and extracranial cerebral and peripheral lower limb vessels are directly accessible to ultrasound examination. The purpose of this study was to assess the cardiovascular status in elderly endurance runners utilizing echo-Doppler technique.

METHODS

Subjects

The study group (group A) consisted of 14 subjects (10 males and four females), aged 60 to 78 years (mean age: 64.7 ± 5.6); they ran seven to 38 km/week and their "run-activity" duration ranged from three to 18 years. They were compared to an age- and sex-matched group (B) of 20 nonathletic subjects (14 males and six females), aged 56 to 81 years (mean age: 63.8 ± 5.9); the sedentary volunteers were in good health and had no historical or clinical evidence of cardiovascular diseases. In all subjects we collected heart rate and blood pressure, and from the clinical profile we detected cardiovascular risk factors; resting electrocardiograms were performed with a Hewlett Packard Page Writer XLe system. Exercise tests (treadmill exercise tests with electrocardiogram monitoring and maximum 0_2 uptake) were not performed in this study.

Anthropometric characterization

In order to characterize our population, the following anthropometric measures were determined: 1) height; 2) body weight; 3) percent body fat: skinfold thickness measurements were made with a Bull plicometer at four sites (triceps, biceps, subscapularis, suprailiac), and percent body fat was estimated from the skinfold measures using the Durnin and Womersley method (Durnin and Womersley, 1974); 4) lean body weight: [body weight - (percent body fat x body weight)] (Chumlea et al., 1986; Pollini, 1984).

Respiratory function evaluation

We also investigated the respiratory function of our subjects with a commercially available spirometer (Cosmed Pony 2.2 spirometer). The following static and dynamic pulmonary volumes were detected: vital capacity, maximal voluntary ventilation, and the forced expiratory volume at the first second. Tiffeneau Index was calculated as the ratio of the forced expiratory volume at the first second to the vital capacity (Brambilla and Pizzamiglio, 1979; Garbagni, 1985).

Ultrasonographic examination of heart

All subjects underwent echocardiographic study at rest; echocardiograms were performed with a Ving Med 750 Color Flow Mapping scanner by using a 3.0 MHz Annular Phased Array Duplex Color transducer. All echocardiographic and cardiac Doppler recordings were made by one observer; tracings of five consecutive cardiac cycles were analyzed, and an average was taken for all measurements. Two-dimensionally directed M-mode echograms were obtained, and measurements of left atrial and left ventricular sizes and left ventricular wall thicknesses were determined according to the recommendations of the American Society of Echocardiography (Sahn et al., 1978). Left ventricular mass was calculated according to the formula of Devereux and Reichek (1977): mass (g) = 1.04 x [(posterior wall thickness + left ventricular end-diastolic diameter + septal wall thickness)^3 - (left ventricular end-diastolic diameter)^3] - 13.6. To assess the overall performance of the left ventricle, percent fractional shortening was calculated: [(left ventricular end-diastolic diameter — left ventricular end-systolic diameter)/ left ventricular end-diastolic diameter] x 100. Two-dimensional echocardiograms of all cardiac chambers were recorded from the apical view. This view allowed assessment of regional wall motion of left ventricle. To assess left ventricular inflow pattern, two-dimensionally guided pulsed-Doppler recordings of transmitral diastolic flow were obtained; peak velocities in early and late diastole and ratio of early-to-late diastolic flow velocities were measured. Validation of Doppler assessment of left ventricular filling was performed by comparison with angiographic and nuclear data (Rokey et al., 1985; Spirito et al., 1986). Color Doppler technique was utilized to study valvular flows; the presence of valvular stenosis and/or insufficiency was confirmed by pulsed and continuous wave Doppler; quantitation of aortic and mitral or tricuspid regurgitation was performed according to the methods of Masuyama et al. (1986) and Helmcke et al. (1987).

Ultrasonographic examination of vessels

Echo color Doppler study of vessels was obtained using a 7.5 MHz Annular Phased Array Duplex Color and a 7.5 MHz Dual Duplex Color transducers. Duplex sonographic assessment of extracranial cerebrovascular system (carotid, vertebral and subclavian arteries) and peripheral vascular system of lower limbs was performed for each subject of both groups. Duplex scanning examination was determined according to the recommendations of Zwiebel (1986) and the Salt Lake City Veterans Administration Medical Center (Cranley et al., 1989). High resolution B-mode imaging (longitudinal and transversal projections), Doppler flow analysis (Rittgers et al., 1983), peak systolic velocity, end-diastolic velocity, index of resistance [(peak systolic velocity - end-diastolic velocity)/(peak systolic velocity)] (Planiol et al., 1973), systole/diastole ratio (peak systolic velocity/end-diastolic velocity) (Courbier et al., 1978) of carotid vessels were obtained. For the lower limbs we recorded high resolution B-mode imaging, ankle/arm systolic index (Yao et al., 1969), and pulsatility index (peak-to-peak velocity difference/mean velocity) (Gosling et al., 1971) of each vessel.

Statistical Analysis

Comparisons between the two groups were made using the Student's t-test and the chi-square test, when appropriate. Statistical significance was defined as $p<0.05$.

RESULTS

Anthropometric characterization

As shown in Table 1, there were no significant differences between runners and controls in mean anthropometric measures.

Respiratory Function Evaluation

Old runners showed greater mean pulmonary values than sedentary volunteers; Tiffeneau Index was similar in the two groups (Table 2).

TABLE 1

Anthropometric Data in 14 Elderly Runners (10 M and 4 F) and 20 Sedentary Controls (14 M and 6 F)

ANTHROPOMETRIC DATA (MV ± SD)	Elderly runners (group A = 14 subjects)	Sedentary controls (group B = 20 subjects)	P
Age (yrs)	64.7 ± 5.6 (M = 65.7 - F = 62.3)	63.8 ± 5.9 (M = 64.8 - F = 61.5)	NS
Height (cm)	170.7 ± 5.7 (M = 172.7 - F = 165.7)	168.3 ± 5.3 (M = 170.4 - F = 163.4)	NS
Body weight (kg)	74.7 ± 10.4 (M = 77.9 - F = 66.7)	72.8 ± 10.5 (M = 76.3 - F = 64.6)	NS
Fat body (%)	24.0 ± 8.1 (M = 24.3 - F = 23.3)	23.9 ± 8.3 (M = 24.2 - F = 23.2)	NS
Lean body weight (kg)	56.8 ± 5.1 (M = 59.0 - F = 51.2)	55.2 ± 4.9 (M = 57.8 - F = 49.6)	NS

F: Females; M: Males; MV ± SD: Mean Value ± Standard Deviation; NS: Not significant

TABLE 2

Repiratory Function Data in 14 Elderly Runners (10 M and 14 F) and 20 Sedentary Controls (14 M and 6 F)

RESPIRATORY FUNCTION DATA (MV ± SD)	Elderly runners (group A = 14 subjects)	Sedentary controls (group B = 20 subjects)	P
VC (l)	3.92 ± 0.53 (M = 4.08 - F = 3.52)	3.52 ± 0.55 (M = 3.70 - F = 3.10)	<0.05
MVV (l/min)	119.7 ± 15.8 (M = 122.9 - F = 111.7)	101.2 ± 10.6 (M = 103.6 - F = 95.5)	<0.001
FEV_1 (l/sec)	3.12 ± 0.42 (M = 3.23 - F = 2.84)	2.67 ± 0.33 (M = 2.78 - F = 2.42)	NS
TI (FEV_1/VC)	0.80 ± 0.07 (M = 0.79 - F = 0.81)	0.76 ± 0.07 (M = 0.75 - F = 0.78)	NS

F: Females; FEV_1: Forced Expiratory Volume at First Second; M: Males; MV ± SD: Mean Value ± Standard Deviation; MVV: Maximal Voluntary Ventilation; NS: Not significant; TI: Tiffeneau Index; VC: Vital Capacity

Ultrasonographic examination of heart

All subjects were in sinus rhythm with heart rate slower than 90 beats/min. Cardiac size: mean end-diastolic left ventricular cavity dimension was superimposable in group A and group B (5.0 ± 0.5 cm.); two runners (one female and one male, 14.3 percent) and three controls (15.0 percent) had left ventricular dilatation of mild degree (left ventricular end-diastolic diameter> 5.6 cm); the others did not exceed the accepted normal limits for adults without heart disease. Eight runners (all males, 57.1 percent) and five controls (25.0 percent) showed left ventricular hypertrophy (left ventricular posterior and/or septal wall thickness > 1.20 cm). Mean end-diastolic left ventricular posterior wall and septal wall thicknesses were respectively 1.16 ± 0.16 cm and 1.22 ± 0.17 cm in elderly runners; in normal controls they were 1.02 ± 0.12 cm and 1.10 ± 0.14 cm. Left atrial enlargement (end-systolic left atrial diameter > 4.0 cm) was present in 35.8 percent of amateurs (five of 14) and in 20 percent of sedentary subjects (four of 20). Table 3 displays the mean morphometric data as detected by echocardiography.

Left ventricular systolic function: the shortening fraction of left ventricular at rest was similar in both groups (32 ± 5 percent); no wall motion abnormalities were present on 2-D echocardiography. Left ventricular diastolic filling: evaluation of left ventricular filling by

TABLE 3

Echocardiographic Data in 14 Elderly Runners (10 M and 4 F) and 20 Sedentary Controls (14 M and 6 F)

Echocardiographic measurements (MV ± SD)	Elderly runners (group A = 14 subjects)	Sedentary controls (group B = 20 subjects)	P
LVIDd (cm)	5.0 ± 0.5 (M = 5.1 - F = 4.9)	5.0 ± 0.5 (M = 5.1 - F = 4.8)	NS
LVIDs (cm)	3.4 ± 0.3 (M = 3.5 - F = 3.3)	3.4 ± 0.5 (M = 3.4 - F = 3.3)	NS
SWT (cm)	1.22 ± 0.17 (M = 1.25 - F = 1.15)	1.10 ± 0.14 (M = 1.12 - F = 1.05)	<0.05
PWT (cm)	1.16 ± 0.16 (M = 1.19 - F = 1.09)	1.02 ± 0.12 (M = 1.04 - F = 0.97)	<0.01
LVM (g)	274 ± 90 (M = 279 - F = 242)	232 ± 56 (M = 246 - F = 200)	NS
LAD (cm)	3.9 ± 0.5 (M = 4.0 - F = 3.7)	3.7 ± 0.5 (M = 3.8 - F = 3.5)	NS

F: Females; LAD: Left Atrial Dimension; LIVIDd: End-diastolic Left Ventricular Internal Dimension; LIVIDs: End-systolic Left Ventricular Internal Dimension; LVM: Left Ventricular Mass; M: Males; MV ± SD: Mean Value ± Standard Deviation; NS: Not significant; PWT: Posterior Wall Thickness; SWT: Septal Wall Thickness.

Doppler showed mitral flow waveform to be similar in the two groups; thirteen runners (92.9 percent) and sixteen controls (80.0 percent) had a Doppler-derived ratio of early-to-late left ventricular inflow velocities <1; mean values of peak velocities of early and late ventricular diastolic fillings are reported in Table 4.

TABLE 4

Cardiac Doppler Data in 14 Elderly Runners (10 M and 4 F) and 20 Sedentary Controls (14 M and 6 F)

Cardiac Doppler measurements (MV ± SD)	Elderly runners (group A = 14 subjects)	Sedentary controls (group B = 20 subjects)	P
Peak E (m/sec)	0.49 ± 0.11 (M = 0.49 - F = 0.50)	0.59 ± 0.13 (M = 0.58 - F = 0.61)	NS
Peak A (m/sec)	0.70 ± 0.10 (M = 0.68 - F = 0.75)	0.72 ± 0.16 (M = 0.71 - F = 0.75)	NS
Peak E/Peak A	0.71 ± 0.15 (M = 0.72 - F = 0.67)	0.82 ± 0.34 (M = 0.82 - F = 0.81)	NS

F: Females; M: Males; MV ± SD: Mean Value ± Standard Deviation; NS: Not significant; Peak A: Peak Velocity of Late Left Ventricular Filling; Peak E: Peak Velocity of Early Left Ventricular Filling; Peak E/Peak A: Ratio of Early-to-Late Left Ventricular Filling

Functioning of cardiac valves: aortic and mitral or tricuspid insufficiency of mild degree was present in 54.3 percent of Group A (nine of 14) and 55 percent of group B (11 of 20); however, no subject of the two groups had valvular disease of hemodynamic relevance.

Ultrasonographic examination of vessels

Vascular Doppler examination: we examined the extracranial cerebral arteries and the peripheral vessels of lower limbs. The flow patterns in the main arteries of the two districts were normal and superimposable in the two groups. All Doppler parameters are shown in Table 5. The only difference between group A and group B related to Doppler waveform of the distal arteries: in 40 percent of our control subjects, the classic triphasic aspect was absent (at least in one distal artery), without any other alteration of Doppler parameters. The absence of triphasic waveform in muscular artery spectrum is an early sign of reduced vascular compliance.

TABLE 5

Vascular Doppler Data in 14 Elderly Runners(10 M and 14 F)
and 20 Sedentary Controls (14 M and 6F)

VASCULAR DOPPLER DATA (MV ± SD)	Elderly runners (group A = 14 subjects)	Sedentary controls (group B = 20 subjects)	P
CAROTID INTERNAL ARTERIES			
Peak systolic velocity (cm/sec)	78 ± 12 (M = 79 - F = 76)	73 ± 11 (M = 74 - F = 71)	NS
End-diastolic velocity (cm/sec)	21.5 ± 8 (M = 21.7 - F = 21.0)	18.5 ± 6 (M = 18.9 - F = 17.6)	NS
Resistance index	0.73 ± 0.08 (M = 0.73 - F = 0.72)	0.74 ± 0.04 (M = 0.74 - F = 0.75)	NS
Systole/diastole ratio	3.63 ± 0.25 (M = 3.64 - F = 3.62)	3.95 ± 0.38 (M = 3.92 - F = 4.03)	NS
LOWER LIMB VESSELS			
Ankle/arm systolic index	1.09 ± 0.11 (M = 1.09 - F = 1.09)	1.11 ± 0.08 (M = 1.10 - F = 1.13)	NS
Pulsatility index of:			
• **Femoral artery**	8.4 ± 4.4 (M = 8.3 - F = 8.7)	7.9 ± 4.1 (M = 7.8 - F = 8.1)	NS
• **Popliteal artery**	7.9 ± 1.3 (M = 7.7 - F = 8.4)	7.4 ± 1.1 (M = 7.2 - F = 7.9)	NS
• **Posterior tibial artery**	15.5 ± 2.1 (M = 15.4 - F = 15.8)	14.8 ± 3.2 (M = 14.6 - F = 15.3)	NS

F: Females; M: Males; MV ± SD: Mean Value ± Standard Deviation; NS: Not significant

Duplex scanning of vessels: echotomography of the cerebro afferent vessels showed: in six elderly runners only an intimal thickening; in seven, an intimal thickening with lamellar calcifications; and in one, an homogeneous plaque with a smooth surface. Eight subjects of the control group had an intimal thickening, seven had an intimal thickening plus lamellar calcifications; in five subjects we found a little, moderately echogenic, homogeneous plaque at level of the carotid bifurcation. Duplex scanning of the iliac-femoral-popliteal vessels pointed out in elderly runners the presence of lamellar calcifications in 85.7 percent of them; the other 14.3 percent had some hyper-echogenic plaques with a smooth surface but without important vessel lumen reduction. All subjects of the control group showed the presence of lamellar wall calcifications; 12 subjects had some hyper-echogenic plaques in femoral bifurcation (bilateral) and three of them also a mild lumen reduction along the superficial femoral artery (Table 6).

TABLE 6

Vascular Echographic Data in 14 Elderly Runners (10 M and 4F) and 20 Sedentary Controls (14 M and 6 W)

VASCULAR ECHOGRAPHIC DATA	Elderly runners (group A = 14 subjects)		Sedentary controls (group B = 20 subjects)		P
	N°	%	N°	%	
CAROTID ARTERIES					
Intimal thickening	6 (M = 4 - F = 2)	42.9	8 (M = 5 - F = 3)	40	NS
Lamellar calcification	7 (M = 5 - F = 2)	50.0	7 (M = 5 - F = 2)	35	NS
Plaques	1 (M = 1 - F = 0)	7.1	5 (M = 4 - F = 1)	25	NS
FEMORAL ARTERIES					
Intimal thickening	0 (M = 0 - F = 0)	0	0 (M = 0 - F = 0)	0	—
Lamellar calcification	12 (M = 8 - F = 4)	85.7	8 (M = 5 - F = 3)	40	<0.05
Plaques	2 (M = 2 - F = 0)	14.3	12 (M = 9 - F = 3)	60	<0.05

F: Females; M: Males; NS: Not significant

DISCUSSION

There are few data currently available on left ventricular dimensions in older non-elite athletes (Heath et al., 1981), although there is the impression that such individuals do not achieve the same degree of cavity enlargement and/or wall thickening as younger runners. In our study, elderly runners showed a normal left ventricular cavity size but an increased left ventricular wall thickness as compared to sedentary subjects. These findings suggest that, during prolonged exercise of mild intensity, the volume overload imposed on the left ventricle might be minimized; on the contrary, it is possible that brief episodes of pressure overload might be sufficient to induce left ventricular wall thickening. The correlation between left ventricular wall thickness or mass and peak systolic blood pressure and the importance of this intermittent stress are supported by the studies of Devereux et al. (1983) and Ren et al. (1985). Left ventricular percent fractional shortening and ejection fraction are usually normal in athletes (Bekaert et al., 1981; Brown et al., 1983; Ehsani et al., 1978; Fegard et al., 1984; Heath et al., 1981; Mumford and Prakash, 1981; Snoeckx et al., 1982; Wieling et al., 1981). Only a few studies found indexes of left ventricular contractility to be mildly increased (Colan et al., 1985; Granger et al., 1985) or decreased (Blair et al.,

1980; Nishimura et al., 1980) in sportsmen. Our amateur runners showed normal left ventricular fractional shortening and no abnormalities of left ventricular wall motion. Abnormalities of left ventricular diastolic performance have been described in hypertrophied hearts due to hypertension, aortic stenosis and hypertrophic cardiomyopathy (Eichhorn et al., 1983; Hanrath et al., 1987; Hartford et al., 1984; Maron et al., 1987; Phillips et al., 1987; Takenaka et al., 1986). On the contrary, physiological increase of left ventricular mass, as seen in endurance athletes, does not impair left ventricular diastolic properties; various studies uniformly show indexes of left ventricular diastolic function to be within normal limits in athletes (Colan et al., 1985; Finkelhor et al., 1985; Granger et al., 1985). In some cases, regular physical activity seems to be associated with a favorable change in early left ventricular filling (Matsuda et al., 1983). In our runners we found an inverted ratio of early-to-late left ventricular diastolic filling but it seems to correlate with age rather than wall hypertrophy: previous studies have suggested that the normal left ventricle becomes stiffer and left ventricular filling is altered with aging (Bryg et al., 1987; Hirota, 1980; Miller et al., 1986); in particular, the relative contribution of atrial systole to overall left ventricular filling increases with age (Gardin et al., 1979).

In our amateurs the scan of cerebro afferent and lower limb vessels showed a lower rank of atherosclerotic lesions in comparison with control population matched for age and sex. Doppler examination of lower limbs in elderly athletes, with the presence of triphasic waveform (typical aspect of muscular artery), reflects the preserved vessel elasticity on distal arteries (posterior tibial, peroneal and anterior tibial). The absence of reversal flow in 40 percent of the control population was the only difference that we recorded between the two groups.

CONCLUSION

Endurance training of mild intensity in elderly runners produces a pattern of left ventricular wall thickening without increase of left ventricular cavity size; it might be the consequence of an intermittent pressure overload, imposed during prolonged exercise. Inverted ratio of early-to-late left ventricular filling in old runners seems to correlate with age rather than left ventricular wall hypertrophy.

REFERENCES

Bekaert I, Pannier JL, Van De Weghe C, Van Durme JP, Clement DL, Pannier R. Noninvasive evaluation of cardiac function in professional cyclist. Br Heart J 1981;45:213-8.

Blair NL, Youker JE, McDonald JG, Jelinek VM. Echocardiographic assessment of cardiac chamber size and left ventricular function in aerobically trained athletes. Aust NZ J Med 1980;10:540-7.

Brambilla I, Pizzamiglio R. ABC dei tests di funzionalita respiratoria. Milano: Masson, 1979:53-78.

Brown S, Byrd R, Jayasinghe J, Jones D. Echocardiographic characteristics of competitive and recreational weight lifters. YCU 1983;2:163-5.

Bryg RJ, Williams JA, Labovitz AJ. Effect of aging on left ventricular diastolic filling in normal subjects. Am J Cardiol 1987;59:971-4.

Chumlea WC, Roche AF, Mukherije D. Some anthropometric indices of body composition for elderly adults. J Gerontol 1986;41:36-9.

Colan SD, Sanders SP, MacPherson D, Borow, KM. Left ventricular diastolic function in elite athletes with physiologic cardiac hypertrophy. J Am Coll Cardiol 1985;6:545-9.

Courbier R, Reggi M, Jausseran JM. Exploration of carotid arteries and vessels of the neck by Doppler techniques In: Dietrich ED, ed. Noninvasive Cardiovascular Diagnosis: Current Concepts. Baltimore: University Park Press, 1978:61-73.

Cranley JJ, Karkow WS, Baldridge ED. Atlas of Duplex Scanning. Philadelphia: W.B. Saunders Company, 1989:86-183.

Devereux RB, Pickering TG, Harshfield GA et al. Left ventricular hypertrophy in patients with hypertension: importance of blood pressure response to regularly recurring stress. Circulation, 1983;68:470-6.

Devereux RB, Reichek N. Echocardiographic determination of left ventricular mass in man. Anatomic validation of the method. Circulation 1977;55:613-8.

Durnin J, Womersley J. Body fat assessed from total body density and its estimation from skin fold thickness measurement on 481 men and women from 16 to 72 years. Br J Nutr 1974;32:77-9.

Ehsani AA, Hagberg JM, Hickson RC. Rapid changes in left ventricular dimensions and mass in response to physical conditioning and deconditioning. Am J Cardiol 1978;42:52-6.

Eichhorn P, Grimm J, Koch R, Hess O, Carroll J, Krayenbuehl HP. Left ventricular relaxation in patients with left ventricular hypertrophy secondary to aortic valve disease. Circulation 1983;65:1395-404.

Fegard R, Aubert A, Staessen J, Van Den Eynde E, Vanhees L, Amery A. Cardiac structure and function in cyclists and runners. Comparative echocardiographic study. Br Heart J 1984;52:124-9.

Finkelhor RS, Hanak LJ, Bahler RC. Diastolic function in endurance trained subjects (abstr). J Am Coll Cardiol 1985;5:540.

Garbagni R. Fisiopatologia respiratoria. Torino: Minerva Medica, 1985;77-110.

Gardin JM, Henry WL, Savage DD, Ware JH, Burn C, Bore JS. Echocardiographic measurements in normal subjects: evaluation of an adult population without clinically apparent heart disease. JCU 1979;7:439-47.

Gosling RG, Dunbar G, King DH et al. The quantitative analysis of occlusive peripheral arterial disease by a noninvasive ultrasonic technique. Angiology 1971;22:52-55.

Granger CG, Karimeddini MK, Smith VE, Shapiro HR, Katz AM, Riba AL. Rapid ventricular filling in left ventricular hypertrophy. I. Physiologic Hypertrophy. J Am Coll Cardiol 1985;5:862-8.

Hanrath P, Mathey DG, Siegert R, Bleifeld W. Left ventricular relaxation and filling pattern of different forms of left ventricular hypertrophy: an echocardiographic study. Am J Cardiol 1987;45:15-23.

Hartford M, Wikstrand J, Wallentin I, Ljungman S, Wilhelmsen I, Berglund G. Diastolic function of the heart in untreated primary hypertension. Hypertension 1984;6:329-38.

Heath GW, Hagberg JM, Ehsani AA, Holloszy JO. A physiological comparison of young and older endurance athletes. J Appl Physiol 1981;51:634-40.

Helmcke F, Nanda NC, Hsiung MC et al. Color Doppler assessment of mitral regurgitation with orthogonal planes. Circulation 1987;75:175-83.

Hirota Y. A clinical study of left ventricular relaxation. Circulation 1980;62:756-63.

Maron BJ, Spirito P, Green KJ, Wesley YE, Bonow RO, Arce J. Noninvasive assessment of left ventricular diastolic function by pulsed-Doppler echocardiography in patients with hypertrophic cardiomyopathy. J Am Coll Cardiol 1987;10:733-42.

Masuyama T, Kodama K, Kitabatake A et al. Noninvasive evaluation of aortic regurgitation by continuous-wave Doppler echocardiography. Circulation 1986;73:460-6.

Matsuda M, Sugishita Y, Koseki S, Ito I, Akatsuka T, Takamatsu K. Effect of exercise on left ventricular diastolic filling in athletes and nonathletes. Appl Physiol 1983;55:323-8.

Miller TR, Grossman SJ, Schectman KB, Biello DR, Ludbrook PA, Ehsani AA. Left ventricular diastolic filling and its association with age. Am J Cardiol 1986;58:531-5.

Mumford M, Prakash R. Electrocardiographic and echocardiographic characteristics of long distance runners. Comparison of left ventricular function with age- and sex-matched controls. Am J Sports Med 1981;9:23-8.

Nishimura T, Yamada Y, Kawai C. Echocardiographic evaluation of long term effects of exercise on left ventricular hypertrophy and function in professional bicyclists. Circulation 1980;61:832-40.

Phillips RA, Coplan NL, Krakoff LR et al. Doppler echocardiographic analysis of left ventricular filling in treated hypertensive patients. J Am Coll Cardiol 1987;9:317-22.

Planiol T, Pourcelot L, Itti R. La circulation carotidienne et cerebrale. La Nouv Pr Med 1973;2:37.

Pollini LM, Elementi di antropometria. Napoli: Idelson, 1984:50-9.

Pyorala K, Karvonen MJ, Taskinen P, Takkunen J, Kyronseppa H, Peltokallio P. Cardiovascular studies on former endurance athletes. Am J Cardiol 1967;20:191-205.

Ren JF, Hakki AH, Kotler MN, Iskandrian AS. Exercise systolic blood pressure: a powerful determinant of increased left ventricular mass in patients with hypertension. J Am Coll Cardiol 1985;5:1224-31.

Rittgers SE, Thornhill BM, Barnes RW. Quantitative analysis of carotid artery Doppler spectral waveforms: diagnostic value of parameters. Ultrasound Med Bio 1983;6:225-264.

Rokey R, Kuo LC, Zoghbi WA, Limacher MC, Quinones MA. Determination of parameters of left ventricular diastolic filling with pulsed Doppler echocardiography: comparison with cineangiography. Circulation 1985;71: 533-50.

Sahn DJ, DeMaria A, Kisslo J, Weyman A. Recommendations regarding quantitation in M-mode echocardiography: results of a survey of echocardiographic measurements. Circulation 1978;58:1072-83.

Sebban C, Berthaux P, Lenoir H et al. Arterial compliance, systolic pressure and heart rate in elderly women at rest and on exercise. Gerontology 1981;27:271-80.

Snoeckx LHEH, Abeling HFM, Lambregts JAC, Schmitz JJF, Verstappen FTJ, Reneman RS. Echocardiographic dimensions in athletes in relation to their training programs. Med Sci Sports Exerc 1982;14:428-34.

Spirito P, Maron BJ, Bonow RO. Noninvasive assessment of left ventricular diastolic function: comparative analysis of Doppler echocardiographic and radionuclide angiographic techniques. J Am Coll Cardiol 1986;7:518-26.

Stephens RB, Stilwell DL. Arteries and Veins of the Human Brain. Springfield: Charles C. Thomas Press 1969:15-26.

Takenaka K, Dabestani A, Gardin JM et al. Left ventricular filling in hypertrophic cardiomyopathy; a pulsed Doppler echocardiographic study. J Am Coll Cardiol 1986;7:1263-71.

Wieling W, Borghols EAM, Hollander AP, Danner SA, Dunning AJ. Echocardiographic dimensions and maximal oxygen uptake in oarsmen during training. Br Heart J 1981;46:190-5.

Yao YST, Hobbs JT, Irvine WT. Ankle systolic pressure measurements in arterial diseases affecting the lower extremities. Br J Surg 1969;56: 676-9.

Zwiebel WJ. Introduction to vascular ultrasonography. Philadelphia: W.B. Saunders Company, 1986:155-6.

Finger Circulation in Younger and Older Men During Prolonged Exercise in Different Thermal Conditions

Juhani Smolander, Ph.D.
Olli Korhonen, M.D.
Ilmari Pyykkö, M.D.

INTRODUCTION

During exercise in a hot environment, skin blood flow increases for heat transfer from the core to the skin. In nonacral areas ("hairy skin"), cutaneous circulation increases mainly through the active vasodilatory reflex (Rowell 1986). In acral areas (fingers, palms, toes, ears), the regulation is different: increase in skin blood flow occurs mainly through the withdrawal of sympathetic nervous activity, i.e., through passive vasodilation (Rowell 1986). In both areas, the increase in skin blood flow is a linear function of core and skin temperature (Wenger et al., 1975a, Wenger et al., 1975b, Hirata et al., 1984). Besides the difference in regulation, the maximal level of flow can reach very high values in acral areas (in fingers ~ 100 ml/100 ml/min) due to the large number of arteriovenous anastomoses, which are relatively rare in nonacral areas (Burton 1939).

Recently, it has been shown that under similar heat stress conditions older adults (50-70 years) have lower skin blood flow in nonacral areas than younger subjects (20-30 years) (Kenney, 1988; Sagawa et al., 1988; Tankersley et al., 1991). The difference persists even when groups of older individuals are matched with younger individuals by body composition, aerobic power, acclimation state, and hydration level (Kenney and Havenith 1991). Whether under heat stress a similar difference between younger and older subjects exists in acral areas is not as well known.

The aim of the present study was to examine the finger circulatory response of younger and older men to prolonged exercise in a thermoneutral, a warm humid, and a hot dry environment.

METHODS

Subjects

Eight young men, aged 28 to 37 years, and six older men, aged 55 to 60 years, participated in the study (Table 1). All subjects were healthy, normotensive, and considered to be unacclimatized to heat. The test procedures followed the Helsinki declaration, and were approved by the Ethics Committee of the Institute of Occupational Health.

TABLE 1

Age and Physical Characteristics of the Subjects (Mean ± SD)

Variable	Younger (N = 8)	Older (N = 6)
Age (years)	34 ± 3	57 ± 2*
Height (cm)	178 ± 6	175 ± 7
Weight (kg)	79 ± 9	87 ± 8*
$\dot{V}O_2$max (ml/min/kg)	41 ± 3	36 ± 4*

* $p<0.05$ as compared to the younger subjects
$\dot{V}O_2$ max, maximum oxygen consumption

Procedures

Before the experiments, the subjects' maximum oxygen consumption and anthropometric characteristics were determined. During the study the subjects performed, in random order, three prolonged treadmill tests in a climatic chamber - once in a thermoneutral (21°C/43 percent), once in warm humid (30°C/80 percent), and once in a hot dry (40°C/20 percent) environment while wearing ordinary work clothing (thermal insulation 0.109 Km^2/W). The treadmill tests consisted of seven 30-minute exercise periods at 30 percent of the individually determined maximum oxygen consumption interspersed by five-minute pauses (total duration four hours). During the tests, water was offered *ad libitum*, and drinking was encouraged. Further details on procedures can be found elsewhere (Smolander et al., 1990).

Measurements

Total blood flow and systolic blood pressure of the left middle finger were measured during each walking period by mercury-in-Silastic strain-gauge plethysmography (Medimatic SP2, Denmark). A small strain-gauge was set around the base of the finger nail to measure changes in circumference. A plastic blood pressure cuff was wrapped around the proximal phalanx. The total finger blood flow was measured by venous occlusion principle utilizing a cuff pressure of 55 mm Hg. In the blood pressure measurement, the cuff pressure was slowly deflated from a suprasystolic pressure, and the point of the first increase in flow was taken as the systolic blood pressure (for further details see Gemne et al., 1986). During the measurement, the forearm was placed on a padded support at heart level. Finger vascular resistance was estimated by dividing the systolic blood pressure by the total blood flow.

Finger skin blood flow was measured with laser-Doppler flowmetry (Nilsson et al., 1980, Gemne et al., 1986) using a Periflux Pfld instrument (Perimed, Sweden). The laser-

Doppler probe was attached on the palmar side of the middle phalanx. A thermistor (YSI 427, Yellow Springs Instruments, USA) taped on the fingertip was used to measure skin temperature. The temperature was recorded from a portable thermometer (YSI 46, USA).

Statistical Analysis

For the analysis, the flow and pressure values were averaged over the entire test period for each subject. A two-way analysis of variance (age group, thermal condition) with repeated measures on thermal condition was used. The differences in background variables between the groups were tested by the Student's t-test. The differences were considered significant when $p < 0.05$.

RESULTS

Whole-Body Responses

In the thermoneutral environment, all subjects were able to perform the four-hour exercise task. At the end of exercise, the heart rate, rectal temperature, and mean skin temperature were not significantly different between the younger and older men in any of the three climatic conditions. (Smolander et al., 1990).

Finger Circulatory Responses

The warm humid and hot dry environment significantly increased finger skin temperature, total finger blood flow, and finger skin blood flow, and significantly decreased finger systolic blood pressure and finger vascular resistance as compared to thermoneutrality (significant thermal condition effects). In addition to the significant main effect of thermal condition, the groups showed different responses with thermal exposures (significant group x thermal condition interaction effects) in all variables.

In the thermoneutral and warm humid environment, the older men had significantly ($p<0.01$) lower finger skin temperatures as compared to younger men (Figure 1), whereas in the hot dry environment the finger skin temperature was at a similar level. Total finger blood flow was similar in both groups in thermoneutrality, but it was at a higher level in older subjects especially in the hot dry environment (Figure 2, upper panel). Older subjects had lower ($p < 0.05$) finger skin blood flow (laser-Doppler flow) than younger men in thermoneutrality, but in both groups the flows did not differ significantly in the warm humid and hot dry environment (Figure 2, lower panel).

In the thermoneutral climate, finger systolic blood pressure ($p<0.01$) and finger vascular resistance ($p<0.05$) were significantly higher in older men in comparison to the younger ones (Figure 3). During exercise in the warm humid (NS) and hot dry environment ($p<0.05$), the older men had higher finger systolic blood pressure than younger men. During exercise in the heat, no significant difference was observed in the finger vascular resistance between the two groups.

DISCUSSION

Several studies have shown age-related structural changes in the cutaneous vasculature, such as loss of papillary capillaries (Ryan 1966, Montagna and Carlisle 1979). These changes indicate that skin blood flow conditions would also be changed with advancing age. Richardson and Schwartz (1985) have demonstrated that older men between 60 and 75

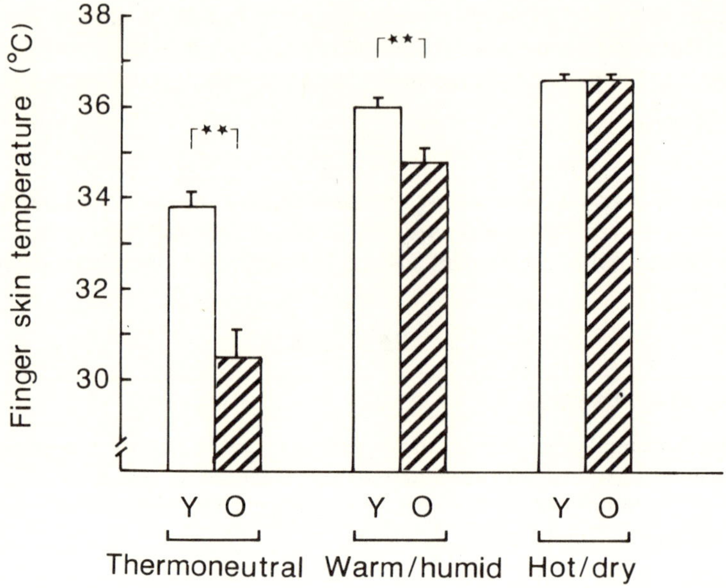

Means ± SE.

** $p < 0.01$ between the groups.

Figure 1. Finger skin temperature in younger (Y) and older (O) men during prolonged exercise in three different climates.

years had lower capillary blood flow in nailfold microcirculation as compared to younger men. Also, the older men had a greater number of tortuous capillaries. Richardson (1989) studied the effect of direct heat on forearm skin blood flow by laser-Doppler flowmetry in young (20 to 39 years), middle-aged (40 to 59 years), and older (60 to 79 years) men. The conclusion was that aging decreases the response of cutaneous blood flow in the forearm to the direct effects of heat via a reduced flow response of individual vessels and a reduced recruitment of flow active vessels.

In addition to these microcirculatory findings, many studies (Kenney 1988, Sagawa et al., 1988, Tankersley et al., 1991) have shown lower forearm blood flow response (an index of skin blood flow) to heat stress in elderly men in comparison to younger men. Because the differences were not caused by differences in body composition, aerobic power, acclimation state, or hydration level (Kenney and Havenith 1991), these data also support the idea of structural changes in cutaneous vascular bed with age. Naturally, age-related regulatory changes, such as an increased vasoconstrictor tone or a reduced vasodilatory response, cannot be ruled out.

In contrast to the above mentioned investigations, in the present study it was found that total finger blood flow in older men was higher in the two hot environments than in younger men. Because in the heat the finger vascular resistance was the same in the two groups of men, the higher total finger blood flow was probably a consequence of higher arterial

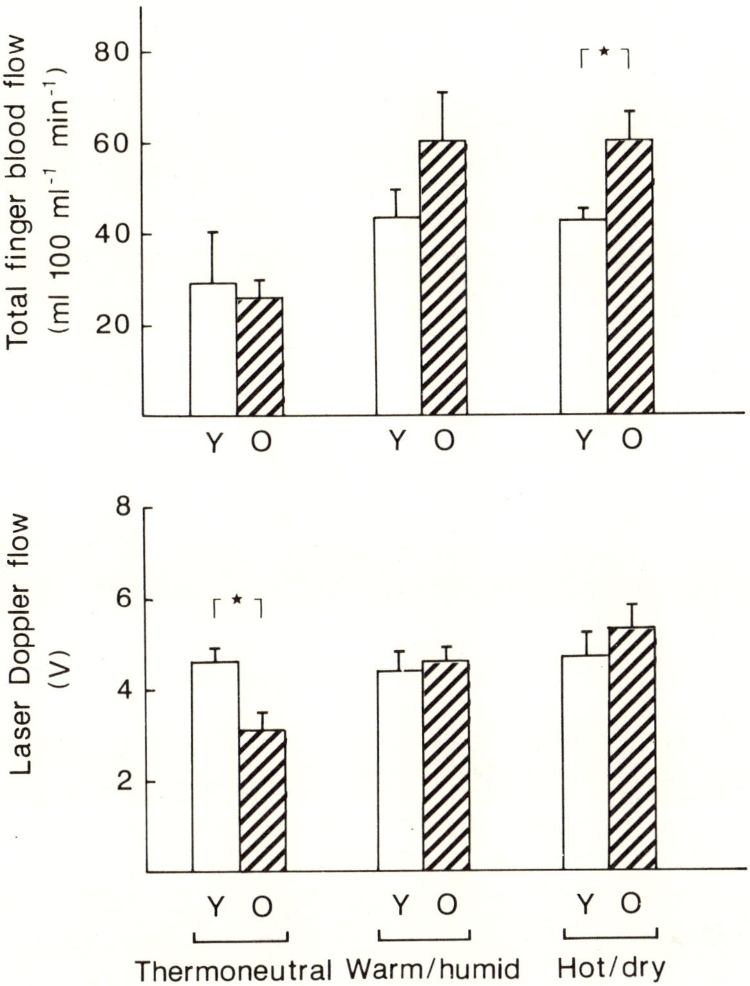

Means ± SE.

* $p<0.05$ between the groups.

Figure 2. Total finger blood flow and laser-Doppler flow of younger (Y) and older (O) men during prolonged exercise in three different climates.

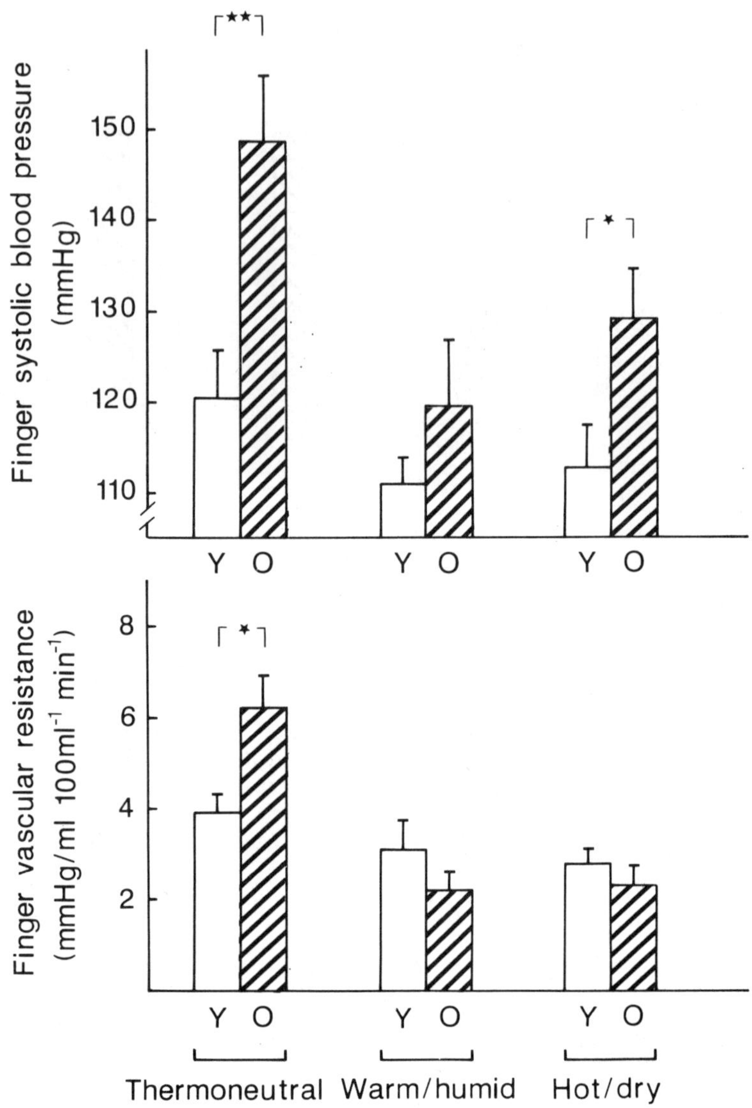

Means ± SE

* $p < 0.05$ between the groups ** $p < 0.01$ between the groups.

Figure 3. Finger systolic blood pressure and figure vascular resistance in younger (Y) and older (O) men during prolonged exercise in three different climates.

blood pressure. However, this conclusion must be made with caution, because we could measure only finger systolic blood pressure by plethysmography instead of mean arterial pressure. The results indicated, however, that the capacity to vasodilate under present heat stress conditions was well maintained in the regional circulation of the fingers in men aged 55 to 60 years. On the other hand, a higher total blood flow in extremities may result in a greater rate of venous pooling of blood, thereby reducing venous return and cardiac filling (Rowell 1986).

In spite of the fact that older men had higher total finger blood flow in the warm humid and hot dry environment, the finger skin blood flow, as measured by laser-Doppler flowmetry, was similar between the two groups. In thermoneutrality, at the same level of total finger blood flow, the finger skin blood flow was significantly lower in the older men. Finger skin temperature was also significantly lower in the thermoneutral and warm humid environment in the older men in comparison to the younger men. Thus, it is possible that older men require a higher level of total finger blood flow in order to attain a similar level of superficial finger skin blood flow and skin temperature as younger men. This may be due to the age-related structural alterations in the cutaneous vessels as found in the microcirculatory studies mentioned above. Westphal and Richardson (1992) have recently made similar findings in a rat tail, in which the structure and regulation of the circulation are similar to those of the human digit.

CONCLUSION

During prolonged exercise in a thermoneutral, a warm humid, and a hot dry environment, older men required a higher total finger blood flow in order to attain a similar level of superficial finger skin blood flow and skin temperature to that of younger men. This may be an indication of age-related structural changes in the cutaneous microvessels of the finger in older men.

ACKNOWLEDGEMENTS

The authors thank Marja Miettinen, M.Sc. and Mr. Matti Kettunen for their help in the analysis of data.

REFERENCES

Burton AC. The range and variability of the blood flow in the human fingers and the vasomotor regulation of body temperature. Am J Physiol 1939;127: 437-53.

Gemne G, Pyykkö I, Starck J, Ilmarinen R. Circulatory reaction to heat and cold in vibration-induced white finger with and without sympathetic blockade - an experimental study. Scand J Work Environ Health 1986;12:371-7.

Hirata K, Nagasaka T, Hirai A, Hirashita M, Takahata T. Peripheral vascular tone during heat load is modified by exercise intensity. Eur J Appl Physiol 1984;51:7-15.

Kenney WL. Control of heat-induced vasodilation in relation to age. Eur J Appl Physiol 1988; 57:120-5.

Kenney WL, Havenith G. Aging, skin blood flow, and heat tolerance. In: Proceedings of the International Conference on Human-Environment System. The Organizating Committee for the International Conference on Human-Environment System, Tokyo, 1991:87-90.

Montagna W, Carlisle K. Structural changes in aging human skin. J Invest Derm 1979;73:47-53.

Nilsson GE, Tenland T, Oberg PA. Evaluation of a laser Doppler flowmeter for measurement of tissue blood flow. IEEE Trans Biomed Eng 1980;27:597-604.

Richardson D. Effects of age on cutaneous circulatory response to direct heat on the forearm. J Gerontol Med Sci 1989;44:M189-94.

Richardson D, Schwartz R. Comparison of capillary blood flow in the nailfold circulations of young and elderly men. Age 1985;8:70-5.

Rowell LB. Human Circulation: Regulation During Physical Stress. New York: Oxford University Press, 1986.

Ryan TJ. The microcirculation of the skin in old age. Gerontol Clin 1966;8:327-37.

Sagawa S, Shiraki K, Yousef MK, Miki K. Sweating and cardiovascular responses of aged men to heat exposure. J Gerontol Med Sci 1988;43:M1-8.

Smolander J, Korhonen O, Ilmarinen R. Responses of young and older men during prolonged exercise in dry and humid heat. Eur J Appl Physiol 1990;61:413-8.

Tankersley CG, Smolander J, Kenney WL, Fortney SM. Sweating and skin blood flow during exercise: effects of age and maximal oxygen uptake. J Appl Physiol 1991;71:236-42.

Wenger CB, Roberts MF, Stolwijk JAJ, Nadel ER. Forearm blood flow during body temperature transients produced by leg exercise. J Appl Physiol 1975a;38:58-63.

Wenger CB, Roberts MF, Nadel ER, Stolwijk JAJ. Thermoregulatory control of finger blood flow. J Appl Physiol 1975b;38:1078-82.

Westphal KA, Richardson DR. Effects of aging on cutaneous regional and superficial capillary blood flows during heat stress in the rat. Age 1992; 15:1-7.

Role of Age-Related Changes of Microcirculation in Evaluating Physical Work Ability of People of Different Ages

Konstantin G. Sarkisov, M.D., Ph.D.
Oleg V. Korkushko, M.D.
Vadim E. Fraifeld, M.D., Ph.D.

INTRODUCTION

Age-related changes in hemodynamics during muscular activity, in particular, arterial and venous pressure in large blood vessels and heart cavities, cardiac rhythm, cardiac output, etc., have frequently been studied (Muravov, 1973; Åstrand, 1968). To define more fully the link between blood and muscle working capacity, however, requires an understanding of the relationships between the regional blood flow, microcirculation and work ability. An association between the number of capillaries and the functional performance of an organ has been discussed since the time of Krogh (1919).

Aging is accompanied by considerable changes in motor activity (Motylyanskaya, 1967; Goldberg and Hagberg, 1990). It is motor activity and its increase in metabolism, particularly in oxygen consumption, that activate the microcirculatory system (Vasiljeva and Stepochkina, 1985).

During muscular activity work, hyperemia is known to be an important adaptation which provides for adequate metabolic expenditures in working muscles. The mechanisms of work hyperemia and its association with local metabolites and factors of neural regulation are still disputed (Skards, 1984; Vasiljeva and Stepochkina, 1985). Analysis of age-related changes in the microcirculation during muscular activity is one of the approaches toward a better understanding of this important compensatory mechanism.

In the present study, we examined the muscle blood flow in the anterior tibial muscle and, simultaneously with the muscular working capacity and carbohydrate metabolism at various types of physical workloads, the skin microcirculation and regional blood circulation in the hand.

METHOD

Muscle blood flow in a portion of the m. tibialis anterior was studied in 170 essentially healthy people, both men and women, aged 18 to 96 years. ^{133}Xe-clearance was determined using the radiometer "Xenon." The counting rate was 300 imp/sec at time constant 2 sec. ^{133}Xe was injected in a small volume (0.1 ml) of physiological solution with an activity of 1850-3700 KBq. Using a thin needle, we injected the solution into the proximal part of the m. tibialis anterior to the depth of 1.5-2 cm and 2 cm outwardly of the os tibialis. The clearance was recorded at rest and after workload under conditions of artificial ischemia. The latter was achieved by creating 250 mm Hg pressure in a cuff placed on the lower one-third of the femur. After a two-minute cessation of blood flow, the patient started intensive flexion-extension movements in the talocrural joint of the ischemic extremity with a rhythm of 60 movements/min until the patient refused because of the onset of pain and fatigue. The reactive hyperemia that followed after cuff release reflected the functional reserve of tissue blood flow in the study muscle, i.e., the physiological maximum of muscle blood flow.

We also studied microcirculatory changes during graded workloads in people of various ages. The study was designed in such a way that a comparison could be made of the pattern of microcirculatory shifts and the pattern of changes in the muscle working capacity, i.e., to relate the change in capillary circulation with the change in function. These series of studies were run together with S.F. Golovchenko and A.Ya. Litoshenko.

The first series consisted of the rhythmic compression by the fingers, at a frequency of 80 metronome strokes per minute, of an elastic rubber tube. The work regimen was as follows: one minute of work, one minute of rest, and an uninterrupted work until the onset of fatigue. For assessment of regional blood circulation of the hand, the occlusive plethysmogram was recorded using the finger capsules placed on distal phalanges of the first and second fingers of the working hand. Skin microcirculation was assessed at the nail bed of the fourth finger of the working hand using capillaroscopy and photocapillarography. For recording muscular performance, the ergogram was registered while the air was passed from the compressed tube to the Marey capsule connected to a recorder. The blood taken from the third finger of the working hand during pauses was analyzed for the lactic acid content.

The second series consisted of working on a handgrip ergometer with load weighing 1, 3, and 6 kg at a frequency of contractions 40 times per minute, with a passage of distance during each contraction equal to 10 cm. The intensity of workload was 4, 12 and 24 kgm/min. Skin microcirculation was assessed by the vital microscopy at the nail bed of the fourth finger of the working hand.

The sensitivity of skin microvessels to adrenalin at a developing fatigue was studied by using the method of adrenalin iontophoresis in various concentrations into the volar surface of the forearm, with the initial dilution being 1×10^{-9} to the final one of 1×10^{-4} g/ml. The area of the positive electrode from which adrenalin was injected was 1 cm^2, the area of the indifferent electrode was 5 cm^2, the current was equal to 1 mA, and the time of introduction was 30 seconds. The reaction was registered as soon as the area of the drug action became pale.

The study of the regional blood flow and skin microcirculation in the hand involved 110 essentially healthy persons aged 20 to 80 years.

RESULTS

We found that muscle blood flow (MBF) decreases in aging. In addition, the age-dependent changes of resting muscle blood flow (RMBF) and maximal muscle blood flow (MMBF) differ from one another in the degree, rate and pattern of decrease in the RMBF and MMBF, as well as in some sex-related peculiarities of the MBF.

The decrease of RMBF was gradual, reaching a fall of 24 percent within the age interval 18-96 years (Figure 1).

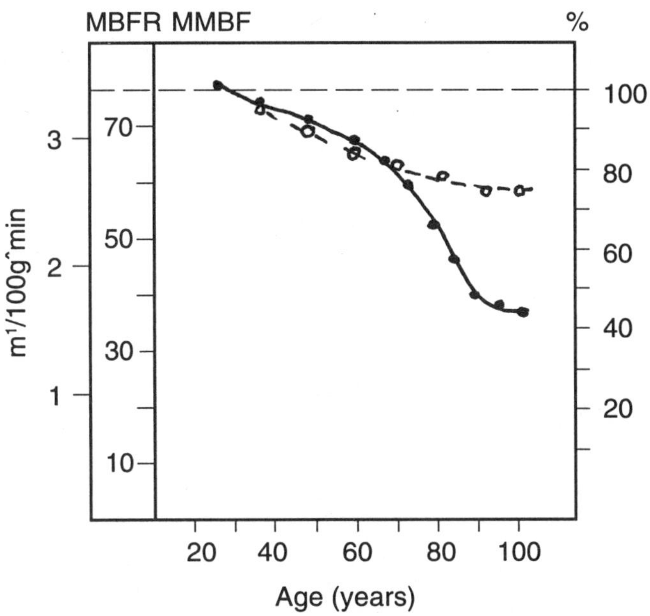

Figure 1. Age-associated dynamics of muscle blood flow at rest (RMBF) and maximal muscle blood flow (MMBF), indicated by closed circles.

Within the same age interval, the fall of MMBF was more than 50 percent. The "RMBF-age" curve approached an exponential curve in its character, with a greater fall in RMBF between 30 and 60 years followed by an insignificant change at subsequent ages. The "MMBF-age" curve was S-shaped, with the age-dependent changes in MMBF distinguished by three clear-cut periods: first, the period of a relative stabilization during the third through sixth decades when the MMBF showed a slight decrease, which averaged four to five percent within each 10 years; second, the period of a steep fall between 60 and 80 years; third, the period of a "plateau" during the ninth and 10th decades. With the beginning of the third period, the rate of fall in MMBF slowed down sharply and maintained a maximally low level in healthy people of the most advanced old ages. The normative values of RMBF may be assumed to be within 2.5-5.0 ml/100 g/min for young subjects and within 1.5-3.5 ml/100 g/min for older people. The majority of individual MMBF meanings within age groups fit in the +20 percent interval of respective average values, which can be recommended as normal values characteristic of healthy people.

With respect to the variables of gender, our data revealed only the tendencies toward differences in average findings of RMBF and MMBF between men and women. At 40 to

80 years, the RMBF was somewhat lower in women than in men. In contrast, there was a delay of five to 10 years in the age-dependent fall of MMBF in the women. After 80 years of age, however, the differences of RMBF and MMBF between men and women leveled off.

During the intermittent workload (compression of a rubber tube), both young and elderly subjects had work hyperemia, as evidenced on the plethysmogram by increased amplitude of pulse waves. Biomicroscopically, there was an extension of arterial and venous branches of capillary loops and an increased number of functioning capillaries. A continued workload presentation resulted, in young subjects, in an enhancement of work hyperemia and skin capillarization (Figures 2A and 2B) but, conversely, in the elderly, in a decrease in the amplitude of pulse waves on a plethysmogram, a narrowing of capillary branches and a reduction of the number of functioning capillaries (Figures 3A and 3B).

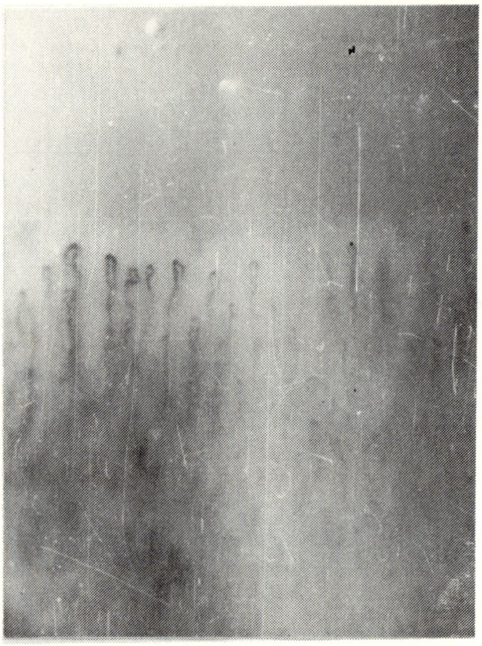

Figure 2A.

a) Microphotogram of capillaries of the nail bed of fourth finger of the left hand of the 28-year-old man before workload.

Capillary loops have a normal shape. There are 9-10 functioning capillaries per 1 linear mm of vision field.

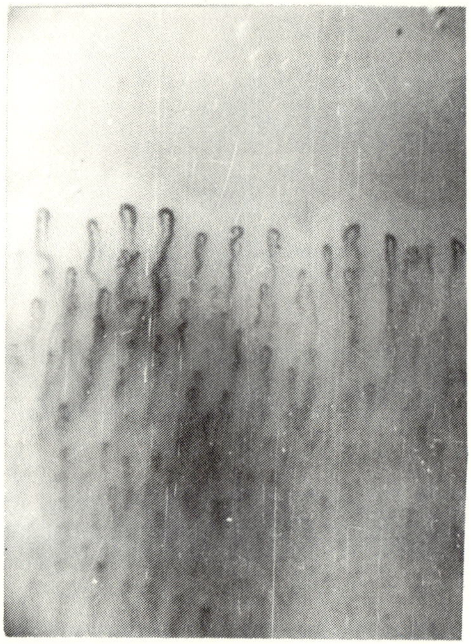

Figure 2B.

b) Microphotogram of capillaries of the nail bed of fourth finger of the left hand of the same person after workload prior to fatigue development (continuous rhythmic compression of the rubber tube for nine minutes). An extension of the arterial and venous branches of the capillary loops and two, three and four rows of capillaries can be seen. There are 11-12 functioning capillaries per 1 linear mm of vision field.

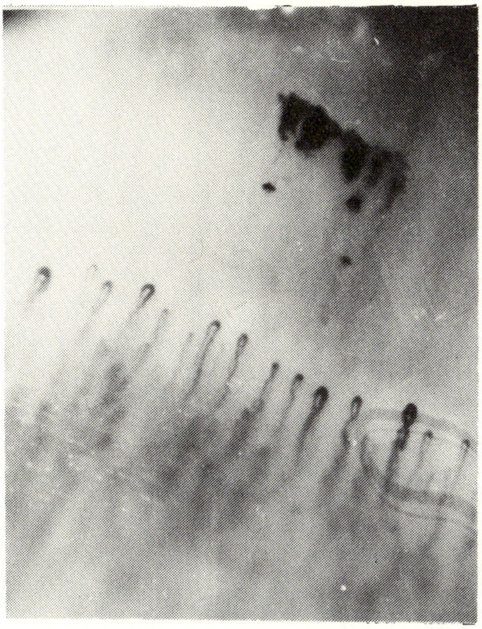

Figure 3A.

a) Microphotogram of capillaries of the nail bed of fourth finger of the left hand of the 70-year old man before workload.

Capillary loops have a spastic-atonic shape. The groups of extravasates can be seen. There are seven to eight functioning capillaries per linear mm of vision field

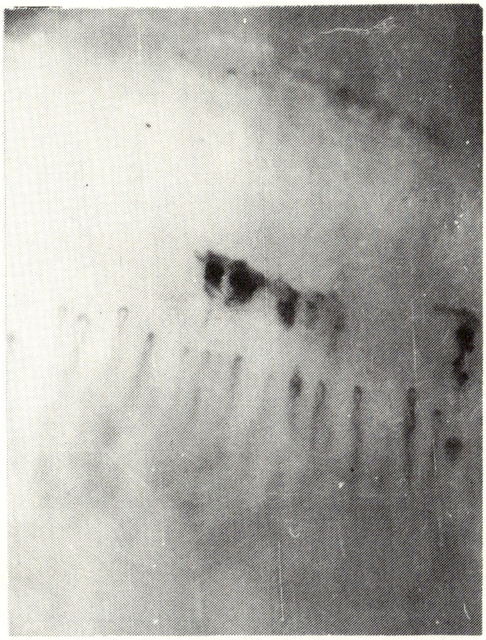

Figure 3B.

b) Microphotogram of capillaries of the nail bed of fourth finger of the left hand of the same person after workload prior to fatigue development (continuous rhythmic compression of the rubber tube for three and five minutes). A narrowing of the arterial and venous branches of the capillary loops can be seen. There are five to six functioning capillaries per 1 linear mm of vision field. The pattern of extravasates shows no changes.

A decline in skin capillarization was observed in young individuals, too, though in fewer cases and in fewer functioning capillaries (Figure 4).

The elderly discontinued working at earlier time periods due to fatigue of the hand (Figure 5).

This was consistent with decreased blood filling of the working muscles as evidenced by the reduced amplitude of pulse waves on a plethysmogram and by the reduced number of functioning capillaries combined with the reduced amplitude on an ergogram. Hand performance on a handgrip ergometer showed a lesser degree of skin capillarization due to workloads of various intensity in elderly and very elderly subjects (Figure 6).

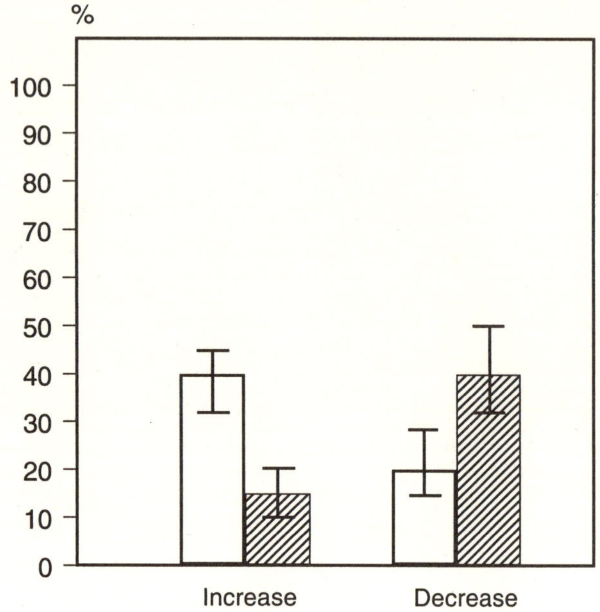

Light bars - young subjects aged 20 to 29 years.

Shaded bars - elderly subjects aged 60 to 79 years.

Figure 4. The dynamics of the diversely directed shifts in the number of functioning capillaries (in relation to the initial level) during performance of an interrupted physical work in the people of different age (in percent).

We tried to clarify the mechanisms causing more frequent narrowing of capillaries during the performance in the elderly. They appeared to have a higher lactate content of the blood compared to the young people. According to data obtained by our collaborator A. Ya. Litoshenko, the blood lactate concentration measured at the first minute of working with a rubber tube exceeded its initial level by 72 percent in young subjects and by only 37 percent in the elderly. However, as work progressed, the lactate concentration decreased in young subjects and at the 10th minute did not differ from the initial value. In contrast, in the elderly and very elderly subjects, the lactate concentration increased and at the third minute exceeded by 80 percent its initial level. Such a high level of lactate concentration of the blood was then sustained in the elderly during the entire rest of the work performance, providing evidence for the prevalence of anaerobic glycolysis.

At the same time, the alteration of regional blood flow during workload might be due, in part, to a change in the sensitivity to adrenergic mediators. Using the method of adrenalin iontophoresis in various concentrations into the volar surface of the forearm, we found that

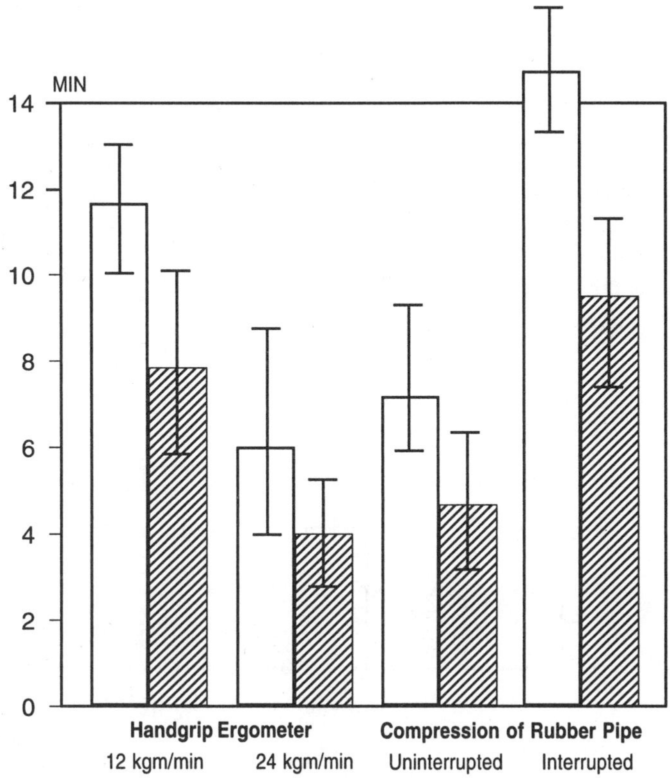

Light bars - young subjects aged 20 to 29 years.

Shaded bars - elderly subjects aged 60 to 79 years.

Figure 5. Work duration (in minutes) before cessation using various workloads.

the sensitivity of skin capillaries to adrenalin increased in elderly subjects, but remained unchanged in the young (Figure 7).

For a deeper study of a possible adrenergic role in the mechanism of capillary narrowing, we have also undertaken an investigation involving an adrenolytic drug, Ornid (bretylium, 5 percent solution), which blocks the release of catecholamines from the presynaptic nerve endings, and dihydroergotamine (0.03 percent solution), which blocks alpha-adrenoreceptors. The drugs were injected intracutaneously in the dose of 0.1 ml solution into the distal phalanx of the finger. It appeared that dihydroergotamine was more effective than Ornid in preventing the narrowing of capillaries and reduction of skin capillarization.

DISCUSSION

The age-related changes of central hemodynamics (decrease of cardiac output) and arterial vessels (physiological arteriosclerosis), level of metabolism, and worsening of rheological

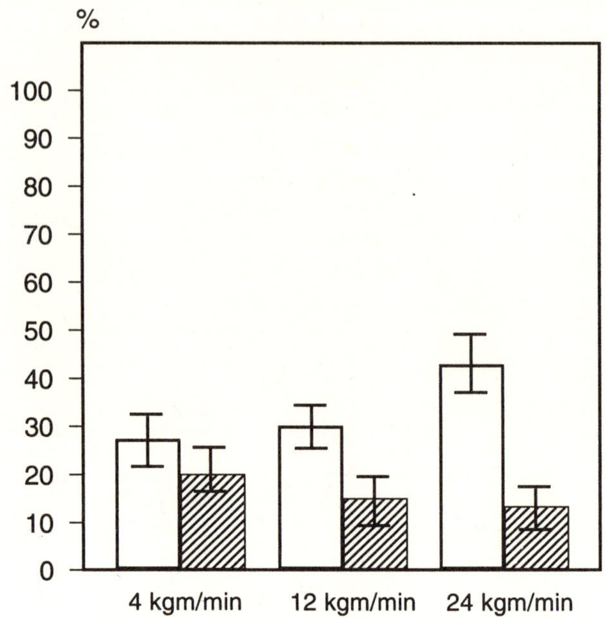

Light bars - young subjects aged 20 to 29 years.

Shaded bars - elderly subjects aged 60 to 79 years.

Figure 6. Percentage of an increase in the number of functioning capillaries with workloads of various intensity (performance on a handgrip ergometer).

properties of the blood (Korkushko, 1983; Frolkis et al., 1984) appear to play a definite role in the reduction of blood flow in skeletal muscles during aging. However, the leading role in this phenomenon has been ascribed to changes in the microcirculation: arteriolar obliteration and reduced capillarization of tissues (Korkushko and Sarkisov, 1976; Sarkisov and Grachev, 1987; Allwood, 1958; Burger, 1960; De Nicola et al., 1983). Relationships have been shown between the working capacity of muscle and the level of muscular capillarization; and the decrease in hyperemia phenomenon in atrophied muscles has been linked to a change of capillary network density, which, in turn, has been linked to the mitochondrial activity in the myocyte (Sullivan and Pittman, 1987; Hoppler et al., 1987; Tyler et al., 1990). In aging, muscle mass decreases with a developing atrophy of the muscular fibres (Berg, 1956; Rubinstein, 1960; Everitt et al., 1985).

The maintenance of RMBF at a sufficiently high level in aging seems to be related to a shunt of blood flow along the arteriolar-venular anastomoses. This was demonstrated in skin and bulbar microvessels (Korkushko and Sarkisov, 1976; Stupina and Sarkisov, 1978; Sarkisov and Grachev, 1987; De Nicola et al., 1983) and is assumed to be the case with blood supply in the muscles. The present finding of age-related decreases in MMBF, which reflects primarily the functional reserves of the terminal blood circulation, provides evidence

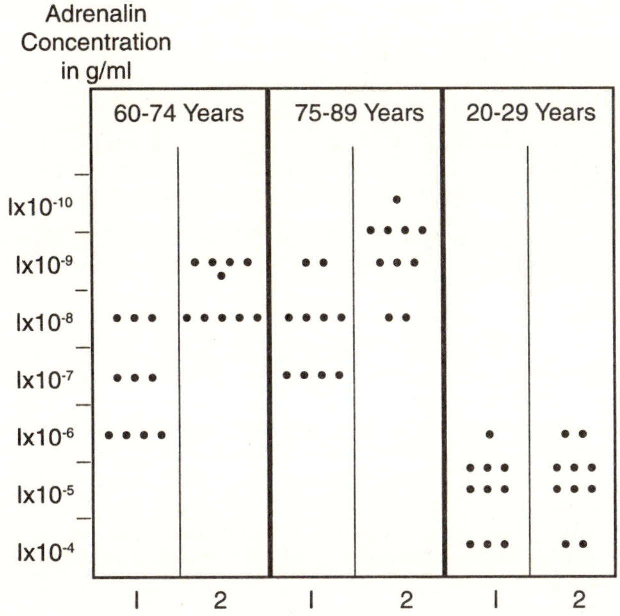

1. initial state before workload

2. at fatigue level

Each point corresponds to one study individual.

Figure 7. The threshold sensitivity of skin capillaries to adrenalin in people of different age at the initial state and at fatigue development during workload (performance on a handgrip ergometer).

for the considerable diminution of these reserves in old age. Apart from the morphological change in microvessels, this may be due, in part, to a disturbance of neurohumoral regulation in aging.

A rather frequent finding in the present study was the constriction of skin microvessels in the elderly when they performed graded muscular workload. The literature has previously reported the constriction of skin microvessels during physical work. Constriction of the venular part of the skin microcirculatory system and hand muscles during physical workload (handgrip ergometer) was described by Tkhorevsky (1981) and Zelis et al. (1969). Data have been reported showing activation of the sympatho-adrenal system (Vasiljeva and Stepochkina, 1985) by an increased content of the lactic acid in the blood during physical work, which may in turn contribute to this constriction. An enhanced sensitivity of the skin microvessels to adrenergic transmitters with increasing age (Frolkis and Verkhratsky, 1963; Sarkisov, 1965) may have contributed to the present finding of a greater prevalence of narrowing of skin vessels in the elderly during their performance of graded physical workloads. The present findings of 1) an increased sensitivity to adrenalin iontophoresis of skin microvessels in older people during fatigue development, and 2) the prevention of this phenomenon by intradermal injections of the adrenolytic drugs, Ornid and dihydroergotamine, point to a neurohumoral contribution to the more marked constriction of skin microvessels during physical workload in old age.

CONCLUSION

Resting blood flow and, especially, maximal muscle blood flow decrease with human aging. Limited adaptive capacities of the microcirculation in older people, perhaps due, in part, to its increased sensitivity to catecholamines, may contribute to the inadequacy of both regional blood flow and aerobic metabolism that accompanies the reduction of muscle performance in old age.

REFERENCES

Alwood MJ. Blood flow in the foot and calf in the elderly: a comparison with that in young adults. Clin Sci 1958;17:331-8.

Åstrand P-O. Physical performance as a function of age. JAMA 1968;205: 729-33.

Berg BN. Muscular dystrophy in aging rats. J Gerontol 1956;11:134-9.

Burger M. Altern und Krankheit als Problem der Biomorphese. Leipzig: Georg Thieme, 1960;24:262.

De Nicola P, Maggi G, Tassi G. Microcirculation. An Atlas. Stuttgart, New York: Schattauer, 1983:22,100.

Everitt AV, Shorey CD, Ficarra MA. Skeletal muscle aging in the hind limb of the old male Wistar rats: inhibitory effect of hypophysectomy and food restriction. Arch Gerontol Geriatr 1985;4:101-15.

Frolkis VV, Verkhratsky NS. Concerning the change in effectors sensitivity to action of neural and humoral stimuli during aging. Dokladi AN SSSR 1963;5:1228-30.

Frolkis VV, Bezrukov VV, Shevchuk VG. Blood Circulation and Aging. Leningrad: Nauka, 1984:20-2.

Goldberg AP, Hagberg JM. Physical exercise in the elderly. In: Schneider EL, Rowe JW, eds. Handbook of the Biology of Aging. San Diego: Academic Press Inc. 1990:407-28.

Hoppeler H, Hudlick O, Uhlmann E. Relationship between mitochondria and oxygen consumption in isolated cat muscles. J Physiol 1987;385:661-75.

Korkushko OV. Cardiovascular System and Age. Moscow: Meditsina, 1983:13-17,22.

Korkushko OV. Age-related peculiarities of microcirculation in old age. Kardiologija 1976;3:19-25.

Krogh A. The number and distribution of capillaries in muscles with calculations of the oxygen pressure head necessary for supplying the tissue. J Physiol (Gr Brit) 1919;52:409-15.

Motylyanskaya RE, Stogova LI, Iordanskaya FA. Physical Culture and Age. Moscow: Fizkultura i Sport, 1967:22-33.

Muravov IV. Physical culture and active rest at various age periods. Kiev: Zdorovja, 1973:83-7.

Rubinstein LJ. Aging changes in muscle. In: Bourne GH, ed. Structure of Muscle. New York: Academic Press Inc., 1960:209-26.

Sarkisov KG. Reactivity of skin capillary blood circulation due to adrenalin action in elderly people In: Problems of Geriatrics in Clinic of Internal Diseases. Kiev: Zdorovja, 1965:57-61.

Sarkisov KG, Grachev ID. Peculiarities of microcirculation in aging and arterial hypertension. Review. Vrachebnoje delo, 1987;8:14-7.

Skards YV. Blood supply of the skeletal muscles. In: Handbook on Physiology. Physiology of Blood Circulation. Physiology of Vascular System. Leningrad: Nauka, 1984:419-45.

Stupina AS, Sarkisov KG. Age-related peculiarities of hemo-microcirculation. In: Gerontology and Geriatrics, 1978. Yearbook. Modern Problems of Gerontology. Kiev:Zdorovja, 1978:91-8.

Sullivan SM, Pittman RN. Relationship between mitochondrial volume density and capillary in hamster muscles. Am J Physiol 1987;252:H149-55.

Tkhorevsky VI. Reaction of venous vessels of the muscles and skin during static contractions of small muscle groups. Fiziol zhurnal SSSR im Sechenova 1981;1:48-55.

Tyml K, Mathieu-Costello D, Budreau CH. Microvascular response to ischemia, and tissue structure in normal and atrophied skeletal muscle. Microvasc Res 1990;39:223-9.

Vasiljeva VV, Stepochkina NA. Muscular Activity. In: Handbook on Physiology. Physiology of Blood Circulation. Regulation of Blood Circulation. Leningrad: Nauka, 1985:335-65.

Zelis R, Mason DT. Comparison of the reflex reactivity of skin and muscle veins in the human forearm. J Clin Invest 1969;48:1870-7.

Is Progressive Resistance Training Beneficial in the Frail Elderly?

Roger A. Fielding, Ph.D.

INTRODUCTION

Human aging is associated with a host of metabolic and physiologic changes and with an increased incidence of several chronic diseases including coronary artery disease, non insulin-dependent diabetes mellitus and osteoporosis. Concurrent with these increased disease states are well documented changes in body composition that include an increased fat mass and a progressive decline in skeletal muscle mass. Together these factors result in age-related decreases in muscle strength and aerobic capacity which contribute to decreases in functional independence. Declines in the functioning of several major organ systems have been observed (Goldman, 1979). Changes in cardiovascular and muscular performance associated with advancing age can affect functional capacity and impinge on an individual's ability to perform activities of daily living. Maximal oxygen uptake declines at a rate of one percent per year after the third decade of life (Åstrand, 1960) and isometric and dynamic muscle strength begin to decrease after the fifth decade (Larsson, 1983). These declines in exercise capacity throughout the life span are in parallel to the declines seen in the musculoskeletal and cardiorespiratory systems. It is unclear whether these changes are an inevitable consequence of aging *per se* or simply a result of age-related declines in voluntary physical activity. The decreased cardiorespiratory function, reduced muscle mass and strength observed with advancing age closely mimic the declines in these parameters which are noted with bed rest or inactivity (Bortz, 1982; Saltin and Rowell, 1980).

That the largest growing segment of our population are those individuals over the age of 60 years is a fact that will cause us to refocus our health care priorities over the next several years. In 1988, 12.4 percent of the United States population was over 65 years, and by the year 2030 this is expected to increase to nearly 22 percent (Spencer, 1989). Perhaps more important, by the year 2020, 15 percent of the over 65 population will be over 85 years. This rapidly growing group of elderly, those over 85 years, may be at the greatest risk for being functionally limited due to declines in muscle mass and the associated loss in muscle strength. Perhaps more than any other limitation, a reduction in muscle strength and mass may place the "oldest old" in jeopardy of losing their functional independence. High intensity strength training has been one counter measure proposed to improve musculoskeletal capacity and preserve functional independence in the elderly. The purpose of this review will be to evaluate the effects of interventions designed to increase muscle strength in the elderly and specifically to address the potential benefits of strength training in the most frail segment of this population.

AGE-RELATED CHANGES IN BODY COMPOSITION

The most visible and, perhaps, the most profound changes which occur with advancing age are the alterations in body composition. Throughout the life span there is a progressive decline in the fat-free mass and a corresponding increase in fat mass. Estimates from several studies have indicated that beyond the third decade fat mass increases and continues to increase into the eighth decade of life (Cohn et al., 1980; Parizkova, 1974). Arm circumference and skinfold thickness measurements from 700 male participants in the Baltimore Longitudinal Aging Study, aged 20 to 92 years, revealed a slow progressive loss of lean tissue until age 65, followed by a more rapid decline (Borkan and Norris, 1977). Fat-free mass or body cell mass as measured by the ratio of total body potassium to nitrogen reveals that non-muscle lean tissue is preserved at the expense of the loss of skeletal muscle mass (Cohn et al., 1980). Based on 24-hour creatinine excretion, Tzankoff and Norris (1977) confirmed that skeletal muscle mass declined on average six percent per decade and that this decline in muscle mass is largely responsible for the age-related decrease in resting metabolic rate. Fleg and Lakatta (1988) have also demonstrated that the decline in muscle mass observed with age as measured by 24-hour urinary creatinine excretion can explain approximately 50 percent of the age-related decline in maximal oxygen uptake. These findings indicate that the alterations in body composition, in particular declines in skeletal muscle mass, have effects on basal metabolism and functional exercise capacity. In addition, loss of lean body or fat-free mass appears to affect disease outcome in patients with chronic illness (DeWyss et al., 1980).

DECLINE IN MUSCLE STRENGTH AS A FUNCTION OF AGE

A decline in dynamic, isokinetic and static muscle strength has been noted with advancing age (Aniansson et al., 1980; Borges, 1989; Rice et al., 1989). However, despite the declines in skeletal muscle mass which begin in the third decade, maximum dynamic and isometric strength and maximum knee extension velocity have been shown to be maintained until the fifth decade of life and then decline precipitously thereafter (Larsson et al., 1979). That there is a selective loss of type II (fast twitch) muscle fibers associated with this decline in strength has been reported by Larsson et al. (1979). Dissections of whole thigh muscles in cross sections from cadavers have also noted an 18 percent decline in total muscle area and a 25 percent decrease in the total number of muscle fibers in older cadavers with a specific decrease in the number of type II muscle fibers (Lexell et al., 1983). However, other studies, using needle biopsy or whole muscle cross sectional analysis, have reported a reduction in mean fiber areas of both type I and type II fiber with no selective reduction in type II muscle fiber populations (Essen-Gustavsson and Borges, 1986; Grimby et al., 1982; Lexell et al., 1988).

Several studies have suggested that, beyond age 50, muscle strength is closely associated with functional activities of daily living. These declines in muscle strength with age are related to impairment in function even in ambulatory free living older individuals. Using a survey questionnaire, Jette and Branch (1981) evaluated the exercise habits of 2,654 men and women aged 55 to 84 years. They reported that 40 percent of the females aged 55 to 64, nearly 45 percent of the females aged 65 to 74, and 65 percent of females aged 75 to 84 responded that they were unable to lift 4.5 kg (approximately ten lbs). The trends reported in this study were similar for men, although of a lower absolute level. In another sample of men and women aged 65 years and older, Bassey et al. (1988) reported a significant inverse relationship between isometric muscle strength of the plantar flexors of the foot and age (men: $R = -0.29$, $p<0.05$; women: $R = -0.37$, $p<0.01$) and lower isometric strength in older women than in men. Customary walking speed was also related to isometric muscle strength (men: $R=0.42$, $p<0.001$; women: $R=0.36$, $p<0.01$). These data suggest, particularly in women, that physical disability is prevalent in a large segment of the population over the age of 55 and this prevalence increases as the population examined becomes older. By far the older age categories encompassed the greatest number of men and women with impairment.

Frontera et al. (1991) examined the relationship between isokinetic knee and elbow joint strength in 200 men and women aged 45 to 78 years. They noted that, at angular velocities of 60 degrees per second, the oldest subjects had significantly lower absolute strength in all muscle groups tested. In addition, when muscle strength was expressed per kilogram of muscle mass, gender and age-related differences were reduced or disappeared completely, suggesting that the reductions in isokinetic strength with age are to a large extent a result of decreased muscle mass.

The loss of muscle mass and strength may not be an inevitable part of the aging process but may, in fact, be more related to changes in activity that accompany advancing age. Klitgaard et al. (1990) have reported that in older men (69 years), who had been strength training approximately 12 to 17 years prior to being studied, maximal isometric torque and muscle mass as measured by computed tomography scan of the upper arm and mid-thigh were significantly greater than in age-matched swimmers or runners and similar to young controls. Their subjects exercised an average of three times per week at approximately 70 to 90 percent of their one repetition maximum. It is also interesting to note that only the older strength-trained men (not the runners or the swimmers) had muscle cross sectional areas and strength similar to the young control subjects. These results suggest that, although aerobic activities such as running and swimming maintain cardiorespiratory fitness, only strength training can effectively maintain skeletal muscle mass.

HIGH INTENSITY STRENGTH TRAINING INTERVENTIONS IN THE ELDERLY

The concept of progressive resistance training for use in injury rehabilitation was first promoted by DeLorme (1945), who proposed that high intensity low repetition weight lifting exercise was necessary to restore muscle power and proper function following injury. Since then, studies on younger individuals have clearly demonstrated that progressive resistance training below 40 percent of the one repetition maximum (1RM) results in no change in muscle strength (MacDougall, 1986). However, there has been a reluctance on the part of investigators and clinicians to allow older subjects to train at a high intensity (70 to 90 percent of the 1RM). Several studies have attempted to examine the effects of dynamic resistance training (weight lifting) in older subjects with the goal of increasing muscle strength and mass and restoring function. In several reports, subjects were trained at low to moderate intensities, or the training was not progressive or was limited in the number of sets performed (Aniansson and Gustafson, 1981; Hagberg et al:, 1989; Larsson, 1982). In general, these studies demonstrated little or no increase in muscle strength with 12 to 26 weeks of training.

Studies employing higher training intensities in older subjects have been more successful. Moritani and deVries (1980) trained five older healthy men (mean age 70 years) for eight weeks at 66 percent of the 1RM of their elbow flexors. They noted a 23 percent increase in isometric strength of the muscle flexors with no change in the upper arm girth. They concluded that changes in neural factors were responsible for the improvements in muscle strength seen in this study. More recently, Frontera et al. (1988) examined the effects of a dynamic high intensity resistance training program in healthy older men (mean age 64 years). Their subjects performed knee flexion and extension exercises three days per week at 80 percent of the 1RM (eight to ten repetitions) for 12 weeks. They found a 107 percent increase in knee extensor strength and a 226 percent increase in knee flexor strength. In addition, they observed an 11 percent increase in mid-thigh cross sectional area as assessed by computed tomography. Muscle biopsy analysis revealed a 33 percent and 27 percent increase in type I and II fiber area, respectively. This was the first study to demonstrate in healthy older men that dynamic high intensity strength training can result in marked increases in muscle strength and muscle hypertrophy. Aerobic capacity ($\dot{V}O_2max$) during leg ergometry increased significantly while $\dot{V}O_2max$ during arm ergometry did not change, suggesting that in previously sedentary older men strength training interventions can also improve aerobic capacity. Along with increases in muscle size and strength, they also noted a 40 percent increase in urinary excretion of 3-methylhistidine, an index of myofibrillar proteolysis, suggesting that strength training increases muscle protein turnover in healthy older men. In this same study, half of the subjects were given a nutritional supplement during the training program which provided an additional 560 kcal per day (17 percent protein, 43 percent carbohydrate, 40 percent fat). There were no differences in strength gains between the supplemented and unsupplemented subjects. However, the subjects who received the supplement had greater increases in body weight, skinfold thicknesses at six sites, creatinine excretion and mid-thigh muscle cross sectional area, suggesting that dietary intake may influence the magnitude of changes in body composition as a result of strength training in the elderly (Meredith et al., 1992).

Two subsequent studies have confirmed the positive impact of strength training in healthy older subjects. Brown et al. (1990) examined a group of healthy older men who performed upper and lower body dynamic resistance training for 12 weeks (70-90 percent 1RM, three times per week) and showed a 48 percent increase in muscle strength, a 17 percent increase in elbow flexor cross sectional area by computed tomography scan and a significant increase in type I and II muscle fiber area. Although the increases in type I fiber area were less than those reported by Frontera et al. (1990), the increases in type II fiber area and total muscle cross sectional area were similar. Recently, Charette et al. (1991) confirmed that dynamic resistance training (upper and lower body) of a similar intensity in healthy elderly women (mean age 69 years) results in significant increases in muscle strength (28 to 115 percent) and a 20 percent increase in type II muscle fiber area. In contrast to Frontera et al., they reported no change in type I fiber area following training. The apparent discrepancies regarding the magnitude of the change in type I fiber area may be related to the differences in the intensity and duration of the warm-up and cool-down period or to the initial pre-training activity patterns of the various subject populations. That the subjects in the study of Frontera et al. were extremely sedentary prior to the start of the study is evidence of the fact that the resistance training resulted in a significant increase in leg maximal oxygen uptake and a 38 percent increase in citrate synthase activity of the vastus lateralis muscle (Frontera et al., 1990). This increased oxidative capacity is consistent with the type I muscle fiber hypertrophy observed. No measures of whole body or cellular oxidative metabolism were reported by Brown et al. or by Charette et al.

These more recent studies suggest that, when the training stimulus is of an appropriate intensity (70 to 90 percent of the 1RM), the gains in muscle strength and size in older healthy individuals are comparable to the gains observed in young individuals. The range of strength gains (28 to 227 percent) reported in these various studies may be related to other factors, including the subjects' initial strength, age and health status, and the choice of muscle groups that were trained. It is clear that the gains in muscle strength are far greater than the observed increases in muscle size, and this must be attributed to the profound neural adaptations which occur with high intensity resistance training. Furthermore, the type of strength training equipment employed has to be considered when evaluating strength gains. Specifically, the relationship between the angle of force and the actual applied force on the muscle can be influenced by the inherent design of the equipment. Regardless of the mechanism, the capacity for senescent muscle to respond to overload persists and is a useful intervention for restoring muscle function in the healthy elderly population.

MUSCLE FUNCTION IN THE FRAIL ELDERLY

It is well established that the frail elderly have by definition deficits in functional capacity that may make them dependent on others for daily care, and that a multitude of factors contribute to their disability. Some studies have shown that muscle weakness is associated with the risk of falling (Nevitt et al., 1989; Whipple et al., 1987) and may be related to functional dependence. There is now reasonable evidence that healthy older subjects respond favorably to strength training interventions. However, there is a lack of information regarding the effects of these interventions on functional capacity or activities of daily living in the frail elderly or individuals over 80 years of age. It is our contention that high intensity resistance training in this population has been underutilized.

In the only study to date in this population, Fiatarone et al. (1990) have reported the results from 10 frail institutionalized elderly men and women (mean age 90 ± 3 years, range 87-96 years) who performed knee extension exercises for eight weeks (three times per week, three sets at 80 percent of their 1RM). These subjects all had a prior history of falls and suffered on average 4.5 chronic diseases and took on average 4.2 medications per day. Seven of the ten subjects studied used an assistive device for ambulation. They noted prior to beginning the intervention a significant inverse relationship between six-meter walk time and the combined leg 1RM of the knee extensors ($R=0.745$, $p<0.01$). Following eight weeks of training, they reported a 174 percent increase in the 1RM of the knee extensors and a significant increase (nine percent) in the mid-thigh muscle cross sectional area by computed tomography. They also noted a 48 percent increase in tandem gait speed after training (Fiatarone, 1990). These data suggest that, even in frail elderly subjects, the capacity for muscle strength increases and hypertrophy is still maintained. In addition, in individuals with marked impairments in functional capacity, strength training interventions may restore some of the age-related loss in function.

While it appears maintenance of muscle strength is an important outcome variable in the oldest old, the ability to generate muscular force over a given period of time (muscle power) may also play an important role in functional independence and fall prevention. For example, making balance corrections when a person stumbles or missteps may be intrinsically related to the ability of that person to generate a large amount of muscle power for brief moments at a time. Muscle power has been shown to decline much more precipitously than the reported declines in dynamic and isometric strength (Bassey, 1990). In a group of nursing home residents with a history of falling, Whipple et al. (1987) reported that lower leg isokinetic power was significantly lower than in a group of age-matched controls. These data imply that muscle weakness is an important factor in gait and balance assessment and may be an underlying cause of falls when other risk factors are absent. Using a specially designed leg power rig, Bassey et al. (1992) evaluated leg extension power in 26 institutionalized frail elderly men and women (mean age 88 years). They reported a significant relationship between both single leg and combined leg extensor power and several functional tests of activities of daily living. The closest relationships were observed between leg extensor power and walking speed ($R=0.80$, $p<0.001$), chair-rising speed ($r=0.65$, $p<0.001$), and stair-climbing speed ($R=0.81$, $p<0.001$). An even stronger relationship to leg extensor power was found when stair climbing power was calculated based on the vertical rise of their body weight during stair climbing ($R=0.88$, $p<0.001$). Future studies will need to examine the specificity of dynamic resistance training in this population and evaluate strategies to improve leg extension power with the aim of improving function.

SUMMARY AND CONCLUSIONS

The changing demographics of the United States population will force us in the next thirty years to design and implement preventive strategies to minimize health care costs and extend the active life span (Katz et al., 1983). However, the present agenda of science and medicine needs to address adequately the requirements of the current elderly population. The well documented declines in muscle function and mass which occur with age appear to be strongly related to the sedentary lifestyle patterns which develop with advancing age. The reversibility of these changes has only recently been documented. In relatively small, well-controlled clinical trials, progressive resistance exercise training has been shown to improve muscle function and size in both healthy free living and frail institutionalized older men and women. These studies imply that progressive resistance training in sedentary older subjects may prevent or delay the need for dependent care. The efficacy of implementing these types of exercise programs for the elderly population as a whole, and in particular the frail elderly, needs to be addressed, with the aim of improving or restoring function. The use of progressive resistance training in the prevention of falls merits further study. Future investigation needs to focus on the complex interaction between health status, nutrient intake, and exercise capacity in both free living and institutionalized older persons and to document the long-term effects of resistance training interventions on health and functional capacity.

ACKNOWLEDGMENT

This study was supported in part by the United States Department of Agriculture, Agricultural Research Service Contract 53-3K06-5-10.

REFERENCES

Aniansson A, Grimby G, Rundgren Å. Isometric and isokinetic quadriceps muscle strength in 70-year-old men and women. Scand J Rehab Med 1980; 12:161-68.

Aniansson A, Gustafsson E. Physical training in elderly men. Clin Physiol 1981;1:87-98.

Åstrand I. Aerobic work capacity in men and women with special reference to age. J Appl Physiol 1960;169:1-92.

Bassey EJ, Bendall MJ, Pearson M. Muscle strength in the triceps surae and objectively measured customary walking activity in men and women over 65 years of age. Clin Sci 1988;74:85-9.

Bassey EJ, Fiatarone MA, O'Neill EF et al. Leg extensor power and functional performance in very old men and women. Clin Sci 1992;82:321-7.

Bassey EJ, Short AH. A new method for measuring power output in a single leg extension: feasibility, reliability and validity. Eur J Appl Physiol 1990; 60:385-90.

Borges O. Isometric and isokinetic knee extension and flexion torque in men and women aged 20-70. Scand J Rehab Med 1989;21:45-53.

Borkan GA, Norris AH. Fat redistribution and the changing body dimensions of the adult male. Human Biol 1977;49:495-514.

Bortz WM. Disuse and aging. JAMA 1982;248:1203-8.

Brown AB, McCartney N, Sale DG. Positive adaptations to weightlifting training in the elderly. J Appl Physiol 1990;69:1725-33.

Charette SL, McEvoy L, Pyka G et al. Muscle hypertrophy response to resistance training in older women. J Appl Physiol 1991;70:1912-6.

Cohn SH, Vartsky D, Yasumura S et al. Compartmental body composition based on total body nitrogen, potassium, and calcium. Am J Physiol 1980;239: E524-30.

DeLorme TL. Restoration of muscle power by heavy resistance exercises. J Bone Joint Surg 1945;27:645-67.

DeWyss WD, Begg C, Lavin PT. Prognostic effect of weight loss prior to chemotherapy in cancer patients. Am J Med 1980;69:491-7.

Essen-Gustavsson B, Borges O. Histochemical and metabolic characteristics of human skeletal muscle in relation to age. Acta Physiol Scand 1986;126:107-14.

Fiatarone MA, Marks EC, Ryan ND et al. High-intensity strength training in nonagenarians. Effects on skeletal muscle. JAMA 1990;263:3029-34.

Fleg JL, Lakatta EG. Role of muscle loss in the age-associated reduction in $\dot{V}O_2$max. J Appl Physiol 1988;65:1147-51.

Frontera WR, Hughes VA, Evans WJ. A cross-sectional study of upper and lower extremity muscle strength in 45-78-year-old men and women. J Appl Physiol 1991;71:644-50.

Frontera WR, Meredith CN, O'Reilly KP, Evans WJ. Strength training and determinants of $\dot{V}O_2$max in older men. J Appl Physiol 1990;68:329-33.

Frontera WR, Meredith CN, O'Reilly KP, Knuttgen HG, Evans WJ. Strength conditioning in older men: skeletal muscle hypertrophy and improved function. J Appl Physiol 1988;64:1038-44.

Goldman R. Decline in organ function with aging. In: Rossman I, ed. Clinical Geriatrics. Philadelphia: Lippincott, 1979.

Grimby G, Danneskiold-Samsoe B, Hvid K, Saltin B. Morphology and enzymatic capacity in arm and leg muscles in 78-81-year-old men and women. Acta Physiol Scand 1982;115:125-34.

Hagberg JM, Graves JE, Limacher M et al. Cardiovascular responses of 70-to-79-year-old men and women to exercise training. J Appl Physiol 1989;66:2589-94.

Jette AM, Branch LG. The Framingham Disability Study: II. Physical disability among the aging. Am J Public Health 1981;71:1211-6.

Katz S, Branch LG, Branson MH et al. Active life expectancy. New Engl J Med 1983;309:1218-24.

Klitgaard H, Mantoni M, Schiaffino S et al. Function, morphology and protein expression of ageing skeletal muscle: a cross-sectional study of elderly men with different training backgrounds. Acta Physiol Scand 1990;140:41-54.

Larsson L. Physical training effects on muscle morphology in sedentary males at different ages. Med Sci Sports Exer 1982;14:203-6.

Larsson L. Histochemical characteristics of human skeletal muscle during aging. Acta Physiol Scand 1983;117:469-71.

Larsson L, Grimby G, Karlsson J. Muscle strength and speed of movement in relation to age and muscle morphology. J Appl Physiol 1979;46:451-6.

Lexell J, Henriksson-Larsen K, Wimblod B, Sjostrom M. Distribution of different fiber types in human skeletal muscles: effects of aging studied in whole muscle cross sections. Muscle Nerve 1983;6:588-95.

Lexell J, Taylor C, Sjostrom M. What is the cause of ageing atrophy? Total number, size and proportion of different fiber types studies in whole vastus lateralis muscle from 15-to 83-year-old men. J Neurol Sci 1988;84:275-94.

MacDougall JD. Adaptability of muscle to strength training - a cellular approach. In: Saltin B, ed. Biochemistry of Exercise VI. Champaign Illinois: Human Kinetics, 1986:501-13.

Meredith CN, Frontera WR, O'Reilly KP, Evans WJ. Body composition in elderly men: effect of dietary modification during strength training. J Am Geriatr Soc 1992;40:155-62.

Moritani T, deVries H. Potential for gross muscle hypertrophy in older men. J Gerontol 1980;35:672-82.

Nevitt MC, Cummings SR, Kidd S, Black D. Risk factors for current nonsyncopal falls: a prospective study. JAMA 1989;261:2663-8.

Parizkova J. Body composition and exercise during growth and development. In: Rarick GL, ed. Physical Activity: Human Growth and Development. New York: Academic Press, 1974.

Rice CL, Cunningham DA, Paterson DH, Rechnitzer PA. Strength in an elderly population. Arch Phys Med Rehabil 1989;70:391-7.

Saltin B, Rowell LB. Functional adaptations to physical activity and inactivity. Fed Proc 1980;39:1506-13.

Spencer G (U.S. Bureau of the Census). Projections of the population of the United States, by age, sex, and race: 1988-2080. In: Current Population Report Series P-25, No.1018, 1989.

Tzsankoff SP, Norris AH. Effect of muscle mass decrease on age related BMR changes. J Appl Physiol 1977;43:1001-6.

Whipple RH, Wolfson LI, Amerman PM. The relationship of knee and ankle weakness to falls in nursing home residents: an isokinetic study. J Am Geriatr 1987;35:13-20.

Exercise, Bone Density and Aging

Paul Kelly, M.D., F.R.A.C.P.
Nicholas Pocock, M.D., F.R.A.C.P.
Philip Sambrook, M.D., F.R.A.C.P.
John Eisman, Ph.D., F.R.A.C.P.

Osteoporosis is a major public health problem in aging communities. It can be defined as a reduction in bone density leading to an increased risk of fracture. Whatever the age of an individual, the risk of fracture is determined not only by bone density but also by the risk of falls and trauma to bone. Osteoporotic fractures typically occur with minor trauma, such as a fall from standing height or less. While much attention has been directed toward the effects of lifestyle and pharmacological interventions in the augmentation of bone density, the role of postural stability and propensity to fall is now receiving critical analysis. Emphasis will be given to the relationship between bone density and physical activity; however, the as yet unexplored role of physical exercise in prevention of falls should not be ignored.

While exercise is often advised in the treatment and prevention of osteoporosis, there are many unresolved questions regarding its effect on bone density that suggest a uniform prescription of exercise in this setting may be premature.

There is little doubt, from cross-sectional studies, that individuals' indices of physical activity, such as physical fitness, correlate positively with bone density. In studies in normal healthy individuals over a wide age range, we (Pocock et al., 1986; Pocock et al., 1989) and others (Aloia et al., 1988; Krolner al., 1982; Sinaki et al., 1986; Chow et al., 1986; Bevier et al., 1989) have found that more physically fit and stronger individuals have greater bone mineral density at both axial and appendicular sites. This effect can account for 20 to 30 percent of the variance in femoral neck bone mineral density. At extremes of physical activity, marked changes in bone density are observed. Weightlessness and immobilization can produce marked bone mineral loss (Mack et al., 1967; Krolner and Toft, 1983; Stewart et al., 1982), and elite athletes tend to have significantly greater bone density than non-athletes (Nilsson and Westlin, 1971; Jones et al., 1977; Nelson et al., 1988). However, studies at such extremes may bear little relevance to the effect of physical activity and muscle strength on bone density in normal individuals and therefore it remains unclear whether *altering* levels of physical activity and strength in an ambulant non-athletic individual can influence bone density in the long term.

Inherent in cross-sectional studies is the probability that the skeletal loading, as measured, has been operative throughout much of that individual's life. Perhaps most importantly this effect may have been operative during adolescence and early adulthood, the time during which peak bone mass is achieved. On the other hand, there is also clear evidence that an excess of physical activity in women leading to estrogen deficiency can have adverse effects on bone mass (Fisher et al., 1986; Drinkwater et al., 1990). There is also some evidence of an adverse effect on lumbar spine density in male marathon runners (Bilanin et al., 1989).

Several prospective studies have demonstrated beneficial effects of exercise on bone mineral density. Dalsky et al. (1988) reported that a 40-week exercise program in postmenopausal women significantly increased lumbar density compared to controls. Orwoll et al. (1989) reported that, in a group of subjects older than 40 who swam at least three times a week over three years, distal radius and lumbar spine bone mineral density was greater in the male but not female swimmers compared to non-exercising controls. The lack of effect in the women could not be explained by differences in duration or amount of swimming undertaken. Chow et al. (1987) assessed the effect of supervised aerobic exercise with or without concomitant strength-building exercise in postmenopausal women. Trunk and upper thigh calcium content increased over 12 months in association with a 25 percent increase in maximal oxygen uptake in both groups. In a four-year study of weight-bearing aerobic exercise for 45 minutes three times per week, Smith et al. (1989) observed a modest (15 percent) increase in fitness and found that bone loss was decreased (but not arrested) compared to controls at the midshaft radius, ulna and humerus. Others have found an even more limited role for exercise in the prevention and treatment of bone loss. Michel et al. (1989) found that exercise in men and women over the age of 50 has been associated with higher levels of spinal density. However, no objective assessment of physical fitness or strength was made and activity was estimated on self reporting of hours per week spent in physical activity. Also they found that higher levels of reported physical activity in some subjects were associated with lower rather than higher bone density at the spine. Interestingly, Bevier et al. (1989) observed a relationship between regional muscle strength and lumbar spine and radial bone density in elderly men but not women. Sinaki et al. (1989) achieved a moderate increase in back extensor muscle strength (mean 25 percent) in postmenopausal women without any increase in lumbar vertebral bone mineral density. Another study in a small group of postmenopausal women found that 12 months of walking exercise did not prevent bone loss (Cavanaugh and Cann, 1988). Why relationships between activity, strength and bone density can be observed in elderly men but not women remains a puzzle. If a threshold effect is operative, whereby increases in bone density are observed only above a critical level of physical activity or strength, this may explain a relationship between strength and bone density that is observed in men who generally have higher levels of strength than women. It is possible that the intervening effect of variability in postmenopausal bone loss obscures a weak effect of physical activity to be observed in women.

Clearly there are inconsistencies in the data on the efficacy of exercise to augment bone mineral density prospectively in either young adult or elderly normal subjects. However, the recent study of Prince may help explain some of these apparent inconsistencies (Prince et al., 1991). They found in early postmenopausal women that the combination of an exercise program with calcium supplementation completely arrested forearm bone loss, while exercise alone was ineffective. An interplay between calcium intake and physical activity is also supported by data in young women. A relationship between physical activity and bone density in adolescent women and those in the third decade was observed by Recker et al. (1992). They observed bone density changes in women in their twenties and found these changes to be related to both their level of physical activity and dietary calcium intake. Interestingly, the data suggest that the effect of moderate physical activity can be augmented by increasing dietary calcium intake.

We and others have proposed that dietary calcium and physical activity are permissive factors that allow bone to reach its inherited potential and that genotype determines the limit of skeletal response to environmental influences (Kelly et al., 1990; Heaney, 1986). Kanders et al. (1988) found a relationship between dietary calcium intake, physical activity and bone density that supports this hypothesis. They found that vertebral bone density was significantly greater in a group of subjects with both greater daily energy expenditure (>970 kcal/day) and dietary calcium intake (>800 g/day). They also found a positive relationship between vertebral bone density and dietary calcium intake in those with calcium intakes less than 1000 mg/day, but in those with higher dietary calcium intake, no such relationship existed. Furthermore the strength of the relationship between dietary calcium intake and bone density was improved with the elimination of the effect of energy expenditure. In examining the effects of an exercise program on postmenopausal women one group could not find any overall significant effect of exercise on vertebral bone loss but there was a trend for the loss in the exercising group to be less in those with the greater dietary calcium intake (Sinaki et al., 1989). In a study of the effect of calcium supplementation with 1500 mg calcium carbonate on bone loss in women, Smith and colleagues (1989) found that, while the rate of loss from the left radius was no different from controls (mean dietary calcium intake 700 mg/day), the rate of loss was decreased by around 50 percent in the right (presumably dominant) radius of the treated subjects. Other data also support an interaction between dietary calcium intake, physical activity and bone density in men (Block et al., 1989). Sinaki et al. (1989) achieved a moderate increase in back extensor muscle strength (mean 25 percent) in postmenopausal women without any increase in lumbar vertebral bone mineral density although there was a trend for bone loss in the exercising group to be less in those with the greatest dietary calcium intake.

It is now well established that there are strong familial and genetic influences on adult bone density with genetic factors estimated to contribute around 80 percent of the total variance in bone density (Pocock et al., 1987; Dequeker et al., 1987; Moller et al., 1978; Smith et al., 1973; Seeman et al., 1989). Analysis of twin data also suggests that a single gene or set of genes is responsible for this genetic effect (Pocock et al., 1987). It is possible that complex interactions between environmental factors and genetic influences may be confounding observations of the role of exercise in osteoporosis treatment and prevention. Since bone mineral density, muscle mass and physical fitness all have genetic determinants (Klissouras et al., 1973; Komi et al., 1976; Lortie et al., 1982; Lesage, et al., 1985; Montoye and Gayle, 1978; Bouchard et al., 1986), it is also possible that these parameters share some common genetic basis. A number of responses to physical training are genetically influenced (Depress et al., 1984; Poehlman et al., 1987), and it remains feasible, although unproven, that the skeletal response to exercise may be similarly affected. The "dose-responsiveness" of the human skeleton to physical loading levels is not established, and whether skeletal adaptation to mechanical strain is genetically influenced or modulated by environmental factors such as current dietary calcium intake has generated interest.

To examine these environmental and genetic interactions and to control for possible genetic sources of variance, we undertook a three-year randomized controlled, cross-over study of the effects of exercise training in a group of identical twins (n=16 pairs, 13 female, 3 male; mean age, 49 years, range 25 to 70 years). Exercise was designed to increase both physical fitness and muscle strength. Bone mineral density (Lunar DPA, SPA), muscle strength (Cibex II ergometer) and physical fitness (predicted maximal oxygen capacity) were measured every six months during each 18-month exercise period.

Despite regular exercise classes and careful follow-up, compliance with exercise was poor. Furthermore, twin pairs' parameters remained highly correlated with no significant within-twin-pair difference in rates of change in bone mineral density, physical fitness or muscle strength in either study period. However, in the group taken as a whole, rates of change in physical fitness, muscle strength and bone mineral density, particularly at the lumbar spine (but not the femoral neck), were correlated within twin pairs (R=0.40-0.60). Moreover, the relatively small within-pair differences in rates of change in physical fitness still predicted within-twin-pair differences in rates of change in femoral neck bone mineral density (R=0.69, $p<0.01$).

Long-term compliance with exercise was poor, even in this motivated highly selected group, as has been observed in other long-term exercise studies (Sinaki et al., 1989). The data support the concept that responses to physical training have strong familial and/or genetic influences. Consistent with our previous observations the study indicates that, while lumbar spine density is strongly influenced by familial-genetic factors, femoral neck density is sensitive to environmental factors, such as physical loading.

The effect of exercise on bone therefore cannot be examined isolated from genetic and other environmental influences. While exercise is widely advised in the setting of prevention and treatment of osteoporosis, we still do not know the optimal regime or exercise frequency. The approach in physical training best suited to increase bone density is also still unclear. Animal studies and computer simulations predict that high frequency, low load strain would be less effective in augmenting bone mineral density than lower frequency, higher skeletal load such as weight training (Lanyon, 1984; Whalen and Carter, 1988). Even if the optimal exercise regime were known, poor compliance with exercise in the long time may limit its use in the community setting.

In conclusion, demonstration of optimal exercise regimens and their positive effect on bone mass and risk of fracture will be essential for more informed, rational implementation of exercise in osteoporosis.

REFERENCES

Aloia JF, Vaswani AN, Yeh JK, Cohn SH. Premenopausal bone mass is related to physical activity. Arch Int Med 1988;148:121-3.

Bevier WC, Wiswell RA, Pyka G, Kozak KC, Newhall KM, Marcus R. Relationship of body composition, muscle strength, and aerobic capacity to bone mineral density in older men and women. J Bone Min Res 1989;4:421-32.

Bilanin JE, Blanchard MS, Russek-Cohen E. Lower vertebral bone density in male long distance runners. Med Sci Sports Exerc 1989;21:66-70.

Block JE, Friedlander AL, Brooks GA, Steiger P, Stubbs HA, Gennat HK. Determinants of bone density among athletes engaged in weight-bearing and non-weight-bearing activity. J Appl Physiol 1989;67:1100-5.

Bouchard C, Lesage R, Lortie G . Aerobic performance in brothers, dizygotic and monozygotic twins. Med Sci Sports Exerc 1986;18:639-46.

Cavanaugh DJ, Cann CE. Brisk walking does not stop bone loss in postmenopausal women. Bone 1988;9: 201-4.

Chow RK, Harrison JE, Brown CF, Hajek V. Physical fitness effect on bone mass in postmenopausal women. Arch Phys Med Rehabil 1986;67:231-4.

Chow R, Harrison JE, Notarius C. Effect of two randomised exercise programmes on bone mass in healthy postmenopausal women. Br Med J 1987; 295:1441-4.

Dalsky GP, Stocke KS, Ehsani AA, Slatopolsky E, Lee WC, Birge SJ. Weight-bearing exercise training and lumbar bone mineral content in postmenopausal women. Ann Int Med 1988;108:824-8.

Depress JP, Bouchard C, Savard R, Prud'Homme D, Bukowiecki L, Theriault G. Adaptive changes to training in adipose tissue lipolysis are genotype dependent. Int J Obesity 1984;8:87-95.

Dequeker J, Nijs J, Verstaeten A, Geusens P, Gevers G. Genetic determinants of bone mineral content at the spine and the radius: a twin study. Bone 1987;8:207-9.

Drinkwater BL, Bruemner B, Chestnut CH III. Menstrual history as a determinant of current bone density in young athletes. J Am Med Assoc 1990; 263:545-8.

Fisher EC, Nelson ME, Frontera WR, Turksoy RN, Evans WJ. Bone mineral content and levels of gonadotropins and estrogens in amenorrheic running women. J Clin Endocrinol Metab 1986;62:1232-6.

Heaney RP. Calcium, bone health and osteoporosis. In: Peck WA, ed. Bone and Mineral Research/4. Amsterdam-New York-Oxford: Elsevier, 1986:255-301.

Jones HH, Priest JD, Hayes WC, Tichenor CC, Nagel DA. Humeral hypertrophy in response to exercise. J Bone Joint Surg 1977;59:204-8.

Kanders B, Dempster DW, Lindsay R. Interaction of calcium nutrition and physical activity on bone mass in young women. J Bone Min Res 1988;3:145-9.

Kelly PJ, Sambrook PN, Eisman JA. The interaction of genetic and environmental influences on peak bone density. Osteoporosis International 1990;1:56-60.

Klissouras V, Pirnay F, Petit J-M. Adaptation to maximal effort: genetics and age. J Appl Physiol 1973;35:288-93.

Komi PV, Viitasalo JT, Havu M, Thorstensson A, Karlsson J. Physiological and structural performance capacity: effect of heredity. In: Komi PV, ed. Biomechanics V. Baltimore MD: University Park Press, 1976:118-23.

Krolner B, Tondevold E, Toft B, Berthelssen B, Pors Nielson S. Bone mass of the axial and the appendicular skeleton in women with Colles' fracture: its relation to physical activity. Clin Physiol 1982;2:147-57.

Krolner B, Toft B. Vertebral bone loss: an unheeded side effect of therapeutic bed rest. Clin Sci 1983;64:537-40.

Lanyon LE. Functional strain as a determinant for bone remodeling. Calcif Tissue Int 1984;36:S56-61.

Lesage R, Simoneau JA, Jobin J, LeBlanc J, Bouchard C. Familial resemblance in maximal heart rate, blood lactate and aerobic power. Human Hered 1985;35:182-9.

Lortie G, Bouchard C, LeBlanc A et al. Familial similarity in aerobic performance. Human Biol 1982;54:801-12.

Mack PB, LaChance PA, Vose GP, Vogt FB. Bone demineralization of foot and hand of Gemini-Titan IV, V and VII astronauts during orbital flight. Am J Roentgenol 1967;100:503-11.

Michel BA, Bloch DA, Fries JF. Weight-bearing exercise, over exercise, and lumbar spine bone density over age 50 years. Arch Int Med 1989;149:2325-9.

Moller M, Horman A, Harvarld B, Hauge M, Henningsen K, Nordin BEC. Metacarpal morphometry in monozygotic and dizygotic elderly twins. Calcif Tissue Res 1978;25:197-201.

Montoye HJ, Gayle R. Familial relationships in maximal oxygen uptake. Human Biol 1978;50:241-9.

Nelson ME, Meredith CN, Dawson-Hughes B, Evans WJ. Hormone and bone mineral status in endurance trained and sedentary postmenopausal women. J Clin Endocrinol Metab 1988;66:927-33.

Nilsson BE, Westlin NE. Bone density in athletes. Clin Orthop 1971;77:179-82.

Orwoll ES, Ferar J, Oviatt SK, McClung MR, Huntington K. The relationship of swimming exercise to bone mass in men and women. Arch Int Med 1989;149:2197-200.

Pocock NA, Eisman JA, Yeates MG, Sambrook PN, Eberl S. Physical Fitness is a major determinant of femoral neck and lumber spine bone mineral density. J Clin Invest 1986;78:618-21.

Pocock NA, Eisman JA, Hopper JL, Yeates MG, Sambrook PN, Eberl S. Genetic determinants of bone mass in adults: a twin study. J Clin Invest 1987;80:706-10.

Pocock NA, Eisman JA, Gwinn TH, Sambrook PN, Kelly PJ, Freund J, Yeates, MG. Muscle strength, physical fitness and fitness and weight but not age predict femoral neck bone mass. J Bone Min Res 1989;4:441-7.

Poehlman ET, Tremblay A, Marcotte M, Perusse L, Theriault G, Bouchard C. Heredity and changes in body composition and adipose tissue metabolism after short-term exercise training. Eur J Appl Physiol 1987;56:398-402.

Prince R, Smith M, Dick I, Price RI, Webb PG, Henderson K, Harris MM. Prevention of postmenopausal osteoporosis: a comparative study of exercise, calcium supplementation, and hormone-replacement therapy. N Engl J Med 1991;325:1189-95.

Recker RR, Davies M, Hinders SM, Heaney RP, Stegman MR, Kimmel DB. Bone gain in young adult women. J Am Med Assoc 1992;268:2403-8.

Seeman E, Hopper JL, Bach LA, . Reduced bone mass in daughters of women with osteoporosis. New Engl J Med 1989;320:554-8.

Sinaki M, McPhee MC, Hodgson SF, Merritt JM, Offord KP. Relationship between bone mineral density of spine and strength of back extensors in healthy postmenopausal women. Mayo Clin Proc 1986;61:116-22.

Sinaki M, Wahner HW, Offord KP, Hodgson SF. Efficacy of nonloading exercise in prevention of vertebral bone loss in postmemopausal women. Mayo Clinic Proc 1989; 64:762-9.

Smith DA, Nance WE, Won Kang K, Christian JC, Johnston CC Jr. Genetic factors in determining bone mass. J Clin Invest 1973;52:2800-8.

Smith EL, Gilligan C, McAdam M, Ensign CP, Smith PE. Deterring bone loss by exercise intervention in premenopausal and postmenopausal women. Calcif Tissue Int 1989;44:312-21.

Stewart AF, Adler M, Byers CM, Segre GV, Broadus AE. Calcium homeostasis inimmobilization: an example of resorptive hypercalciuria. N Engl J Med 1982;306:1136-40.

Whalen RT, Carter DR. Influence of physical activity on the regulation of bone density. J Biomech 1988;21:825-37.

Exercise Prescription for Prevention of Osteoporosis in Elderly Women

Harri Suominen, Ph.D.

INTRODUCTION

According to the consensus statement presented at the International Conference on Exercise, Fitness and Health in Toronto 1988 (Bouchard et al., 1990), "Physical activity is important both for the prevention of osteoporosis and for the rehabilitation of the osteoporotic patient. However, more research is required to establish optimal exercise programs that are attractive as well as beneficial, programs that avoid the possible deleterious effects of fatigue, starvation diets, or altered sex hormone activity. Prevention of osteoporosis also requires attention to overall good health."

Recently, the national consensus meeting on the prevention and treatment of osteoporosis in Finland (The Academy of Finland, 1992) went one step further by stating that "bones are most affected by strength-demanding, fast and unusual movements, also short term if repeated enough. Weight-bearing essentially enhances the effect of active muscle work. Suitable types of exercise, for example, are work with diverse loading, weight-training, vigorous gymnastics, aerobics, brisk walking, jogging, cross-country skiing, and stair climbing. To prevent osteoporotic fractures, exercise should particularly load the hip, lumbar spine and forearms." It was also stated that "exercise can improve coordination and muscle performance and thus reduce the risk of accidents."

It is not certain that a consensus exists concerning the current knowledge regarding exercise prescription for the prevention of osteoporosis. Ideas differ according to the viewpoints and personal interests of different scientists and practitioners and the age, sex and other characteristics of those being studied. The purpose of this paper is to review the effects of exercise on bone mineral density in elderly women and to look for existing evidence in support of prescribing exercise for older age groups.

CROSS-SECTIONAL STUDIES

The most extensive indirect evidence in support of the effects of exercise comes from cross-sectional studies among young and middle-aged athletes. The original results by Nilsson and Westlin (1971) together with other studies of men since then have shown differences in bone mineral density (BMD) between athletes and controls extending to above 40 percent in bones exposed to weight-bearing and lower limb loading. Studies of older male athletes and on non-weight-bearing exercise and bones have, however, generally reported BMD values less than 20 percent higher than those in their controls (Suominen, 1993).

While elderly male athletes from various sports have significantly higher BMD values in several bone sites when compared to controls, many studies of women have found nonsignificant differences between athletes and nonathletes (Suominen 1993). Jacobson et al. (1984), however, found bone mineral content (BMC) to be 12 to 17 percent higher in the spine and radius in athletic women, and Lane et al. (1986) found BMD to be even 35 percent higher in the spine in long-distance runners compared to controls.

Our recent study of 66- to 85-year-old females (Suominen et al., unpublished) showed no significant differences in BMD in the calcaneus between a population sample and those active in endurance sports such as long-distance running and skiing or other types of sports such as sprinting, jumping, throwing, and gymnastics. However, BMD correlated with body mass, which was significantly greater among the controls. When the effect of body mass was controlled by means of the analysis of covariance, the difference in BMD between the athletic women and the controls became significant.

This result is illustrated in Figure 1 which shows the values for body mass and the regression estimates for BMD in the athletes and controls. Even though there were no differences in BMD between the two groups as such, for a given level of body mass, BMD was clearly higher among the athletes.

In our recent population study of 75-year-old women (Cheng et al., 1993), BMD correlated with body mass and fat content but not with current physical activity. Similarly, Reid et al. (1992) found that body mass was more closely related to BMD than any of the lifestyle parameters in postmenopausal women. These studies also indicated that fat mass is less important as a determinant of BMD in men. These results, together with the smaller differences in BMD between athletes and controls in females than in men, suggest that, in elderly females doing less exercise, body weight and fat mass become relatively more important determinants of BMD and source of mechanical stress for weight-bearing bones.

When the BMD values of the female athletes in our study (Suominen et al., unpublished) were related to the number of training kilometers in running and/or skiing during the preceding year, no significant differences were found between the given training categories. If anything, there was a tendency towards lower BMD among those having the greatest number of training kilometers. Although studies in athletes generally indicate positive training effects, there are studies of both adult and elderly males (Bilanin et al., 1989; MacDougall et al., 1992; Michel et al., 1989; Suominen and Rahkila, 1991; Vico et al., 1993) as well as elderly females (Michel et al., 1989) which show a tendency for BMD to decrease in those groups with the highest volumes of training, especially long-distance running, thus suggesting that the effects of exercise on bones can be non-linear.

PROSPECTIVE EXERCISE STUDIES

In spite of the considerable number of papers published on exercise and osteoporosis, only a few randomized controlled experimental trials have been conducted on the effects of exercise on bones (Table 1). For a further review see Gutin and Kasper, 1992; Smith and Gilligan, 1991; Snow-Harter and Marcus, 1991. Conducting prospective studies using exercise programs of sufficient duration and intensity is notoriously difficult, particularly in elderly women. The longer the training periods the more problematic they are with regard to the exercise compliance and the follow-up.

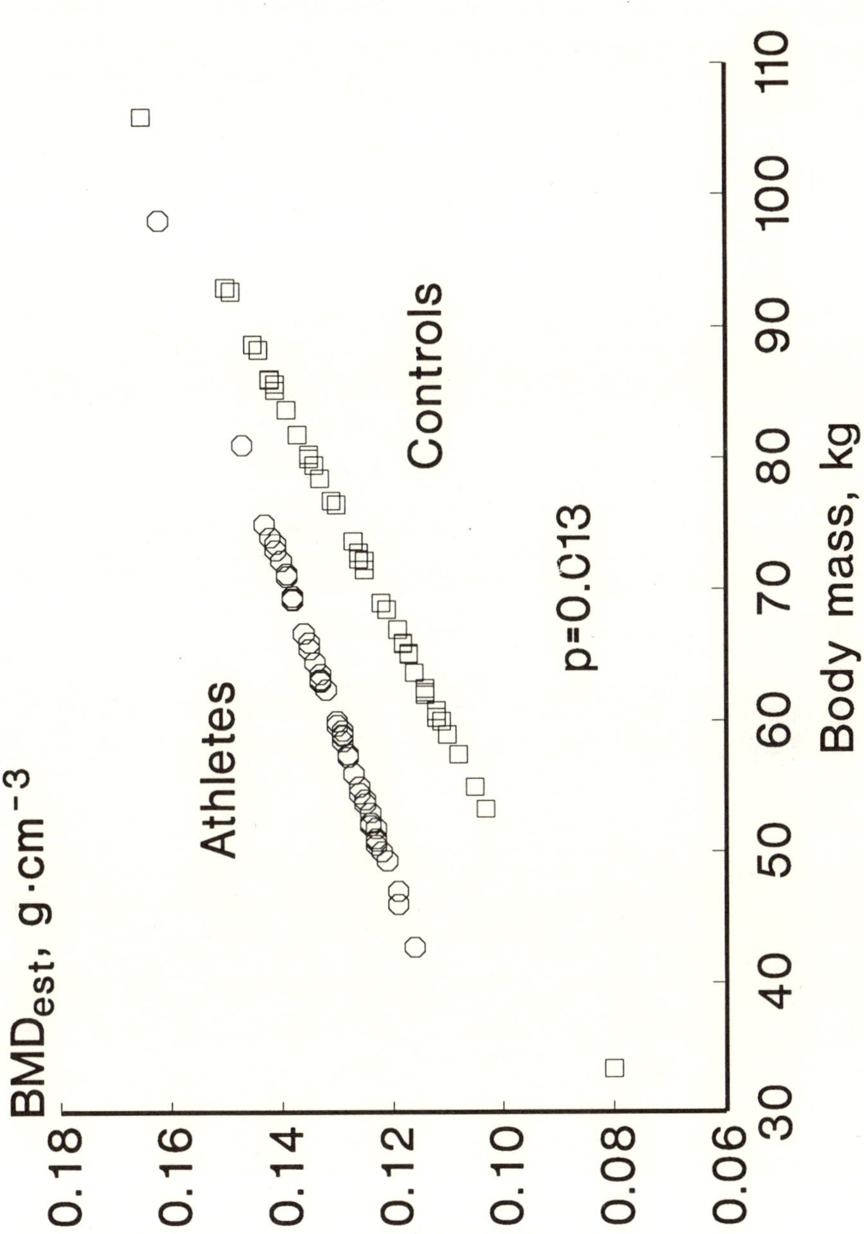

Figure 1. Body mass and regression estimates for calcaneus bone mineral density (BMD_{est}) in elderly female athletes and population controls (Suominen et al., unpublished).

TABLE 1

Prospective Studies on the Effects of Exercise on Bones in Elderly Women

Reference	Age[a] (years)	Training duration	Technique/bone	Change[b] (%)
Aloia et al., 1978	53 ± 6	1 year	NAA TBCa	+ 5*
			SPA Radius	+ 1
Cavanaugh and Cann, 1988	49-64	1 year	QCT Spine	- 2
Chow et al., 1987	50-62	1 year	NAA CaBI	+ 9*RT
Dalsky et al., 1988	55-70	22 months	DPA Spine	+ 7*
Dilsen et al., 1989	39-80	6 months	QCT Spine	+ 7*
Grove and Londeree, 1992	56 ± 5	1 year	DPA Spine	+ 7*RT
Krolner et al., 1983	54 ± 4	8 months	DPA Spine	+ 6*
			Forearm	+ 4
Pruitt et al., 1992	54 ± 4	9 months	DPA Spine	+ 5*
			Femur	- 2
			DPA Wrist	+ 2
Rikli and McManis, 1990	57-83	10 months	SPA Radius	+ 4*
Rundgren et al., 1984	63-84	9 months	DPA Calcaneus	+ 6*
Sandler et al., 1987	49-65	3 years	QCT Radius	0 RT
Simkin et al., 1987	53-74	5 months	CST Radius	+ 6*
			SPA Radius	- 6
Sinaki et al., 1989	49-65	2 years	DPA Spine	- 1 RT
Smidt et al., 1992	55 ± 8	1 year	DPA Spine	+ 1 RT
			DPA Hip	+ 1
Smith et al., 1989	35-65	4 years	SPA Radius	+ 4*
			Ulna	+ 4*
			Humerus	+ 1
Smith el al., 1981	69-95	3 years	SPA Radius	+ 6*
White et al., 1984	50-63	6 months	SPA Radius	+ 1

Symbols and abbreviations: a = mean ± SD or range; b = difference in change between exercisers and controls; * = statistically significant ($p<0.05$); CaBI = calcium bone index; CST = compton scattering technique; DPA = dual photon absorptiometry; NAA = neutron activation analysis; RT = randomized trial; QCT = quantitative computed tomography; SPA = single photon absorptiometry; TBCa = total body calcium

Even though several exercise interventions have suggested positive effects on bones after training periods which in some cases have extended up to three years in elderly and even four years in slightly younger women (Smith et al., 1989, 1981), prospective studies do not seem to confirm the "training effects" indirectly obtained in the athlete studies where intensive exercise has been practiced over periods of years.

The net results in the exercise interventions performed so far in middle-aged and elderly women range from a -6 percent BMC (Simkin et al., 1987) to a + 9 percent calcium bone index (Chow et al., 1987) difference in change between exercisers and controls. Several studies in elderly women, however, report no significant training-induced changes in BMC or BMD. In the studies where the effects attributable to exercise were statistically significant, the differences in changes usually remained at the level of four to seven percent.

EXERCISE PRESCRIPTION

So, what can be said about exercise prescription? There is a general agreement that immobilization results in rapid bone loss and that bone responds to the physical stress of exercise. When considering women, regular physical activity is likely to contribute to the attainment of peak bone mass and also to slow the decline in bone mineral density in middle-aged and elderly women. However, it is not clear whether exercise commenced at older ages has any major effects on bone mass and can thus help to prevent osteoporosis and related fractures.

As shown, short-term exercise interventions have failed to confirm the marked differences obtained in BMD between athletes and controls in some studies. In addition to the unrealistic aims of generally applying the intensive exercise practiced by athletes, it has also been suggested that exercise has non-linear effects, i.e., increasing the volume of intensive endurance training such as long-distance running may not result in a gain in bone mass, but, in fact, may even be rather detrimental to bone health (Suominen, 1993).

The question thus remains as to whether a small percentage gain of bone mineral density possibly achieved by moderate exercise is of clinical significance for bone strength or whether there are other changes in bone structure and general physical performance which could inhibit the occurrence of fractures. The studies performed so far on the association between physical activity and fracture risk have reported conflicting results (Law et al., 1991). Our recent study among the 75- and 80-year-olds in Jyväskylä showed that calcaneus BMD was significantly related to the occurrence of fractures studied retrospectively for 25 to 30 years and prospectively for 2.5 to 3 years (Cheng et al., 1994). The fracture risk was not, however, associated with self-reported physical activity or other living habits.

When reviewing the literature to date, it is clear that no randomized prospective studies have systematically examined how the type, duration, frequency, and intensity of exercise affect the magnitude of response of bones. There is not, then, enough evidence for a specific exercise prescription for bone health in elderly women.

Nonetheless, on the basis of current knowledge, it is possible to offer several general guidelines on the use of exercise. The first decision which has to be made is whether there is any reason to start a short-term but still laborious training regimen purely on account of the bones, when no marked changes in BMD are likely to occur. It may even be reasonable to design a program mainly to improve muscular performance and cardiovascular fitness and to be enjoyable, and trust that the exercise will also be osteogenic. The statements issued by the consensus meetings cited at the beginning of this paper might well be applicable, provided that elderly women at imminent risk for fracture are identified in order to minimize the possibility of falls and to avoid excessive mechanical loading of the bones.

As stated by Notelovitz in his article a few years ago (Notelovitz, 1989), sedentary individuals need a gradual introduction to a formal exercise program. Any aerobic exercise program - walking, biking, jogging, etc. - must be preceded by a careful assessment of each individual's health and cardiovascular fitness, especially the ability of the heart to withstand physical stress. In supervised muscle strengthening exercises, care should be taken to establish the individual's repetition maximum. Once the maximum performance is assessed and possible contraindications taken into account, an exercise prescription can be based on accepted criteria as to the intensity, duration and frequency of aerobic and strengthening exercises.

REFERENCES

Aloia JF, Cohn SH, Ostuni JA, Cane R, Ellis K. Prevention of involutional bone loss by exercise. Ann Intern Med 1978;89:356-8.

Bilanin JE, Blanchard MS, Russek-Cohen E. Lower vertebral bone density in male long distance runners. Med Sci Sports Exerc 1989;21:66-70.

Bouchard C, Shephard RJ, Stephens T, Sutton JR, McPherson BD, eds. Exercise, Fitness, and Health. A Consensus of Current Knowledge. Champaign, Il: Human Kinetics Publishers, 1990:22.

Cavanaugh DJ, Cann CE. Brisk walking does not stop bone loss in postmenopausal women. Bone 1988;9: 201-4.

Cheng S, Suominen H, Era P, Heikkinen E. Bone density of the calcaneus and fractures in 75- and 80-year-old men and women. Osteoporosis Int 1994;4:48-54.

Cheng S, Suominen H, Heikkinen E. Bone mineral density in relation to anthropometric properties, physical activity and smoking in 75-year-old men and women. Aging Clin Exp Res 1993;5:173-80.

Chow R, Harrison JE, Notarius C. Effect of two randomized exercise programmes on bone mass of healthy postmenopausal women. Br Med J 1987;295:1441-4.

Dalsky GP, Stocke KS, Ehsani AA, Slatpolsky E, Lee WC, Birge SJ. Weight-bearing exercise training and lumbar bone mineral content in postmenopausal women. Ann Intern Med 1988;108:824-8.

Dilsen G, Berker C, Oral A, Varan G. The role of physical exercise in prevention and management of osteoporosis. Clin Rheumatol 1989;8(Suppl 2):70-5.

Grove KA, Londeree BR. Bone density in postmenopausal women: high impact vs low impact exercise. Med Sci Sports Exerc 1992;24:1190-4.

Gutin B, Kasper MJ. Can vigorous exercise play a role in osteroporosis prevention? A review. Osteoporosis Int 1992;2:55-69.

Jacobson PC, Beaver W, Grupp SA, Taft TN, Talmage RV. Bone density in women: college athletes and older athletic women. J Orthop Res 1984;2:328-32.

Krolner B, Toft B, Nielsen SP, Tondevol E. Physical exercise as prophylaxis against involutional vertebral bone loss: a controlled trial. Clin Sci 1983;64:541-6.

Lane NE, Bloch DA, Jones HH, Marshall WH, Wood PD, Fries JF. Long-distance running, bone density, and osteoarthritis. JAMA 1986;255:1147-51.

Law MR, Wald NJ, Meade TW. Strategies for prevention of osteoporosis and hip fracture. Br Med J 1991;303: 453-9.

MacDougall JD, Webber CE, Martin J et al. Relationship among running mileage, bone density, and serum testosterone in male runners. J Appl Physiol 1992;73:1165-70.

Michel BA, Bloch DA, Fries JF. Weight-bearing exercise, overexercise, and lumbar bone density over age fifty. Arch Inter Med 1989;149:2325-9.

Nilsson BE, Westlin NE. Bone density in athletes. Clin Orthop Rel Res 1971;77:179-82.

Notelovitz M. Osteoporosis: screening and exercise. Prog Clin Biol Res 1989;320:225-52.

Pruitt LA, Jackson RD, Bartels RL, Lehnhard HJ. Weight-training effects on bone mineral density in early postmenopausal women. J Bone Miner Res 1992;7:179-85.

Reid IR, Ames R, Evans MC, Sharpe S, Gamble G et al. Determinants of total body and regional bone mineral density in normal post-menopausal women - a key role for fat mass. J Clin Endocrinol Metab 1992;75:45-51.

Rikli RE, McManis BG. Effects of exercise on bone mineral content in postmenopausal women. Res Q 1990;61:243-9.

Rundgren Å, Aniansson A, Ljungberg P, Wetterqvist H. Effects of a training programme for elderly people on mineral content of the heel bone. Arch Gerontol Geriatr 1984;3:243-8.

Sandler RB, Cauley JA, Hom DL, Sashin D, Kriska AM. The effects of walking on the cross-sectional dimensions of the radius in postmenopausal women. Calcif Tissue Int 1987;41:65-9.

Simkin A, Ayalon J, Leichter I. Increased trabecular bone density due to bone-loading exercises in postmenopausal osteoporotic women. Calcif Tissue Int 1987;40:59-63.

Sinaki M, Wahner HW, Offord KP, Hodgson SF. Efficacy of nonloading exercises in prevention of vertebral bone loss in postmenopausal women: a controlled trial. Mayo Clin Proc 1989;64:762-9.

Smidt GL, Lin SY, O'Dwyer KD, Blanpied PR. The effect of high-intensity trunk exercise on bone mineral density of postmenopausal women. Spine 1992;17:280-5.

Smith EL, Gilligan C. Physical activity effects on bone metabolism. Calcif Tissue Int 1991;49:S50-4.

Smith EL, Gilligan C, McAdam M, Ensing CP, Smith PE. Deterring bone loss by exercise intervention in premenopausal and postmenopausal women. Calcif Tissue Int 1989;44:312-21.

Smith EL, Reddan W, Smith PE. Physical activity and calcium modalities for bone mineral increase in aged women. Med Sci Sports Exerc 1981;13:60-4.

Snow-Harter C, Marcus R. Exercise, bone mineral density, and osteoporosis. In: Butler JP, ed. Exercise and Sport Sciences Reviews, Vol. 19. Baltimore: Williams & Wilkins, 1991:351-88.

Suominen H. Bone mineral density and long term exercise. An overview of cross-sectional athlete studies. Sports Medicine 1993;16:316-330.

Suominen H, Rahkila P. Bone mineral density of the calcaneus in 70-to-81-year-old male athletes and a population sample. Med Sci Sports Exerc 1991;23:1227-33.

The Academy of Finland, The Finnish Medical Society Duodecim, Ministry of Social Affairs and Health: Prevention and Treatment of Osteoporosis. Consensus Meeting, Hanasaari March 30 - April 1, 1992. Helsinki: Hakapaino 1992:7 (in Finnish).

Vico L, Bourrin S, Chatard J-C et al. Possible nonlinear effects of exercise on bone in male subjects over age 60 years. Anat Rec 1993;235:206-14.

White MK, Martin RB, Yeater RA, Butcher RL, Radin EL. The effects of exercise on the bones of postmenopausal women. Int Orthop 1984;7:209-14.

The Effect of Exercise on Bone Mineral Density and Physical Fitness in Osteoporotic and Osteoarthritic Women

Niamh M. Murphy, M.A.
Simon A. Henderson, B.Sc., M.D.

INTRODUCTION

As the proportion of elderly in the population rises (CSO, 1989), so too do the demands on the health service. Elderly women with osteoporotic fracture of the hip or with primary osteoarthritis requiring total hip replacement form the majority of orthopedic patients requiring surgery.

Osteoporosis, a metabolic bone disease in which the mineral density of the bones is decreased, thereby increasing their fragility and susceptibility to fracture, has a high incidence in the over-65 age group, especially among women. In England and Wales, 40,000 people sustain hip fractures annually and it has been estimated that 84 percent of them have significant osteoporosis (Aitken, 1984). Osteoarthritis of the hip is a more common disorder in women than in men, particularly after age 55 (Goodacre, 1984), and frequently results in the need for total hip replacement.

The quality of life for elderly women following hip surgery depends largely upon their capability for independent living. Reduction in levels of habitual physical activity with age and following surgery is likely to lead to a deterioration in both exercise capacity and physical condition, setting up a vicious cycle which will eventually jeopardize the capacity for independent living (Bassey, 1978). A loss of functional fitness may result from inactivity during the operative period, rendering individuals close to their "thresholds of independence" (The Lancet, 1986). The social and economic consequences of supporting a dependent elderly population are an important public health concern.

Regular physical activity can improve physiological functioning in the elderly, just as it can in the young. Improvements in cardiovascular fitness (Moray et al, 1989; Smith, 1989) and skeletal muscle strength (Fiatarone et al., 1990) with exercise have been well documented. Perceived psychological functioning may also be positively affected by exercise (Emery and Blumenthal, 1990).

Exercise also appears to have a beneficial effect on the skeleton (Rikli and McManis, 1990; Dalsky et al., 1988). Athletes have been found to have higher bone density than non-athletes (Nilsson and Westlin, 1971). In tennis players the dominant radius has been shown to have significantly greater bone mineral density than the non-dominant radius (Huddleston et al., 1980; Pirnay et al., 1987). Although few longitudinal studies have been conducted, in general the results indicate that exercise training can result in increased bone density (Krolner et al., 1983; Ayalon et al., 1987). However, the results of such studies are highly dependent on the bone site measured, the exercise type and duration, the age of subjects, and the measurement instruments used.

The ability to produce improvements in functional fitness and bone health in elderly patients following hip surgery using an exercise program would be of major significance, especially if it resulted in prolonged independence and improved quality of life. A prospective, longitudinal study to investigate the effects of a twice weekly six-month exercise regime on 26 elderly women who had undergone hip surgery was therefore undertaken to ascertain whether fitness and bone health benefits occurred.

SUBJECTS

Forty-two women aged 64-83 years (mean 73 years) were recruited from orthopedic outpatient clinics. Twenty-six consented to take part in regular exercise classes. Of these, 13 had undergone surgery following osteoporotic fracture of the neck of the femur and 13 had total hip replacement for primary osteoarthritis. In the non-exercising control group, there were seven fracture and nine osteoarthritis patients. To be included in the study, subjects had to be at least four months post-surgery, mentally alert, and independently mobile without a walking aid. Criteria for exclusion included causes of secondary osteoporosis (i.e., post-gastric surgery, high alcohol intake, drugs, etc.).

Informed consent was obtained from all subjects. Approval was obtained from the Medical Ethical Committee, The Queen's University of Belfast.

METHODS

Bone Mineral Density

Bone mineral density was measured in the lumbar spine before and after the six-month exercise program using quantitative digital radiography (Hologic QDR 1000 Bone Densitometer). The measurement precision of the machine is quoted to be better than 0.01 g/cm^2. Prior to each scanning session a quality control scan of the Hologic X-CALIBER model QDR-1 anthropomorphic spine phantom supplied with the machine was performed. The coefficient of variation (standard deviation expressed as a percentage of the mean) for the quality control scans performed during the study was 0.42 percent. Each scan was analyzed as laid down in the instruction manual to give a figure for bone mineral density for L2-L4 in g/cm^2. The scan is compared with a reference database of volunteers from the University of California, San Diego.

Anthropometry

Body mass was measured on a chair scales (Avery, England). Heavy clothing and shoes were removed. Height was measured, without shoes, using a stadiometer.

Skinfold over the biceps, triceps, subscapular and suprailiac sites was measured using Harpenden skinfold calipers (John Bull Ltd., England) according to the Eurofit protocol (Council of Europe, 1988). Percentage body fat was calculated according to the formula of Durnin and Rahaman (1976). Lean body mass was calculated as body mass less fat mass.

Grip Strength

Grip strength was measured using an analogue hand grip dynamometer (Kyoshi, Japan). The dynamometer was held in the preferred hand by the side of the thigh, with the subject standing, and squeezed as hard as possible for several seconds. The better of two attempts was recorded as the subject's score.

Cardiorespiratory Fitness

A submaximal test of Physical Working Capacity equivalent to 85 percent of age-related maximum heart rate (PWC 85 percent) (Cooke, 1986) was performed on an electronically-braked cycle ergometer (Seca, Germany). The protocol was designed to raise the subject's heart rate to 85 percent of age-predicted maximum over an exercise period of six to eight minutes. Following a habituation period, the subject rested for 10 minutes before commencing the test. The initial workload was set at 0.7 watts per kilogram of lean body mass. The subject cycled for two minutes at the initial workload, after which time heart rate was measured using a heart rate monitor (Sportstester 2000, Polar Electro, Finland).

A second workload was calculated based on heart rate response to the first workload:

The increments were calculated in accordance with Eurofit protocols (Council of Europe, 1988). Scores were converted into predicted maximum oxygen uptake ($\dot{V}O_2max$) values according to the formula of Shephard (1970).

Statistical Analysis

All fitness data were entered and stored on ICL 3930 main frame computer and analyzed using SPSS. Bone density analyses were calculated using the Statgraphics V2.6 (Statistical Graphics Corporation) on Opus II Advanced Personal Computer. Paired t-tests were used to measure changes in fitness and bone variables over the study period. Independent samples t-tests measured differences between exercise and control groups.

RESULTS

Anthropometric and cardiorespiratory fitness characteristics of the exercise and control groups are shown in Table 1. The groups' bone characteristics are shown in Table 2. There was no significant difference between the mean weight of the subjects and the controls. The difference between the mean ages of the subjects and controls of 4.75 years was statistically significant ($p=0.007$).

Bone mineral density was measured in the lumbar spine using quantitative digital radiography. The changes in bone mineral density for the study period are shown in Table 2. There was no significant difference in initial spine bone mineral density between the exercise and control groups. During the study period, an increase in lumbar spine bone mineral density ($p=0.0078$) was found in the exercise group, but no significant change occurred in the control group. The greatest increases occurred in those subjects with the highest initial bone mineral density (3.5 percent vs. 0.5 percent. $p<0.05$)

There were no significant changes in height, weight, body fat, grip strength, physical working capacity, or physical fitness tests, with the exception of walking speed, over the six-month period. Figure 1 shows the improvement in walking speeds for the total hip replacement subjects (n=13), fracture subjects (n=13) and the whole group (n=26) over

TABLE 1

Anthropometric, Fitness and Bone Characteristics of the Exercise and Control Groups [Mean (SD)]*

	Exercise Group	Control Group	Significance Level and p-value
n	26	16	
Age (years)	71.5(5.4)	75.9(4.9)	0.007
Height(cm)	159(10.4)	-	-
Weight(kg)	64.2(12.4)	63.2(10.6)	N.S.
Body Fat(%)	28.2(0.8)	-	-
Physical work capacity (85% max HR) (watts)	63.2(7.7)	-	-
Estimated $\dot{V}O_2$ max (ml/kg/min)	21.3(7.1)	-	-
Grip strength (kg)	18.1(1.0)	-	-

* An independent samples t-test was performed to determine whether differences existed between groups.

TABLE 2

Changes in Lumbar Spine Bone Mineral Density Over the Study Period [mean(SD)]

	Exercise Group		
	Fracture Group	Osteoarthritis Group	Control Group
n	13	13	16
BMD1	0.720(0.18)	0.870(0.19)	0.839(0.16)
BMD2	0.723(0.18)*	0.890(0.19)*	0.842(0.16)

Key: BMD1 Initial lumbar spine bone mineral density (g/cm^2)
BMD2 Poststudy lumbar spine bone mineral density (g/cm^2)
*$p<0.05$

the course of the study. Mean walking speed increased by 50 percent between 0 and three months, and increased by a further 21 percent between three and six months ($p<.05$).

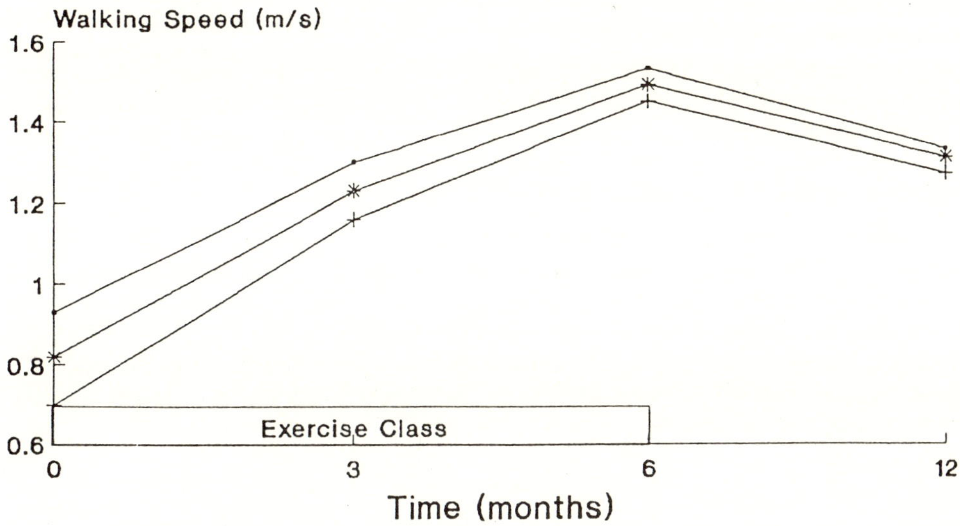

·Total hip replacement group (n=13)
+Fracture group (n=13)
*Total group (n=26)

Figure 1. Walking speed before, during and after completion of exercise programs. Speeds for the total hip replacement group, fracture group and total group shown.

DISCUSSION

A six-month general exercise program was associated with significant improvements in lumbar spine bone mineral density and walking speed in a group of elderly women who had undergone hip surgery. No significant changes in anthropometry, cardiorespiratory fitness, measured on a cycle ergometer, or grip strength were observed.

On entry to the study only three out of 26 subjects were able to achieve the minimum recommended walking speed of 1.07 m/sec required to safely negotiate a pelican crossing (Department of Transport, 1987). On completion of the exercise period, however, 25 of the 26 subjects were able to exceed this requirement. On average, a 50 percent increase in mean walking speed occurred between 0 and three months, with a further 21 percent increase between three and six months.

The significant increase in mean walking speed from 0.82 m/sec on entry to 1.49m/sec at the completion of the study suggests not only that full walking rehabilitation following surgery is possible but also that present post-operative rehabilitation may be inadequate. Uncorrected walking speed has been shown to be a reliable clinical method of monitoring gait rehabilitation for hospitalized elderly (Friedman et al., 1988).

The total hip replacement subjects had a higher walking speed on entry to the study group than the fracture group. Both groups had a significant rise in walking speed during the first three months, and the difference between the groups was maintained. It is not clear whether the initial differences in walking speed between fracture patients and total hip replacement patients were due to differences in post-operative rehabilitation or to the differing underlying pathology of the patients. The fact that both groups had similar walking speeds after six months of exercise supports the hypothesis that initial poor performance may reflect inadequate post-operative rehabilitation.

It has been calculated that walking at 1.38 m/sec is maximum aerobic exercise for the average 70 to 75-year-old female (The Lancet, 1986; Saltin, 1980). Despite the fact that the exercise involvement of the study group fell short of the recommended guidelines for developing cardiorespiratory fitness in healthy adults (American College of Sports Medicine, 1990), the walking speed achieved at the completion of the study exceeded this proposed minimum level. However, no significant improvements in physical working capacity or estimated maximum oxygen uptake as assessed on the bicycle ergometer were observed.

The cycle ergometer test was found to be an insensitive measure of improved submaximal function in this group, and alternative protocols and tests need to be considered.

The rise in mean lumbar spine bone mineral density is of the same order as that reported in other exercise intervention studies, although these were mainly in younger post-menopausal subjects (Krolner et al., 1983). In this population who were in excess of 15 years post-menopause, the annual rate of bone loss would be expected to be 0.5 to one percent. The lack of this fall in the present control group may reflect either the low initial bone mineral density of the subjects or the short study period relative to the small expected change.

CONCLUSION

In summary, exercise was associated with significant improvements in lumbar spine bone mineral density and walking speed in elderly hip replacement and fracture patients. The mechanism for these improvements is, however, unclear. The required intensity and mode of activity necessary to elicit a positive response to exercise in elderly patients following surgery must also be established.

ACKNOWLEDGEMENTS

The assistance of the following is gratefully acknowledged: Dr. T.R.O. Beringer and Mrs. O. Finlay, Department of Geriatric Medicine, Dr. Colin Boreham, Physical and Health Education Unit, and Professor R.A.B. Mollan, Department of Orthopaedic Surgery, The Queen's University of Belfast.

REFERENCES

Aitken JM. Relevance of osteoporosis in women with fracture of the femoral neck. Br Med J 1984;285:585-8.

American College of Sports Medicine. The recommended quantity and quality of exercise for developing and maintaining cardiorespiratory and muscular fitness in healthy adults. Med Sci Sports Exerc 1990;22:265-74.

Ayalon J, Simkin A, Leichter I, Raifman S. Dynamic bone loading exercises for post-menopausal women: effect on density of distal radius. Arch Phys Med Rehab 1987;68:280-3.

Bassey EJ. Age, inactivity and some physiological responses to exercise. Gerontology 1978;24:66-77.

Cooke CB. Welsh Heart Programme Directorate. Clinical Survey Manual. Heart Beat Report No. 3, Cardiff, 1986.

Council of Europe. Eurofit, European tests of physical fitness. Council of Europe, Rome, 1988.

CSO Social Trends 19. Central Statistics Office, HMSO London, 1989.

Dalsky GP, Socke BS, Ehsani AA, Slatopoloskey E, Lec WC, Birge J. Weight bearing exercise training - lumbar bone mineral content in post-menopausal women. Ann Intern Med 1988;108:624-828.

Department of Transport. Highways and traffic. A departmental standard. Transport Department 28/87, 1987.

Durnin JVG, Rahaman MM. The assessment of the amount of fat in the human body from measurement of skinfold thickness. Br J Nutr 1976;21:681-9.

Emery CF, Blumenthal JA. Perceived change among participants in an exercise program for older adults. The Gerontologist 1990;30:516-21.

Fiatarone MA, Marks PC, Ryan ND, Meredith CN, Lipsitz LA, Evans WJ. High intensity strength training in nonagenarians; effects on skeletal muscle. JAMA 1990;263:3029-34.

Friedman PJ, Richman DE, Baskett JJ. A prospective trial of serial gait speed as a measure of rehabilitation in the elderly. Age Aging 1988; 17:227-35.

Goodacre J. Osteoarthritis. Introductions to Clinical Rheumatology. London: Churchill Livingstone, 1984.

Huddleston AL, Rockwell D, Kuland DN, Harrison RB. Bone mass in lifetime tennis athletes. JAMA 1980;244:1107-9.

Krolner P, Toft B, Nielson SP, Tandevold E. Physical exercise as prophylaxis against involutional vertebral bone loss: a controlled trial. Clin Sci 1983;64:541-6.

The Lancet. Physical activity in old age (Editorial), 1986, Dec 20/27:1431.

Moray MC, Cowper PA, Feussner JR, et al. Evaluation of a supervised exercise programme in a geriatric population. J Am Geriatr Soc 1989;37:348-54.

Nilsson BE, Westlin NE. Bone density in athletes. Clin Orthop Rel Research 1971;77: 179-82.

Pirnay F., Bodeux M, Cruliard JM, Franchimont P. Bone mineral content and physical activity. Int J Sports Med 1987;8:331-5.

Rikli RE, McManis BG. Effects of exercise on bone mineral content in post menopausal women. Res Quart Ex Sport 1990;61:243-9.

Saltin B. Iysisk vedligeholdelse hos ældre I. Aerob arbejdsevne. Månedsskr Prakt Læg 1980;58:193-216.

Shephard RJ. Computer programs for solution of the Åstrand nomogram and the calculation of body surface area. J Sports Med Phys Fitness 1970;10:206.

Smith WDF. Fitness training for the elderly: Canadian experience. Geriatr Med 1989;11:55-61.

Women, Sports, Exercise, and Nutrition

Jeannie Crane Sykes, Ph.D., R.D.

INTRODUCTION

Nutrition concerns for the older athlete are similar to those of younger athletes. There is evidence that prolonged and high-intensity training increases protein needs. For most athletes whose daily diets include animal products, meeting increased protein demands is not likely to be problematic. Poorly planned meat-free diets may provide inadequate protein, however, especially if caloric intake is also insufficient. The protein requirement of the older population is controversial, and studies of older athletes are required to evaluate protein needs specific to this population. For all athletes, adequate hydration is crucial to performance and health. A purposeful plan for fluid replacement is recommended. Sports drinks providing a source of carbohydrate may be beneficial in endurance events lasting 60 minutes or longer. If the diet is chosen judiciously, electrolyte supplementation is unnecessary except in extremely prolonged events such as ultramarathons. Studies of noninstitutionalized older people suggest that there is a wide spectrum of dietary adequacy with respect to vitamins and minerals. Physical activity may add another dimension of variability in both nutrient needs and intake. The increased energy expenditure of physically active older women allows a greater caloric intake without weight gain. Most studies of the general population indicate a reduction of food intake with increasing age, which makes nutritional adequacy more difficult to achieve. Exercise, therefore, offers a distinct nutritional advantage in this respect.

DIETARY REQUIREMENTS

Dietary requirements for the physically active must take into account both the effects of aging and of exercise. Exercise-related nutrient needs depend on training intensity and duration, fitness level, and type of activity. Aging-related dietary needs can be as diverse as the older population itself; there is tremendous individual variation in body composition, physiologic function, and health status, reflecting genetic differences as well as accumulated histories of individual lifestyle practices. There are, however, some generalizations that can be made with regard to nutrient needs and dietary recommendations for older persons involved in sports and fitness activities.

For the purposes of this discussion, "physically active" refers to the moderately active as well as elite athletes. This seems especially appropriate in light of the evaluation of participants in the 1985 World Masters Games: more than 90 percent of the Masters athletes reported that they were involved in sports more for social than competitive reasons, and the training regimen of most of the athletes was modest (Kavanagh et al., 1989).

Protein

Prolonged and high-intensity exercise increases the need for dietary protein due to the depression of protein synthesis (Richardson and Birchenall-Sparks, 1983) and to increases in muscle breakdown, amino acid oxidation, and gluconeogenesis (Grandjean, 1989). Although the United States Recommended Dietary Allowance for protein for adults is 0.8 g per kg of body weight (National Research Council, 1989), athletes' protein requirement may be as high as 1.0 to 1.5 g/kg body weight (Tarnpolsky et al., 1988). For athletes whose diets include daily consumption of animal protein sources (meat, fish, poultry, dairy), even the higher protein recommendation can be easily met. It should be emphasized that these higher protein requirements reflect the demands of training at a high intensity and/or duration, and are, therefore, not universal to all physically active persons.

Vegetarian athletes should be encouraged to incorporate adequate plant protein sources into their diets, making use of legumes, grains, nuts, and seeds. Appropriate food combinations enhance protein availability, such as grains with legumes or legumes with seeds. Meeting protein needs is much easier with the inclusion of dairy and egg products (lacto-ovo vegetarianism), and such high-quality protein may be preferable to plant sources for older athletes due to declining renal function with age (Roe, 1992; Shephard, 1986).

In evaluating protein adequacy, it is important to assess calorie intake because energy deficiency decreases nitrogen balance (Göranzon and Forsum, 1985). Risk for protein inadequacy increases, therefore, in endurance athletes whose caloric intake is marginally sufficient to meet the energy demands of training, and especially when dietary protein is minimal and of poor quality (plant source). Protein requirements of the older population have been controversial. The United States National Research Council (1989) recommends a greater protein intake per unit of lean body mass for adults above age 50. Protein needs may be increased due to impaired digestive function, disease states, decreased efficiency of protein utilization, and abnormal metabolic states associated with aging (Young et al., 1976).

It is arguable that protein needs decline with age due to decreased total body protein synthesis and a reduction of lean body mass. This conjecture may not apply, however, to those persons with a higher level of lean tissue maintained through continued activity during adulthood.

Fluid and Electrolytes

Adequate hydration is crucial to both athletic performance and to health. A purposeful plan for fluid replacement is essential, rather than allowing thirst to dictate water consumption. Five-hundred ml of fluid should be consumed pre-exercise, and 200-400 ml every 20 minutes during activity (American Dietetic Association, 1987). In addition to preventing heat injury, muscle cramps may be prevented by adequate hydration (Benda, 1989).

If a sound, well-balanced diet is consumed, electrolyte replacement is necessary only in severe conditions: electrolyte replacement is recommended for events lasting four hours or more (Frizzell et al., 1986). Exercise-induced sweating activates electrolyte conservation mechanisms in the body, which are enhanced as the individual becomes acclimatized to heat. Salt tablets are unnecessary in most situations, and can even be harmful, especially if consumed in the absence of water (Williams, 1985). Due to sweat losses, electrolyte concentrations actually increase during exercise; therefore, electrolyte replacement should occur following exercise, and should be accompanied by water (Williams, 1985). The presence of electrolytes in sports drinks consumed during exercise is useful primarily for their role in enhancing the rate of fluid and carbohydrate uptake rather than for the actual electrolytes provided.

Carbohydrate

Pre-exercise carbohydrate loading is generally not necessary for events that are 90 minutes or shorter in duration. A fluid replacement containing carbohydrate is advised during activity, however, if exercise exceeds one hour. Maintenance of blood glucose and muscle glycogen levels and endurance are enhanced with consumption of sports drinks containing four to ten percent carbohydrate of any type, if consumed every 20 minutes during exercise (Davis et al., 1990). Simple sugars and glucose polymers have been shown to have similar effects on both substrate utilization and fluid replenishment.

Vitamins and Minerals

Studies of noninstitutionalized indicate a wide spectrum of dietary adequacy with respect to vitamins and minerals. There is evidence that older women may be at increased risk of deficiencies of vitamin A (Chandra et al., 1991), vitamin B6 (Ribaya-Mercado et al., 1991), vitamin C (Chandra et al., 1991; Heseker and Kübler, 1992), and vitamin D (Chandra et al., 1991).

Minerals of particular concern are calcium and magnesium (Pao and Mickle, 1981; Morgan et al., 1985), zinc (Sandstead et al., 1982; Vaughan and Manore, 1988), and iron (Chandra et al., 1991).

Nutrient needs among athletes depend in part upon the type of activity (for example, endurance, speed, or strength). Dietary iron requirements are believed to increase with prolonged, high-intensity training due to sweat losses as well as red blood cell hemolysis that can occur in sports such as endurance running (Hunding et al., 1981). The existence of a so-called "sports anemia" remains controversial, however. The apparent anemia may be due to the normal expansion of plasma volume that occurs with training rather than a reduction in absolute cell mass (Eichner, 1986). Riboflavin requirements may be elevated in physically active young women (Belko et al., 1983). Electrolytes, most notably sodium and chloride, are needed in greater amounts with chronic high-intensity training (Murray et al., 1987).

Increased food intake to meet energy demands of training, if chosen judiciously, provides additional nutrients, including those that are needed in greater amounts by athletes. As previously indicated, high-level athletic training is most likely to raise nutrient needs, and therefore necessitates greater attention to sound food choices.

DIETARY RECOMMENDATIONS

The following dietary recommendations for physically active older individuals are based on three dietary objectives: disease prevention, weight control, and optimal athletic performance. The recommendations are compatible with each of these objectives, and are similar to recommendations for the general athletic population (Leaf and Frisa, 1989).

1. Limit dietary fat to 25 percent of total calories.

2. Obtain 60-70 percent of total calories from carbohydrate.

3. Moderate dietary protein (10-15 percent of total calories), and emphasize:

    a. lean types of meat, fish, and poultry.

    b. high-quality sources (animal protein or complementary plant sources such as rice and beans or hummos (garbanzos and sesame seeds).

4. Choose a well balanced diet with special attention to foods rich in

    a. Calcium (low-fat milk, yogurt, and buttermilk; canned fish with the bones, such as salmon or mackerel; broccoli; tofu; sesame meal [tahini]).

    b. Iron (lean red meats; legumes; dried fruit; dark green, leafy vegetables).

    c. Magnesium (nuts; green vegetables; whole grains).

    d. Zinc (lean meats; eggs; seafood; whole grains).

    e. Vitamin B6 (lean pork; legumes; whole grains).

5. Drink before thirst: 6-8 cups of water daily, more if training or heat is excessive.

6. Limit sodium intake to 3,000 mg per day.

CONCLUSION

Nutritional needs of physically active older women vary according to level and type of activity, age, and health status. The older female athlete benefits from an increased energy expenditure that allows greater food consumption, thereby increasing nutrient intake. A diet that is geared toward optimizing athletic performance is also compatible with and complementary to one designed for disease prevention.

Exercise is of obvious benefit (Åstrand, 1992), even when begun later in life (Cunningham and Paterson, 1990). Women, formerly excluded from sports and exercise participation in many cultures, are becoming increasingly active. The increase in participation by older women has prompted questions regarding exercise risks, benefits, and specific needs of this population. More research into nutrient and dietary needs of this population will further support women's fitness participation well into old age.

REFERENCES

American Dietetic Association. Position of the American Dietetic Association: nutrition for physical fitness and athletic performance for adults. J Am Diet Assoc 1987;87:933-9.

Åstrand P. Physical activity and fitness. Am J Clin Nutr 1992;55:1231-6.

Belko AZ, Obarzanek E, Kalkwarf HJ et al. Effects of exercise on riboflavin requirements of young women. Am J Clin Nutr 1983;37:509-17.

Benda C. Outwitting muscle cramps—Is it possible? Physician Sportsmed 1989;17:176-8.

Chandra RK, Imbach A, Moore C, Skelton D, Woolcott D. Nutrition of the elderly. Can Med Assoc J 1991;145:1475-87.

Cunningham DA, Paterson DH. Discussion: exercise, fitness, and aging. In: Bouchard C, Shephard RJ, Stephens T, Sutton JR, McPherson BD, eds. Exercise, Fitness, and Health. Champaign, IL: Human Kinetics Books, 1990:699-704.

Davis JM, Burgess WA, Slentz CA, Bartoli WP. Fluid availability of sports drinks differing in carbohydrate type and concentration. Am J Clin Nutr 1990;51:1054-7.

Eichner ER. The anemias of athletes. Physician Sportsmed 1986;14:122-30.

Frizzell RT, Lang GH, Lowance DC, Lathan SR. Hyponatremia and ultramarathon running. J Am Med Assoc 1986;255:772-4.

Göranzon H, Forsum E. Effect of reduced energy intake versus increased physical activity on the outcome of nitrogen balance experiments in man. Am J Clin Nutr 1985;41:919-28.

Grandjean AC. Macronutrient intake of U.S. athletes compared with the general population and recommendations made for athletes. Am J Clin Nutr 1989;49:1070-6.

Heseker H, Kübler W. Vitamin requirements of the Elderly. In: Munro H and Schlierf G, eds. Nutrition of the Elderly, Vol. 29. New York: Raven Press,1992:129-43.

Hunding A, Jordal R, Paulev PE. Runner's anemia and iron deficiency. Acta Med Scand 1981;209:315-8.

Kavanagh T, Mertens DJ, Matosevic V, Shephard RJ, Evans B. Health and aging of Masters athletes. Clin Sports Med 1989;1:72-88.

Leaf A, Frisa KB. Eating for health or for athletic performance? Am J Clin Nutr 1989;49:1066-9.

Morgan KJ, Stampley GL, Zabik ME, Fischer DR. Magnesium and calcium dietary intakes of the U.S. population. J Am Coll Nutr 1985;4:195-206.

Murray R, Eddy DE, Murray T, Seifert JG, Paul GL, Halby GA. The effect of fluid and carbohydrate feedings during intermittent cycling exercise. Med Sci Sports Exerc 1987;19:597-604.

National Research Council. Recommended Dietary Allowances, 10th edition. Washington, DC: National Academy Press, 1989:60.

Pao EM, Mickle SJ. Problem nutrients in the United States. Food Technol 1981;35:58-62,4,6-9.

Ribaya-Mercado JD, Russell RM, Sahyoun N, Morrow FD, Gershoff SN. Vitamin B6 requirements of elderly men and women. J Nutr 1991;121:1062-74.

Richardson A, Birchenall-Sparks MC. Age-related change in protein synthesis. Rev Biol Res Aging 1983;1:255-73.

Roe, DA. Geriatric Nutrition. Englewood Cliffs, NJ: Prentice-Hall, 1992:72.

Sandstead HH, Henriksen LK, Greger JL, Prasad AS. Zinc nutriture in the elderly in relation to taste acuity, immune response, and wound healing. Am J Clin Nutr 1982;36:1046-59.

Shephard RJ. Nutrition and the physiology of aging. In: Young EA, ed. Nutrition, Aging, and Health. New York: Alan R. Liss, 1986:1-23.

Tarnpolsky MA, Mac Dougall JD, Atkinson SA. Influence of protein intake and training status on nitrogen balance and lean body mass. J Appl Physiol 1988;4:187-93.

Vaughan LA, Manore MM. Dietary patterns and nutritional status of low income, free-living elderly. Food and Nutrition News 1988;60:27-30.

Williams MH. Nutritional aspects of human physical and athletic performance, 2nd edition. Springfield, IL: Charles C. Thomas Publisher, 1985:226-53.

Young V, Perera W, Winterer J, Scrimshaw N. Protein and amino acid requirements of the elderly. In: Winick M, ed. Nutrition and Aging, New York: Wiley, 1976:77-118.

Section 2

Physical Activity and Performance

Functional Performance Assessment in Old Age

Archie Young, B.Sc., M.B. Ch.B., M.D., F.R.C.P.
Jose Botella, M.B. Ch.B.
Carolyn A. Greig, M.Sc., Ph.D.
Dawn A. Skelton, B.Sc.

INTRODUCTION

Illness in old age highlights the elderly person's lack of safety margins. The ability to perform everyday physical tasks is one of many areas where this is evident (Young, 1986). Increasing age brings with it reductions in strength, power and maximum oxygen uptake (Young, 1992; Greig and Young, 1992), so that some everyday tasks require maximal effort for their performance. It then needs only a minor intercurrent illness to take an elderly person across the threshold from being just able to being just unable to perform a functionally important task without assistance (Figure 1).

In clinical practice, the efficacy of therapeutic interventions must be judged not only by improvements in specific, disease-related impairments, but also (and more importantly) in terms of the patient's ability to function. This also solves the problem of evaluating the net effect of multiple, possibly conflicting, interventions in the patient with multiple pathology. In his Gifford Lectures of 1937/8, Sir Charles Sherrington emphasized that human existence depends on functional performance, which, in turn, depends on muscle contraction (Sherrington, 1963). As both a geriatrician and a physiologist, my interest in functional performance reflects both my view of geriatric medicine as a function-oriented specialty and Sherrington's view of the central role of muscle. I shall not attempt a comprehensive review of the methodology of functional performance assessment: these are available elsewhere (Applegate et al., 1990; Kane and Kane, 1981; Wade, 1992). Instead, I shall highlight selected areas which strike me as particularly important, interesting, or controversial. They can be considered in four broad categories: those of particular relevance to clinical practice in hospital, those more applicable to a community-based approach to health in old age, pitfalls in the use of functional performance assessment, and, finally, research questions being addressed in our laboratory concerning mechanisms limiting the functional performance of healthy elderly people.

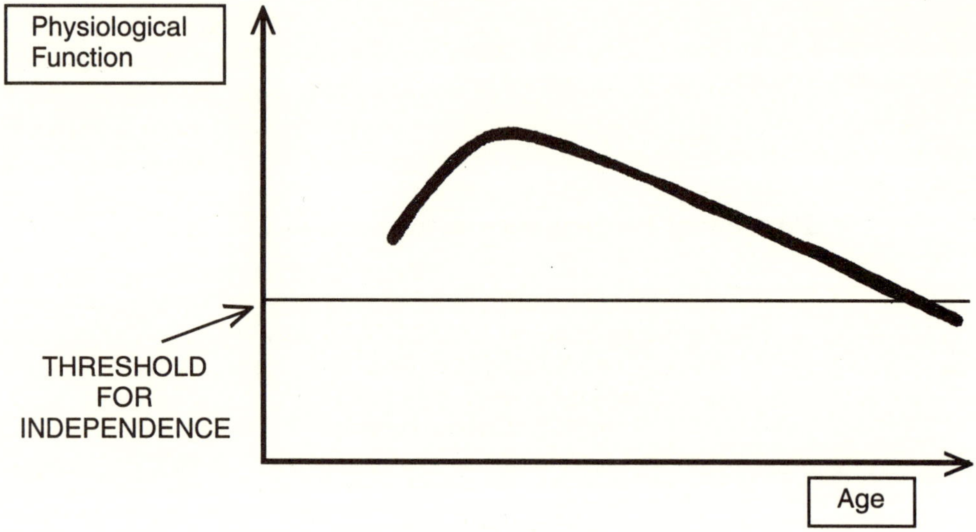

Figure 1. Age-associated reductions in strength, power, and maximum oxygen uptake bring elderly people closer to functional "thresholds"

IN HOSPITAL PRACTICE

Clinical Recording

In general, doctors are not good at recording their patients' functional abilities. Even the most detailed "medical" account of a patient would be grossly incomplete without an account of selected functional abilities. This is especially true in old age; it is in older patients that information about functional performance makes the greatest contribution to diagnosis, treatment and prognosis. Despite the very large and very rapidly rising number of elderly people in the population (and their particular prevalence among those admitted to hospital), the gathering of such information is still not part of standard teaching for medical students. In an attempt to rectify this, we have emphasized that functional information relevant to severely disabled elderly people can be readily incorporated into both the conventional clinical history and the conventional clinical examination (Dickinson and Young, 1990). A degree of scaling is possible for each activity, recording whether the patient is able to perform the activity independently, with supervision, with prompting, with the physical help of one person or with the physical help of two people. Overall, however, this is not intended as a measurement tool. Rather, it should be seen as an aid to the structured collection and recording of clinically important information.

Other instruments which can be used for the structured gathering of clinically important information about functional performance include well-known scales such as the Barthel scale (Mahoney and Barthel, 1965; Collin et al., 1988) or Katz's index of activities of daily living (ADL) (Katz et al., 1963). These scales are less sensitive to small changes in function, which can make an enormous difference to the individual patient, such as the transition from needing the help of two people to needing the help of only one person. Their usefulness extends, however, to levels of function higher than those which will produce a "ceiling" effect on our recording system.

The Barthel score can be readily adopted into routine clinical practice even on a busy acute admitting ward for elderly people (Stone et al., 1992). Data recording is the responsibility of the nurse in charge of the ward. Each week the information is gathered from her staff and then discussed on the multidisciplinary ward round. While the total score for each patient, e.g., on discharge, provides a convenient shorthand for describing the overall level of disability, the greatest value of this approach has been the structure which it provides for informed discussion and improved recording of important clinical information. A report from the Royal College of Physicians of London and the British Geriatrics Society (1992) has recommended that the Barthel scale should be adopted as a standardized record of the functional performance of elderly people. Whether or not the recommendation is honored in practice will probably depend more on its value for the structured collection of the component information than on its ability to allocate an overall score to a patient.

Clinical Trials

The overall score on a standardized scale, however, is important for clinical research. A well-known example is the Northwick Park trial of hospital-based rehabilitation for stroke patients living at home (Smith et al., 1981). An ADL index was developed and validated specifically for this study (Sheikh et al., 1979).

In the Northwick Park study, patients attending a rehabilitation department for four full days each week were compared with patients attending three half-days each week and with patients visited regularly at home by a health visitor. Treatment was for six months. Mean entry scores were comparable for the three groups, but statistically significant group differences had emerged by three months and were sustained at one year (Table 1). The mean improvements in the score were small and concealed quite large differences in the number of patients deteriorating in each group (Table 1). One of the difficulties which must be addressed when using a functional performance rating scale is that the intervals in the scale need not be of equal size; a two-point change in one part of the scale may well not be equivalent to a two-point change elsewhere in the scale. Thus, it is statistically more secure to use the scores to identify those who have improved or deteriorated rather than trying to compare the extent of such changes.

Another approach to this difficulty may be to recognize that the amount of attainable functional recovery available to a patient will depend on his/her pre-event level of functional performance. Therefore, future trials of rehabilitation should stratify patients before randomization according to a historical assessment of their functional performance before the acute illness.

Pre-event functional performance may also have considerable potential as a stratification device for clinical trials where functional performance is not itself an outcome measure. This possibility is well illustrated by a retrospective study of predictors of the mortality of older patients within six months of treatment in a medical intensive care unit (Mayer-Oakes et al., 1991). In the absence of pre-acute functional limitation, patients aged 75 and over were no more likely to die than those aged 50 to 64. Among those who already had a

TABLE 1

The Effects of Different Intensities of Out-Patient Rehabilitation on Functional Performance After a Stroke (Smith et al., 1981)

	4 days/week	3 x 1/2-days/week	none
Mean score on entry	22	22	21
Mean change after 3 months	-3.5	-2.9	-1.5
Mean change after 1 year	-3.5	-2.9	-0.6
Number deteriorated after 3 months	1 of 41	4 of 40	10 of 42
Number deteriorated after 1 year	2 of 36	4 of 36	8 of 35

Functional performance in activities of daily living was scored on a scale from 17 (not disabled) to 51 (severely disabled).

degree of functional limitation, however, not only was mortality higher, there was also a significant age effect. This implies that, when testing the effect of a new treatment on the mortality of older patients receiving intensive care, stratification according to the pre-illness level of functional performance is at least as important as stratification by age.

Case-Mix

Just as the details of functional performance are necessary for a full description of the individual elderly patient, they are also necessary when describing a group of patients. For example, in the Geriatric Medicine service at the Royal Free Hospital, very few of our patients are so severely disabled and/or medically unstable that they require permanent hospital care. A summary of their principal diagnoses (Table 2) gives only a very vague impression of the nature of their needs. A much more informative picture emerges from a summary of their functional abilities (Table 3). This goes some way towards identifying the workload involved in providing care for such patients, although some caution is still necessary (see "Pitfalls," below).

Older patients have a much longer mean length of hospital stay than younger patients. There is a three to fourfold increase in the mean length of stay between ages 60 and 85 (Office of Population Censuses and Surveys, 1986). While reduction of the length of stay to the shortest which is compatible with the needs of the individual patient is a legitimate aim, mounting financial pressures tend to encourage the pursuit of a short mean length of stay as an end in itself. If a reduction in the mean length of stay could result only from

TABLE 2

Commonest Diagnoses Among Patients Receiving Permanent Hospital Care (N = 42, mean age = 89, 25 percent men, Royal Free Hospital, March 1990)

DEMENTIA	86 percent
STROKE	48 percent
ARTHRITIS	35 percent
SKIN PROBLEMS	28 percent
HEART FAILURE	20 percent

TABLE 3

Selected Functional Performance Indicators of Patients Receiving Permanent Hospital Care (Royal Free Hospital, March 1990)

	I **%**	**S/P** **%**	**+1** **%**	**+2** **%**	**+3** **%**	**Not at all** **%**
Walking	-	-	10	17	3	52
Transfers *	-	3	27	63	8	-
Dressing	-	-	85	15		-
Feeding **	55	20	25	-	-	-

I Independent
S/P With supervision or verbal prompting
+1 With physical help of one person
+2 With physical help of two people
+3 With physical help of three people

* Mean of sit-to-stand, toilet, and bed transfers.
** "Feeding" does not include cutting or spreading.

improved treatment or from improved efficiency in the organization of investigations and discharge arrangements, this would be entirely legitimate. Unfortunately, a reduction in the mean length of stay can also result from an increased early death rate or from the premature discharge of patients without adequate rehabilitation. These anomalies are well recognized; when comparing two departments (or one department over time), one would routinely assess whether any differences in mean length of stay might be explained on such a basis. But there is another, more subtle, way that the mean length of stay may be reduced; there may be a change in the nature of the patients entering the department. Mean lengths of stay and other group outcome measures cannot be justifiably compared unless the input case-mixes are demonstrably equivalent. This is very difficult, but pre-illness functional assessment (by history) and post-acute functional assessment (by observation at, say, seven to ten days post-admission) offer a promising approach.

IN THE COMMUNITY

Case-Finding

Various "instruments" have been used for case-finding and screening among elderly people. In one study (Carpenter and Demopoulos, 1990), 539 people aged 75 and over were randomly allocated to a control or a study group. Those in the study group were each visited by a lay volunteer every three or six months (six for those with less severe disability) for three years. At each visit their functional performance was assessed, by interview, according to a disability rating scale. An increase in an individual's disability rating by ≥5 points between successive visits was the trigger for referral to their primary care physician. The most striking difference in outcome between the two groups was that members of the study group spent a much lower total number of days in residential care (Figure 2). In terms of individual people, this corresponds to 14 members of the control group having admissions to residential care lasting at least six months, compared to only four members of the study group. It seems that functional performance assessment, even just by lay volunteers, may have led to a substantial reduction in institutionalization. On the other hand, there is only circumstantial evidence that the use of the scale (or, indeed, the referral to the doctor) caused the outcome. It may just be that frail, elderly people who are visited every three months by an interested volunteer are less likely to choose to enter residential care. Despite these uncertainties, this study highlights an area well worth further study; what benefits may there be when functional performance is assessed by people other than health professionals?

An Elder-Friendly Environment

Environmental discrimination against elderly people is not uncommon. In Sweden, Lundgren-Lindquist and her colleagues (1983) demonstrated that barely a third of healthy 79-year-old women were able to match the walking speed ($1.4 m \cdot s^{-1}$) considered by planners to be the norm for users of pedestrian crossings. In the United Kingdom, the principal users of long-distance coaches are young adults and elderly adults. The former are now bigger, on average, than they used to be, and the latter are now more numerous than they used to be. There is a persuasive argument, therefore, for updating the national standards upon which the knee room provided between coach seats is based. The greater size of young adults and the lesser agility of older adults both require an additional three inches knee room (Jeffs, 1991). The platform of many London Transport buses is ≥40cm above

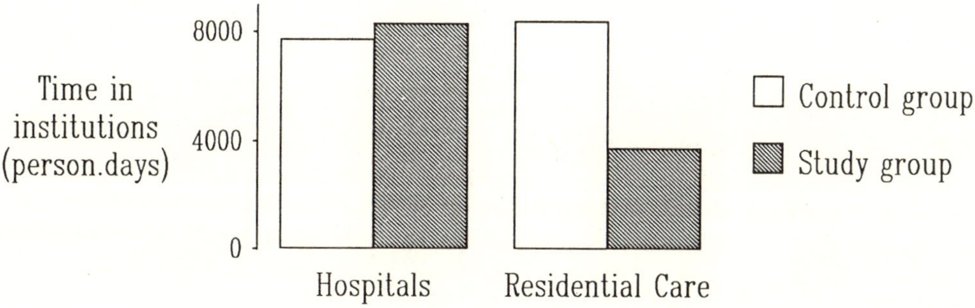

Figure 2. Total person-days of non-hospital, institutional care was lower for elderly people whose functional ability was monitored by lay volunteers than for a control group (Carpenter and Demopoulos, 1990)

the road. Even in perfect health, only 80 percent of women aged 80 to 84 can negotiate a 40cm step without using a handrail (Skelton et al., 1992a).

There is an urgent need for both epidemiological and laboratory-based information upon which to base new national design standards, to produce an environment more appropriate to the ergonomic limitations of elderly people.

Active Life Expectancy

It is not merely the length of life that is important. Nor is it merely the quality of life. It is some combination of the two. "Active Life Expectancy" (Katz et al., 1983) is an objective approach to such a combination. It appears to offer a means of differentiating between interventions which postpone the onset of physical dependence, and those which prolong life by prolonging the period of terminal dependence. From a two-year follow-up of 89 percent of 1625 non-institutionalized people aged 65 and over, Katz and his colleagues developed age-specific predictions of the average number of further years individuals could expect before they would either die, enter an institution, or become unable to satisfy one of four functional performance criteria, concerning bathing, dressing, bed to chair transfers, and eating. There has been surprisingly little evidence of enthusiasm for this approach but the time is surely right for the development of more refined versions of this approach, taking alternative cut-off points for the functional performance criteria by which to define the end of "active" life (Suzman et al., 1992).

In Katz' study elderly men and elderly women of the same age had similar active life expectancies. Their substantial differences in total life expectancy were due to the much greater length of terminal dependence experienced by women (Figure 3). This is a phenomenon that has not been adequately addressed. It is also seen in the greater prevalence of disability amongst elderly women and in the age-related decline in the percentage of elderly women using public transport on their own (Figure 4) (Green et al., 1989). It is tempting to suppose that the greater vulnerability of elderly women to physical dependence is related to their lower power/weight ratios and a correspondingly smaller safety margin for the retention of functional independence (Skelton et al., 1992a,b). (See discussion in "Limiting Mechanisms?" below).

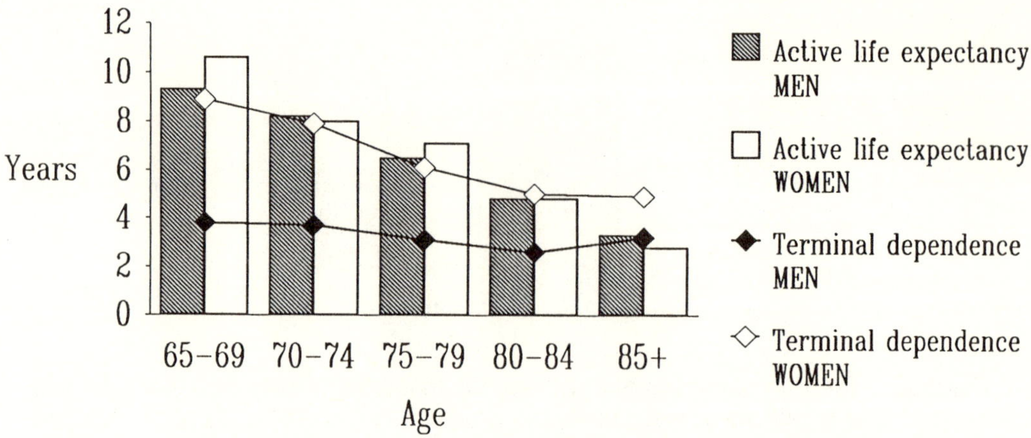

Figure 3. The life expectancy of elderly people, divided into "active life expectancy" and subsequent "dependent life expectancy" (Katz et al., 1983)

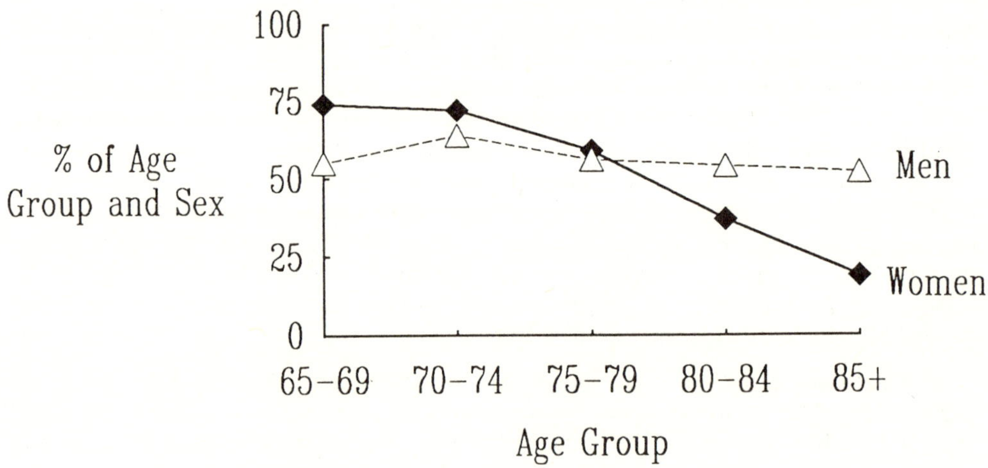

Figure 4. Independent use of public transport by elderly men and women (Green et al., 1989)

PITFALLS

There is enormous potential for the misuse of scales that measure functional performance. Their simplicity is deceptive. They are not interchangeable and they vary in their appropriateness for different purposes, different degrees of severity of disability, different populations and different cultures. Only a few have been adequately validated, and in only a few of the situations where they might be used. They measure discontinuous variables and are constructed with unequal intervals; parametric statistical techniques are not appropriate for such data. All are subject to "ceiling" and "floor" effects; failure of a scale to detect improvement or deterioration need not mean that there has been no change.

Dependence rating scales are sometimes used to calculate the number of nurses required to staff a ward. In an acute ward, dependence may be a valid proxy for workload. In a rehabilitation setting, on the other hand, this assumption is not always valid. The patient who is completely incontinent of urine and has this managed by the application of pads is more dependent than the patient receiving continence training and being assisted to walk to and from the toilet every hour. The latter patient, however, requires many more minutes of nurse time. Similar arguments can be applied to feeding, dressing and even general mobility. It is important to guard against uncritical assumptions of equivalence between workload and dependence, especially in a rehabilitation setting.

LIMITING MECHANISMS

The studies in our Human Performance Laboratory attempt to understand the mechanisms limiting the functional performance of healthy, elderly people. As yet, we have not been able to define specific "threshold values" of strength, power, or oxygen uptake at which the healthy person's ability to perform specific important functions is threatened. Our work, however, has provided substantial information about the functional abilities of very healthy elderly people, which could be used as standards against which to judge the performance of more typical elderly people. The concept of normative data, based on a random sample of the population, is appropriate when studying younger age groups. The high prevalence of chronic disease in the elderly population, however, means that what is "usual" may not be "normal." In old age, it may be preferable to use "ideal" standards based on highly selected people who meet predetermined health criteria.

We are also attempting to establish whether safety margins can be increased or thresholds recorded by physical training; that is, do improvements in strength, power and oxygen transport necessarily result in corresponding improvements in functional performance? We hope to be able to report the results of current training studies to the Fourth International Conference on Physical Activity, Aging and Sport.

Contrary to our expectations (Young, 1986), we have identified only a few very elderly people who are healthy but have major functional limitations in everyday life. We speculate that a decline in muscle function which crosses a functionally important threshold may be incompatible with continuing health; that is, perhaps a functionally important reduction in strength, power, or maximal oxygen uptake may greatly increase susceptibility to injury or disease. This might also explain the surprise finding of an eight-year follow-up study of the quadriceps strength of healthy people aged 82 at follow-up (Greg et al., 1993). Those who were still healthy at follow-up showed no significant loss of quadriceps strength, despite the fact that cross-sectional studies suggest that they should have lost at least 12 percent of their strength over that period. Perhaps a slow loss of muscle is yet another physiological function which fits Rowe and Kahn's model for successful aging (Rowe and Kahn, 1987). To remain healthy in advanced old age, perhaps one must either have an intrinsically slow loss of muscle function or follow such an active lifestyle that, despite the loss of muscle with increasing age, the crossing of important thresholds is substantially postponed.

ACKNOWLEDGEMENTS

Supported by grants from The Violet M. Richards Charity Trust (London) and from Research into Ageing (London).

We thank The Violet M. Richards Charity Trust and Research into Ageing for their support. Professor Young gratefully acknowledges the intellectual stimulus afforded by collaboration in the Morris W. Stroud III Program ("Scientific approaches to quality of life in health and ageing").

REFERENCES

Applegate WB, Blass JP, Williams TF. Instruments for the functional assessment of older patients. N Engl J Med 1990;322:1207-14.

Carpenter GI, Demopoulos GR. Screening the elderly in the community: controlled trial of dependency surveillance using a questionnaire administered by volunteers. Br Med J 1990;300:1253-6.

Collin C, Wade DT, Davies S, Horne V. The Barthel ADL index: a reliability study. Int Disabil Studies 1988; 10:61-3.

Dickinson EJ, Young A. Framework for medical assessment of functional performance. Lancet 1990;355:778-9.

Green H, Milne A, Rauta I, Eldridge J, Wilmot A, Levy G. General Household Survey 1986. London: Her Majesty's Stationery Office, 1989.

Greig C, Young A. Aerobic exercise. In: Evans JG, Williams TF, eds. Oxford Textbook of Geriatric Medicine. Oxford: Oxford University Press, 1992:601-4.

Greig CA, Botella J, Young A. The quadriceps strength of healthy elderly people remeasured after eight years. Muscle Nerve, 1993;16:6-10.

Jeffs S. Ergonomic requirements of passengers in coach transport. University of London: M.Sc. Thesis, 1991.

Kane RA, Kane RL. Assessing the Elderly: a Practical Guide to Measurement. Lexington, Mass.: Lexington Books, 1981.

Katz S, Ford AB, Moskowitz RW, Jackson BA, Jaffe MW. Studies of illness in the aged. The index of ADL: a standardized measure of biological and psychosocial function. J Am Med Assoc 1963;185:914-9.

Katz S, Branch LG, Branson MH, Papsidero JA, Beck JC, Greer DS. Active life expectancy. N Engl J Med 1983;309:1218-24.

Lundgren-Linquist B, Aniansson A, Rundgren Å. Functional studies in 79-year-olds. III. Walking performance and climbing capacity. Scand J Rehabil Med 1983;15:125-31.

Mahoney FI, Barthel DW. Functional evaluation: the Barthel index. Maryland State Medical Journal 1965;14: 61-5.

Mayer-Oakes SA, Oye RK, Leake B. Predictors of mortality in older patients following medical intensive care: the importance of functional status. J Am Geriatr Soc 1991;39:862-8.

Office of Population Censuses and Surveys. Hospital In-Patient Enquiry 1984; Summary Tables. London: Her Majesty's Stationery Office, 1986.

Rowe JW, Kahn RL. Human ageing: usual and successful. Science 1987;237:143-9.

Royal College of Physicians of London, British Geriatrics Society. Standardised Assessment Scales for Elderly People. London: Royal College of Physicians of London and British Geriatrics Society, 1992.

Sheikh K, Smith DM, Meade TW, Goldenberg E, Brennan PJ, Kinsella G. Repeatability and validity of a modified Activities of Daily Living (ADL) index in studies of chronic disability. Int Rehabil Med 1979;1:51-8.

Sherrington C. Man on His Nature, 2nd edition. Cambridge: Cambridge University Press, 1963;102.

Skelton DA, Greig CA, Davies JM, Young A. Muscle function in healthy women aged 65 to 84. Med Sci Sports Exerc 1992a;24:S75 (abstr).

Skelton DA, Greig CA, Davies JM, Young A. Muscle function in healthy men aged 65 to 84. Age Ageing 1992b;21(Suppl.2):P8 (abstr).

Smith DS, Goldenberg E, Ashburn A et al. Remedial therapy after stroke: a randomised controlled trial. Br Med J 1981;282:517-20.

Stone SP, Herbert P, Chrisostomou J, Vessey C, Horwood C. The assessment of disability in patients on an acute medical ward for elderly people. Disabil Rehabil 1992:15:35-7.

Suzman R, Kinsella KG, Meyers GC. Demography of older populations in developed countries. In: Evans JG, Williams TF, eds. Oxford Textbook of Geriatric Medicine. Oxford: Oxford University Press, 1992:3-14.

Wade DT. Measurement in Neurological Rehabilitation. Oxford: Oxford University Press, 1992.

Young A. Exercise physiology in geriatric practice. Acta Med Scand 1986; Suppl 711:227-32.

Young A. Strength and power. In: Evans JG, Williams TF, eds. Oxford Textbook of Geriatric Medicine, Oxford: Oxford University Press, 1992:597-601.

Feasibility of Assessing Physical Functional Capacity in Elderly Subjects

Pertti Era, Ph.D.

INTRODUCTION

The lack of standardized ways of assessing physical functional capacity in the elderly is demonstrated by the considerable variation in the methods and tests used in different studies. This is true for muscle strength: due to the heterogeneity of methods and protocols for testing muscular functions in different laboratories, cross comparison studies may be impossible (Viljanen et al., 1991). The use of often submaximal measures in unstandardized ways makes it difficult to compare the findings of different studies. Medical risks and contraindications may also limit the use of certain measures, not to mention problems in motivating the subjects to maximal effort within the tests applied (Era et al., in press).

This report is based on a study in which the physical functional capacity of 75- and 80-year-old men and women was studied using maximal tests of power (bicycle ergometer test), isometric muscular strength in five muscle groups (hand grip, arm flexion, knee extension, body extension, and body flexion), walking speed (10-meter track) and a stair-mounting test. The study of the 75-year-olds forms the Finnish contribution to an ongoing comparison of 75-year-old people in three Nordic localities, namely Glostrup in Denmark, Gothenburg in Sweden and Jyväskylä in Finland (Schroll et al., 1993). In Jyväskylä an additional group of 80-year-olds was also studied. In this report the feasibility of the methods to assess physical functional capacity among the Finnish subjects is analyzed.

SUBJECTS AND METHODS

The subjects consisted of all persons of relevant age resident in the city of Jyväskylä at the time of data collection (October 1989 - March 1990). The study protocol included an interview carried out in the respondents' homes and laboratory examinations made after the interview. These examinations focused on body structure, physical functions mentioned above, sensory and psychomotor functions, cognition and memory. The participation rate in the laboratory examinations in the younger age group was 82.4 percent among the men and 75.3 percent among the women; in the older group the corresponding figure for the men was 78.9 and for the women 70.0 percent (Table 1).

TABLE 1

Participation Rates in Different Stages of the Study Among 75-and 80-Year-Old Men and Women

	Age group			
	75-year-olds		80-year-olds	
	Men	Women	Men	Women
Number of eligible subjects	125	255	76	207
Home interview	119 95.2%	231 90.6%	70 92.1%	185 89.4%
Medical examination	105 84.0%	202 79.2%	63 82.9%	150 72.5%
Entered the laboratory	103 82.4%	192 75.3%	60 78.9%	145 70.0%

The most usual reasons for non-participation in laboratory tests were poor self-evaluated functional capacity and unwillingness to participate. In some cases the non-participants also indicated that they were so healthy that they did not need any medical examinations.

A thirty-minute medical examination, including blood pressure measurement and electrocardiographic recording at rest, preceded the tests of functional capacity. In some cases a physician did the medical examination in the respondent's home if he/she was not able to enter the laboratory. During this examination the physician evaluated the possibilities for performing the tests in each subject individually. The evaluation was based on the recommendations of the American College of Sports Medicine (1986).

Maximal power was assessed using an indirect continuous stepwise bicycle ergometer test. The first load was set at 25w in all subjects, and it was increased after every two minutes' step by 15 or 30w depending on the performance of each subject. The aim was to reach the subjective maximal power in eight to 12 minutes. The test was continued until exhaustion unless it was terminated earlier due to medical problems or the subject's unwillingness to continue. A mechanically loaded bicycle ergometer (Monark 90814E) was used. The pedaling frequency (60 rpm) was presented to the test subject both as a tone and a flashing light, and the actual work carried out during each minute of the test was afterwards calculated on the basis of load and number of revolutions.

Electrocardiographic responses were followed throughout the test (lead V5), and blood pressure was measured during the last seconds of every minute of the test. The bicycle test was conducted by a group including a physician, a laboratory nurse, and an exercise physiologist.

Maximal isometric strengths of hand grip, elbow flexion, and knee extension were measured on the side of the dominant hand in a sitting position using an adjustable dynamometer chair constructed at the Department of Health Sciences, University of Jyväskylä (Heikkinen et al., 1984, Sipilä et al., 1991). Hand grip strength was measured by a dynamometer fixed to the arm of the chair and adjustable according to the size of the hand. Elbow flexion strength was measured at an angle of 90 degrees in a neutral position (thumb up) with the elbow supported comfortably and the wrist attached by belts to a strain-gauge system. Knee extension strength was measured at a knee angle of 60 degrees from full extension towards flexion. The ankle was fastened by a belt to a strain-gauge transducer. Maximal isometric trunk flexion and extension were measured in a standing position according to Viitasalo et al. (1977).

For each strength test the testee was allowed two or three practice trials, after which three formal trials were performed with a one-minute interval between each. The best result of the three was accepted as the result.

Maximal walking speed over 10 meters was measured in the laboratory corridor using a regular stop-watch. A three-to-four-meter distance preceded the start line of the 10 m track so that the subject could accelerate his/her speed before the actual track began.

A stair-mounting test was used to study the climbing ability of the subjects. This test was developed in the Department of Geriatric Medicine, University of Gothenburg, Sweden (Aniansson et al., 1980). The test was carried out using five 10-cm-high boxes, which could be combined to form steps with heights of 10, 20, 30, 40, and 50 cm. The subject was asked to step up and down each step once. The highest step reached, without and with support if needed from the hand-rail, was recorded as the result.

RESULTS

On the basis of the medical examination preceding the functional tests, contraindications for the bicycle test were found in 20 to 30 percent of cases in the younger group, and the test was possible immediately in about 70 percent of men and in 64 percent of women. In the older group contraindications for the bicycle test were found in nearly 50 percent of both men and women (Table 2). For about five percent of the cases, after evaluation, it was ascertained that the test could be carried out later.

TABLE 2

Feasibility of the Bicycle Test in 75- and 80-Year-Old Men and Women. Physician's Rating if It Was Possible to Perform the Test Immediately, Later, or Not at All

Feasibility of the bicycle test	Age group			
	75-year-olds		80-year-olds	
	Men n=105	Women n=202	Men n=63	Women n=150
Yes, immediatelly	73 69.5%	129 63.8%	28 45.2%	68 45.6%
Yes, later	9 8.6%	11 5.5%	4 6.5%	8 5.1%
No	23 21.9%	62 30.7%	31 48.3%	74 49.3%

The most usual reasons for excluding a subject from these tests were musculoskeletal problems, cardiovascular symptoms and diseases, and poor cooperation.

The participation in different phases of the bicycle test in the younger age group is presented as a kind of survival curve in Figure 1. The starting point of the curve, 100 percent level, indicates the birth cohort in the year 1914, when the people aged 75 in 1989 were born. Half of the women and 75 percent of men in this cohort had died before reaching this age. The participation figures shown here are calculated in relation to the size of the birth cohort. These lines show that a greater proportion of women than of men born 75 years earlier could be examined and tested, and the difference between the sexes levels off only at the highest levels of exercise, where the number of subjects is very low for both sexes.

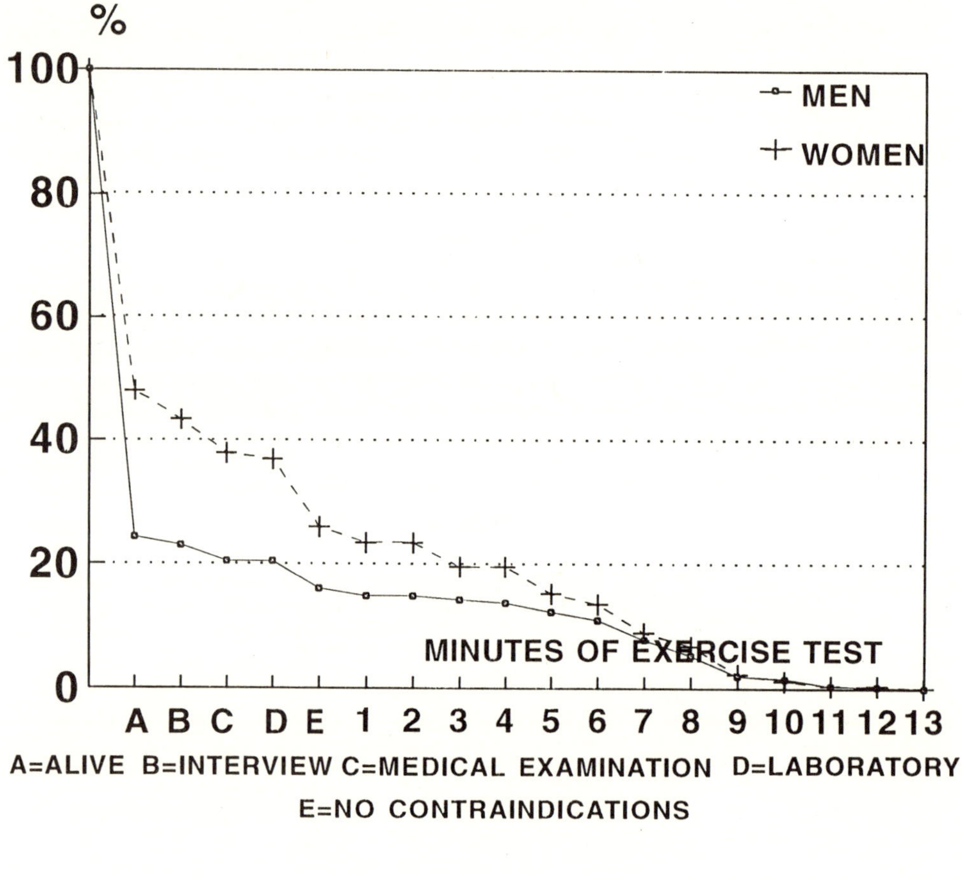

Figure 1. Participation in the bicycle ergometer test and different phases preceding the test among 75-year-old men and women. The figures have been calculated in relation to the survival of the birth cohort born 75 years earlier.

If the differences in mortality between men and women, however, are not taken into account, a different picture is seen. In Figure 2 the corresponding lines are calculated in relation to the survivors for both sexes. It appears that a higher proportion of men than of women could be examined and tested, and the men also tolerated the exercise test better.

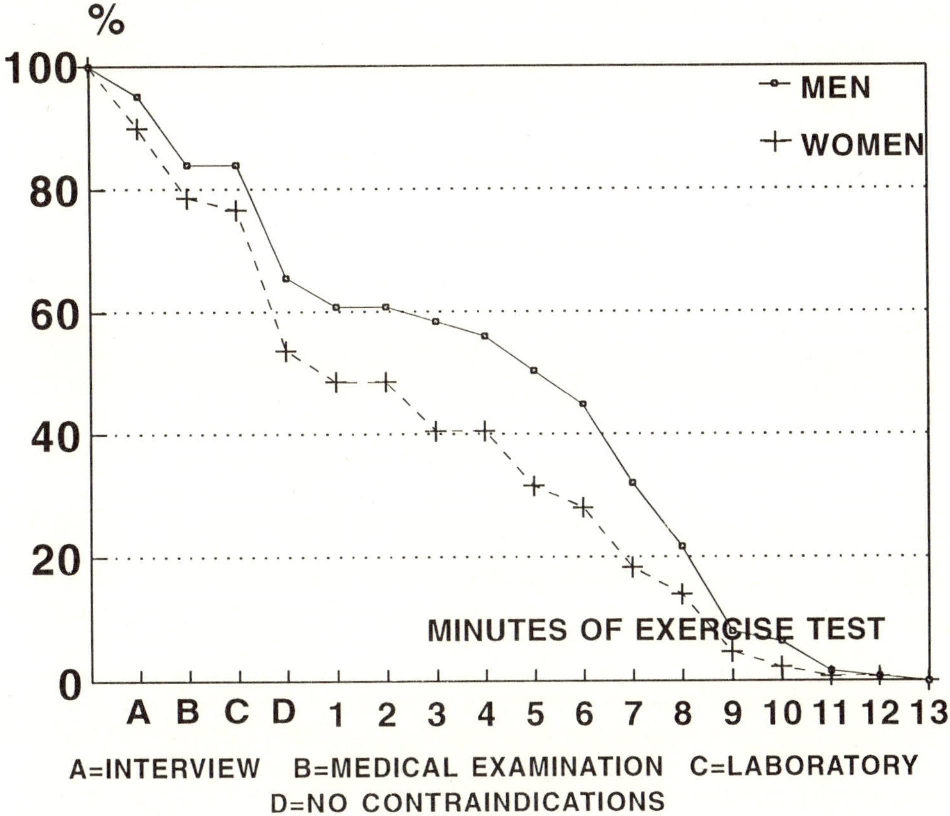

Figure 2. Participation in the bicycle ergometer test and different phases preceding the test among 75-year-old men and women. The figures have been calculated in relation to the number of the 75-year-old men and women living in the study area during the data collection.

The survival curves for the 80-year-olds had a similar pattern. When the differences in mortality between men and women are taken into account, women born 80 years earlier seemed to survive better than men, and a higher proportion of them could be tested 80 years later. When only the remaining subjects are looked at, however, men seemed to manage better than women in the exercise test.

Of those in the younger group who started the test, the bicycle test was interrupted before exhaustion in 57 percent of the men and 41 percent of the women. In the older group these figures were 69 percent for men and 40 percent for women. The most common reasons for interruption were electrocardiographic changes, systolic blood pressure elevation above 250 mm Hg or decline in blood pressure.

For the muscular strength tests contraindications were less common than for the bicycle test, showing about five percent in the younger group and 15 to 20 percent in the older group (Table 3).

TABLE 3

Feasibility of the Isometric Strength Tests in
75- and 80-Year Old Men and Women.
Physician's Rating if It Was Possible to Perform the Tests
Immediately, Later, or Not at All.

Feasibility of the isometric strength tests	Age group			
	75-year-olds		80-year-olds	
	Men n=105	Women n=202	Men n=63	Women n=150
Yes, immediatelly	99 94.2%	188 93.0%	52 82.0%	126 83.9%
Yes, later	1 1.0%	1 0.5%	0 0.0%	1 0.7%
No	5 4.8%	13 6.5%	11 18.0%	23 15.4%

The step test proved possible for nearly all the subjects in the younger group, whereas in the older group four to eight percent found it impossible to complete. Similarly, the maximal walking speed test was performed for nearly all subjects in the younger group, whereas for 13 percent of the men and nine percent of the women in the older group the test could not be carried out.

DISCUSSION

These results demonstrated that tests of isometric muscular strength, maximal walking speed and the step test were performable for the vast majority (80 to 100 percent) of the 75- and 80-year-old subjects who entered the laboratory. Maximal power measured by the help of the bicycle test was assessable for about 30 percent of the subjects in the younger group and 20 to 25 percent in the older group. There were no medical contraindications to start the bicycle test in the majority of the subjects (70 percent of men and 64 percent of women in the younger age group, and about 50 percent of both men and women in the older group), but the test was interrupted before exhaustion in many cases.

When evaluating the results, it must be emphasized that selective drop-out may have occurred in many phases. The role of mortality was clearly demonstrated here when the "survival curves" of the bicycle test were analyzed. Among the men in the 75-year-old group, only a quarter of those born 75 years earlier still existed; among the women, one-half. Although the participation rate in the study was rather high, the drop-out in this phase was to some extent selective as well; mobility was lower among those who participated only in the home interview but did not enter the laboratory (Rantanen et al., in press).

The more efficient selection due to mortality among men was seen in the "survival curves" of the bicycle test. If difference in mortality between men and women was not taken into account, the usual observation indicating more active participation and better physical functioning among men was repeated here also. When, however, the mortality difference was taken into consideration, it appeared that actually women born 75 or 80 years earlier had a greater possibility of participating in a study like this at old age and they were also probably better able physically to tolerate loading tests than men. Naturally this mortality difference between the sexes exists through the whole life span. Thus it is not possible to state that men would tolerate aging itself less than women, but instead that there is a greater possibility that they will die at an earlier age from life-shortening diseases and accidents.

In about 60 percent of men and 40 percent of women, the bicycle test was interrupted either due to medical problems or to the respondent's unwillingness to continue. The symptoms leading to interruption were most often in locomotive organs. Thus, the result obtained rarely reflected cardiorespiratory capacity of the subject and the result was not expressed in terms of aerobic capacity, absolute or relative, but as voluntary maximal power in riding a bicycle as such. This measure may give valuable information concerning the subject's potential to carry out physically demanding tasks. By careful medical control before and during the test, it has been possible to avoid serious complications among the total of one to two thousand subjects aged 70 and over tested in our laboratory.

The isometric muscular strength tests together with simple measures resembling daily tasks (maximal walking speed, stair-mounting test) were feasible within the groups studied. The necessary equipment to make these tests is quite simple and, as a consequence, also rather inexpensive compared with apparatus to assess muscle strength in well controlled dynamic conditions. However, the standardization of the test conditions, instructions and motivation of the test subjects may also be a problem in these rather simple tests, and the testers must be well qualified (Era et al., in press). The results obtained using these methods have also been shown to correlate with the abilities of elderly subjects to carry out everyday tasks demanding mobility, thus suggesting ecological validity (Rantanen et al., in press). Although the bicycle test could not be carried out in many subjects and, in a great number of those who started the test, it was interrupted before exhaustion, its use is still recommended as a useful tool to evaluate the ability of an elderly person to tolerate long-lasting physical loading. The result rarely reflects the aerobic capacity of the subject in a way that could reasonably be described in terms of maximal oxygen consumption but rather describes voluntary maximal power in riding a bicycle in test conditions lasting several minutes.

REFERENCES

American College of Sports Medicine. Guidelines for Exercise Testing and Prescription, 3rd edition. Philadelphia: Lea & Febiger, 1986.

Aniansson A, Rundgren Å, Sperling L. Evaluation of functional capacity in activities of daily living in 70-year-old men and women. Scand J Rehab Med 1980;12:145-54.

Era P, Rantanen T, Avlund K et al. Maximal isometric muscle strength and anthropometry in 75-year-old men and women in three Nordic localities. Scand J Med Sci Sports, in press.

Heikkinen E, Arajärvi RL, Era P et al. Functional capacity of men born in 1906-1910, 1926-30 and 1946-50. Scand J Soc Med 1984;suppl.33:1-93.

Rantanen T, Era P, Heikkinen E. Maximal isometric strength and mobility among 75-year-old men and women. Age and Ageing, in press.

Schroll M, Steen B, Berg S et al. NORA-Nordic Research on Ageing. Functional capacity of 75-year-old men and women in three Nordic localities. Den Med Bull, 1993;40:618-24.

Sipilä S, Viitasalo JT, Era P, Suominen H. Muscle strength in male athletes aged 70-81 years and a population sample. Eur J Appl Physiol 1991;63:399-403.

Viitasalo JT, Komi PV, Karvonen MJ. Physical health and performance capacity, and physical activity habits in conscripts in the beginning of service at Air Communications School. Research Reports from the Department of Biology of Physical Activity, University of Jyväskylä, 19/1977.

Viljanen T, Viitasalo JT, Kujala U. Strength characteristics of a healthy urban adult population. Eur J Appl Physiol 1991;63:43-7.

Past Participation in Sport and Old Age Performance

Achim Conzelmann

INTRODUCTION

One frequently encounters reports about outstanding performances of aged athletes, which are still superior to average performances of people at their best age. When explaining such performances, it is often suspected that, in addition to certain genetic prerequisites and systematic training, participation in sport throughout one's entire life represents a significant influencing factor. However, comprehensive empirical investigations on this topic with representative samples of older competitive athletes have not yet been undertaken. Within the framework of a study of 620 of the most successful Master athletes in the Federal Republic of Germany, the importance of past participation in sport for achieving great performances in old age was assessed. The results reveal that different patterns of past participation in sport exist for successful Master athletes. In particular, considerable differences occur when differentiating the sample according to the discipline group in track and field. While the best performances are often achieved by late beginners in middle- and long-distance running, former top-level throwers are most successful in the throwing disciplines. These results are due to social rather than biologic reasons.

The average course of physical performance capacity during adulthood is characterized by a plateau at some point in early adulthood followed by a continuous decrease in performance (Israel et al., 1982; Israel and Weidner, 1988; Willimczik 1981; Winter 1987). In contrast to this, one frequently encounters reports about outstanding performances of athletes in their seventies or even eighties, especially in track and field, which are still superior to average performances of people at their best age (Table 1).

It is now generally assumed that, apart from certain genetic predispositions and systematic training, physical activity throughout the entire life and especially a training specific to a type of sport during early adulthood are necessary prerequisites for achieving outstanding performances in old age (Diem, 1954). Even for the performance factor "aerobic endurance," which is frequently characterized as being relatively stable over time, Liesen and Hollmann (1981) assume that commencing training in early adulthood is a necessary prerequisite for reaching "maximal" aerobic capacity in old age. However, a comprehensive investigation testing this hypothesis with a representative sample of competitive Masters athletes has not yet been undertaken.

In an extensive study of 620 of the most successful Masters athletes in the Federal Republic of Germany, data were collected on past participation in sport performance

TABLE 1

Unofficial World Records in Masters Track and Field (7/91)*

Age	100 m (in sec)		5000 m (in min)		Long Jump (in m)		Javelin (in m)			
	Men	Women	Men	Women	Men	Women	Men		Women	
35-39	10,28	11,49	13.16,38	15.15,2	8,50	6,50	82,62	800	67,00	600
40-44	10,52	12,03	13.45,6	16.02,88	7,57	6,21	75,28	800	51,84	600
45-49	11,05	12,63	14.23,6	16.17,5	7,27	5,49	66,26	800	47,74	600
50-54	11,40	13,29	14.55,60	17.46,2	6,66	5,25	64,00	800	44,90	400
55-59	11,65	13,93	15.42,35	18.49,0	6,10	4,70	57,70	800	40,48	400
60-64	11,8	14,40	16.33,3	20.04,0	6,07	4,44	58,48	600	32,34	400
65-69	12,56	14,90	17.13,8	21.58,26	5,46	4,47	51,26	600	26,54	400
70-74	13,00	16,41	18.43,61	23.58,0	5,03	3,41	48,08	600	24,96	400
75-79	14,06	16,87	20.50,73	25.43,39	4,78	3,22	40,88	600	23,02	400
80-84	15,59	18,10	21.57,88	30.21,85	4,04	2,40	29,70	600	19,12	400
85-89	16,98	33,1	26.50,2	41.56,2	2,77		22,94	600	4,40	400
90-94	20,67		37.39,38		2,39		17,43	600		
95-99	20,82		50.23,53		2,15		21,16	600		

* This list was produced on the basis of a table published by Olavi Niemi for the IX World Veterans' Championships in 1991 in Turku, Finland and of the official results of this event.

development, training programs, etc. Within the framework of this paper, some of the most important results regarding the significance of past participation in sport are presented.

METHODS

The design of this empirical investigation is a combined cross-sectional and (retrospective) longitudinal study of top-level German Master track and field athletes. The study was conducted by mail.

Research Design

Due to the inadequacy of cross-sectional designs for examining individual developments and due to practical and methodic problems of longitudinal studies, especially for the long period of adulthood (Petermann, 1987; Trautner, 1978; Wohlwill, 1977), alternative research strategies are required. A combined cross-sectional and longitudinal (retrospective) design was selected to examine the sample of competitive Master athletes in this study.

Data collection

Data collection was undertaken with the help of a questionnaire which contained the following subject areas: qualitative and quantitative training variables, planning of training and competition, conditions of training and competition, general habits, personal data, development of athletic performance in track and field, volume of training and methods of training, history of involvement in athletics, medical history, and other so-called "critical life events."

The method of a written questionnaire mailed out to the subjects appeared to be most adequate, since the athletes usually required old personal notes for answering the questions and since considerable organizational problems could be avoided (the Master athletes live all across Germany). Considering the length and complexity of the questionnaire, the return rate of 76 percent was surprisingly high, a tribute to the choice of method for data collection.

POPULATION/SAMPLE/CREATION OF SUBSAMPLES

Population

The population selected for this study has the following characteristics:

- Gender: male

- Age: born 1943 and before (Age Groups M45-M75, as of 1988)

- Sport Activities: successful participation in track and field competitions (place 1 - 10) in the unofficial Master rankings of the German Track and Field Federation in a "common" track and field discipline in the years of 1986-1988 (Reckemeier 1987-1989) (Table 2).

Sample

To ensure a sufficient number of subjects in the subsamples, the aim was measuring the population. From the total of 964 Master athletes who fulfilled the required criteria, 620 (64 percent of the subjects) were included in the sample. The sample contains at least half of the athletes in each age group and discipline: 90 percent of the best athletes in their age group in the disciplines (1988), 74 percent of German Masters record holders (1/1989),

TABLE 2

Minimum Norms Required for Inclusion in the Population and Average Performances of Subjects Differentiated According to Age Group and Discipline

	Minimum norms							Average Performance						
	M 45	M 50	M 55	M 60	M 65	M 70	M 75	M 45	M 50	M 55	M 60	M 65	M 70	M 75
100m	11,7	12,0	12,7	13,1	13,9	15,0	17,5	11,43	11,78	12,43	12,76	13,57	14,17	15,58
400m	54,8	57,1	62,0	65,2	76,3	80,3	80,1	53,08	54,86	58,68	61,26	69,00	71,08	74,67
1500m	4:20,1	4:29,7	4:51,5	5:20,0	5:59,3	6:50,0	7:17,0	4:14,3	4:25,4	4:36,3	5:01,5	5:31,5	6:09,3	6:33,6
10000m	33:35	34:29	36:31	39:55	43:10	51:22	61:51	32:34	33:39	35:38	38:08	40:42	45:59	49:50
42,2km	2:33:00	2:41:23	2:51:34	3:06:45	3:28:37	4:19:07	5:10:56	2:28:46	2:36:08	2:42:55	2:56:55	3:16:55	3:42:27	4:10:33
Long Jump	6,08	5,63	5,18	4,93	4,52	3,80	3,54	6,29	5,87	5,43	5,15	4,76	4,31	3,90
Shot put	13,71 (7,25)	12,99 (6,25)	11,66 (6,25)	12,06 (5)	11,27 (5)	10,60 (4)	9,53 (4)	14,99 (7,25)	13,93 (6,25)	12,36 (6,25)	12,54 (5)	12,45 (5)	11,59 (4)	10,78 (4)
Javelin	51,34 (800)	45,50 (800)	38,94 (800)	37,14 (600)	33,72 (600)	25,62 (600)	19,58 (600)	57,24 (800)	49,79 (800)	43,42 (800)	42,52 (600)	38,60 (600)	30,88 (600)	28,08 (600)

and 27 current or former holders of unofficial Masters world records were included in the sample.

Therefore, the sample is very likely to be representative for the majority of the research questions examined in this study.

Subsamples

The differentiation of the total sample according to the main criteria "age group" and "discipline group" (Figure 1) resulted in sufficient subsample sizes between 11 (throwing, M70) and 53 (running, M50).

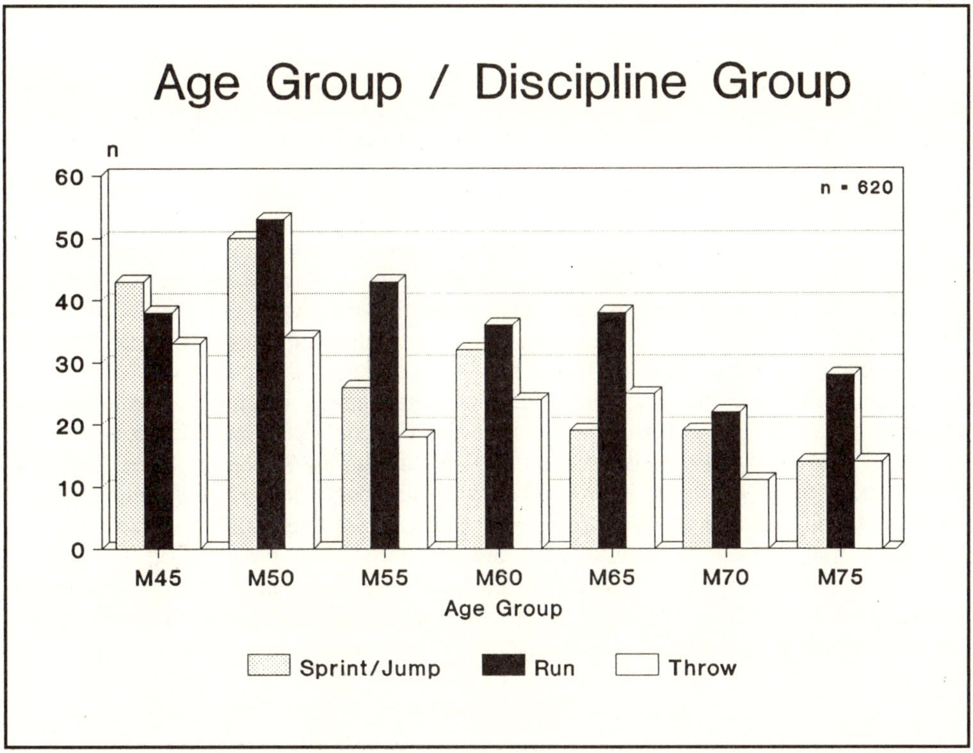

Figure 1. Total sample differentiated according to Age Groups.

RESULTS

(1) In light of the hypotheses formulated in the introduction, the results of this investigation are surprising. The history of sport activities varied considerably for Masters athletes. Of the 620 interviewed athletes, 179 (28.9 percent) had competed successfully in track and field during early adulthood (at least third place at state championships, WLA-I). Another 159 (25.6 percent) Masters athletes had participated in track and field competitions without noteworthy success (WLA-II). Of 156 Masters who had taken part in competitions in other sports during early adulthood, 36 (5.8 percent) were successful (W-I) and 120 (19.4 percent) had little success (W-II). One hundred and twenty-six subjects (20.3 percent) had not participated in athletic competition between the ages of 20 and 40, and often (n = 65) they had not been physically active at all (beginner).

Large differences occurred when examining single cases. While one 80-year-old athlete had competed in various track and field disciplines for 74 years, today's most successful marathon runner in the world in the age group "90 years or older" did not begin to take part in physical activities until the age of 74.

(2) There is a highly significant correlation between age group and history of athletic participation (Cramer's V = 0.16; $p<0.001$). In the higher age groups, with the exception of the class M75, the number of former track and field athletes decreases and the number of late beginners increases (Figure 2).

(3) Of special interest are the results on the history of sport activities specific to the discipline groups (Figure 3), where significant differences were found (Cramer's V = 0.36: $p<0.001$). The results for the groups running and throwing were completely different. While more than 80 percent of the athletes in the throwing disciplines participated in track and field competitions in early adulthood and 55.3 percent of them were very successful, former track and field athletes were underrepresented in the discipline of middle- and long-distance running. Surprisingly, the majority of Masters endurance athletes who are successful today had not started running until late adulthood (69 percent). The discipline group "sprint/jump" is located in the middle, with a tendency towards the group "throw." A differentiated examination of the influence of the competitive discipline reveals that the disciplines "javelin" and "marathon" mark the two extreme positions. While 46.6 percent of marathon runners who are successful today are beginners and only 7.2 percent are former top runners, the proportions are reversed for the javelin throw: 69.4 percent are former top-level javelin throwers and only two percent are late beginners.

DISCUSSION

For middle- and especially for long-distance runners, where the proportion of beginners is clearly above that of middle-distance runners, it appears that a later commencement with competition is not a disadvantage. An early start of training and competition in street running (25 km/marathon) and the following decades of training can possibly represent a barrier for good performances in old age. A satisfactory answer cannot be given as to what extent competitive experience in the disciplines oriented towards power and higher coordinative demands are a necessary prerequisite for achieving outstanding performances in old age. The results indicate that (discipline-specific) involvement in sport during early adulthood has a positive effect; however, social reasons could also be responsible for the dominance of former athletes. Although many opportunities exist for participating in recreational endurance activities, giving everybody a chance to become involved in competitive running via fun runs and recreational sporting events, late beginners in disciplines oriented towards power have to overcome great barriers.

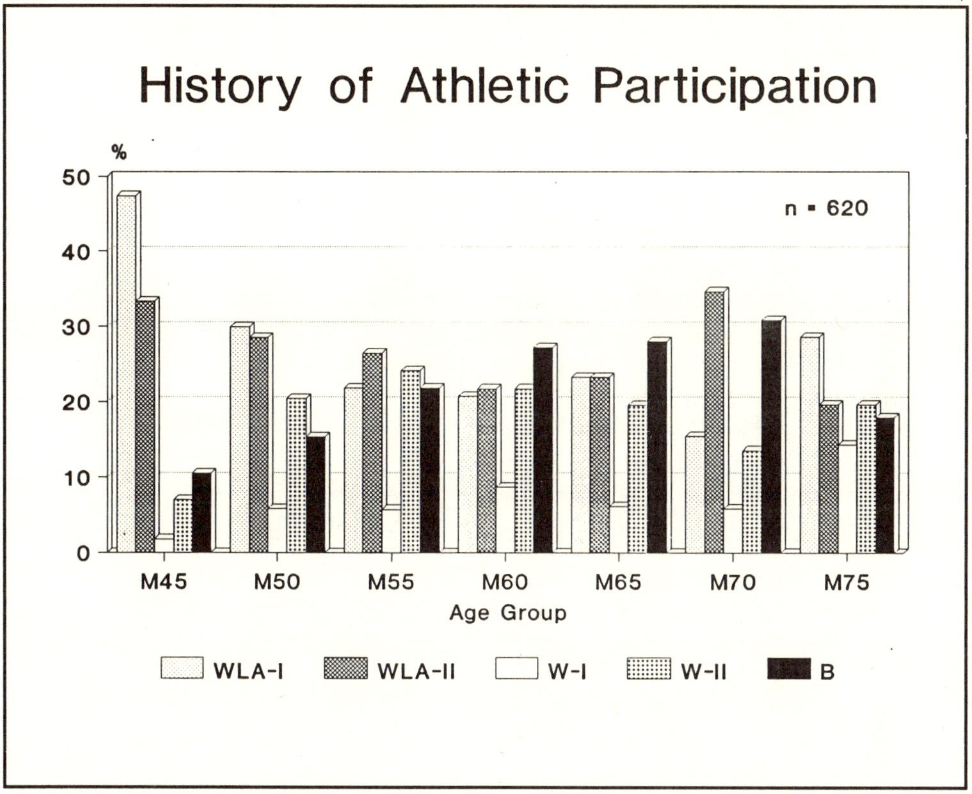

WLA-I: Competitive athletes in track and field with success on state or higher level
WLA-II: Competitive athletes in track and field without notable success
W-I: Competitive athletes with success on state or higher level
W-II: Competitive athletes in other sports without notable success
B: Beginner, i.e., no participation in competitive sport during childhood

Figure 2. History of athletic participation differentiated according to age groups.

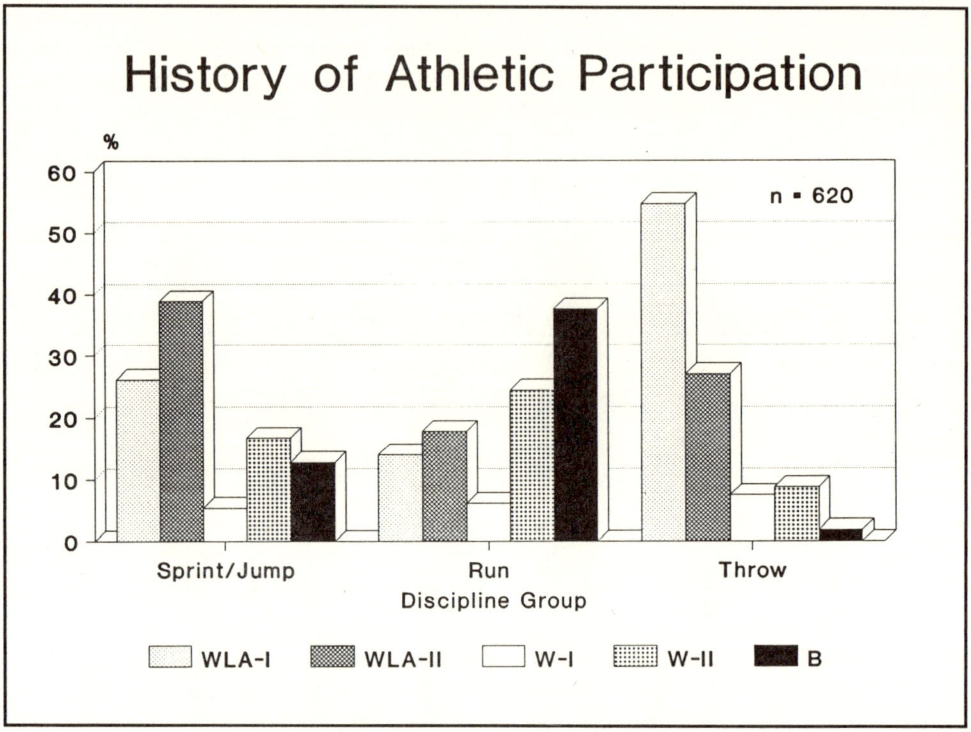

WLA-I: Competitive athletes in track and field with success on state or higher level
WLA-II: Competitive athletes in track and field with notable success
W-I: Competitive athletes in other sports with success on state or higher level
W-II: Competitive athletes in other sports without notable success
B: Beginner, i.e. , no participation in competitive sport during early adulthood

Figure 3. History of athletic participation differentiated according to discipline groups

CONCLUSION

The differences regarding the history of athletic involvement in the individual age groups can essentially be explained with effects due to changes over time. It can be assumed that the proportion of late beginners will increase in the future. However, this does not mean that beginning with training and competition in the second half of life hinders outstanding performances in old age. It is likely that in the future more and more late beginners, especially from endurance disciplines, will be able to achieve extraordinary performances in old age.

REFERENCES

Diem C. Geleitwort (Foreword). In: Jokl E, ed. Alter und Leistung (Age and Performance) Berlin/Göttingen/ Heidelberg: Springer-Verlag, 1954.

Israel S, Buhl B, Purkopp K-H, Weidner A. Körperliche Leistungsfähigkeit und organismische Funktionstüchtigkeit im Alternsgang (Physical performance capacity and the functioning of the organism throughout the course of life). In: Wissenschaftliche Zeitschrift der Deutschen Hochschule für Körperkultur Leipzig 23, 1982;1:19-62.

Israel S, Weidner A. Korperliche Aktvität und Altern (Physical Activity and Aging). Leipzig: VEB J.A. Barth, 1988.

Liesen H, Hollmann W. Ausdauersport und Stoffwechsel - insbesondere beim älteren Menschen (Endurance Sport and Metabolism - Especially of Older People). Schorndorf: Hofmann-Verlag, 1981.

Petermann F. Daten, Dimensionen, Verfahrensweisen (Data, dimensions, procedures). In: Oerter R, Montada L, eds., Entwicklungspsychologie (Developmental psychology). München/Weinheim: Psychologie Verlags Union, 1987:1017-60.

Reckemeier J. Seniorenleichtathletik (Masters track and field). Ausgaben 1986-1988. Oldenburg 1987, 1988, 1989.

Trautner HM. Lehrbuch der Entwicklungspsychologie (Text Book on Developmental Psychology). Göttingen/ Toronto/Zürich: Verlag Hogrefe, 1978.

Willimczik, K. Die (sport-)motorische Entwicklung beim älteren Menschen (Sport-motor development of older people). In: Singer R, ed. Alterssport - Versuch einer Bestandsaufnahme (Sport for the Aging - Attempt of an Inventory). Schorndorf: Hofmann-Verlag, 1981:91-108.

Winter R. Die motorische Entwicklung des Menschen von der Geburt bis ins hohe Alter (Überblick) (Motor development of the human being from birth until old age (overview). In: Meinel K, Schnabel G, eds. Bewegungslehre - Sportmotorik (Movement Theory - Sport Motor System). Berlin (Ost): Volkseigner Verlag, 1987:275-397.

Wohlwill JF. Strategien entwicklungspsychologischer Forschung (Strategies of Research in Developmental Psychology). Stuttgart: Ernst Klett Verlag, 1977.

The Relationship Between Physical Activity and Physical Fitness in the Older Age Group

Marieke J.G. van Heuvelen, M.Sc.
Piet Rispens, M.D., Ph.D.
Koen A.P.M. Lemmink, M.Sc.
Wiebo H. Brouwer, Ph.D.

INTRODUCTION

The decline in physical fitness with increasing age is a well-known phenomenon. Many investigations have demonstrated the age-dependent decrease in endurance, strength, flexibility, balance, reaction time, and manual dexterity (Buskirk and Hodgson, 1987; Dehn and Bruce, 1972; Wilkinson and Allison, 1989; Gottsdanker, 1982; Rikli and Busch, 1986; Ekdahl et al., 1989; Pearson et al., 1985). There is much evidence that exercise of high and moderate intensity improves physical fitness in the elderly (Seals et al., 1984; Haber et al., 1984; Morey et al., 1991; Badenhop et al., 1983;, Makrides et al., 1990; Blumenthal et al., 1989; Hagberg et al., 1989; Steinhaus et al., 1990; Morey et al., 1989; Sidney and Shephard, 1978). Recent research has shown that even low intensity exercise can enhance physical performance (Brown and Holloszy, 1991; Hopkins et al., 1990; Agre et al., 1988; Raab et al., 1988). However, the nature of the relationship between physical activity, physical fitness, and age is not quite clear.

On the one hand, results of several investigations support the assumption that physical activity can counteract the age-dependent decline in fitness. A significant interaction between age and activity, in which differences between inactive and active groups increased with age, was found in several reaction time studies (Spirduso, 1975; Spirduso and Clifford, 1978; Clarkson and Kroll, 1978; Sherwood and Selder, 1979). Rikli and Busch (1986) found significant age-activity interaction effects for choice reaction time, balance, and shoulder flexibility. In these tests the differences between inactive versus active were higher in old groups than in young groups. However, for simple reaction time, grip strength, and trunk flexibility, they found no significant age-activity interaction. Rogers (1994; see pages 15-23 of the present volume) showed that regular vigorous exercise allows the decline in maximum oxygen uptake of 12 percent per decade in sedentary men to be reduced to 5.5 percent per decade in former Master athletes who continued to be physically active.

On the other hand, several investigations found no evidence supporting the assumption that the decline in fitness can be retarded by means of physical activity. Kozma et al. (1991) found a significant age-activity effect for push-ups in which the differences between inactive and active were smaller in old people than in young people, and they suggest that there is an age limit to the effects of physical activity. Suominen et al. (1980) found a higher rate of decline with age in maximal aerobic capacity and grip strength age in trained men than in sedentary men. Buskirk and Hodgson (1987) concluded after a review study that there is no clear distinction in the rate of change in maximal oxygen uptake when comparing active and inactive populations. In a study on the effects of age and experience on a cognitive spatial task, Salthouse (1991) found no support for the assumption that the age-related decline should be attributed to disuse or lack of experience.

In all these studies the examined age range was from twenty to thirty years and up to sixty to seventy years. No information is available about the nature of the relationship between physical activity and physical fitness in old age. The purpose of this study is to investigate whether physical activity can retard the age-dependent decline in old age in a wide range of components of physical fitness, including endurance, strength, flexibility, balance, reaction time, and manual dexterity, and subjective experiences regarding these components of physical fitness.

METHOD

Subjects

The subjects of this study were 466 volunteers from the northern provinces of The Netherlands. In general they were quite healthy and all were retired and living independently. Their mean age was 66 years (range 55 to 85 years).

Assessment of Physical Activity

The level of physical activity was assessed with a self-administered questionnaire. Subjects were asked how much time they spent doing sports, walking and bicycling as recreation during the last twelve months. After weighing scores with intensity codes (Table 1), a total activity score was obtained. The questionnaire was adapted from the Minnesota Leisure Time Physical Activity Questionnaire (Taylor et al., 1978). It was adjusted to the Dutch situation and self-administered rather than given as an interview. A preliminary study showed that the strength of the relation between the self- administered form and the interview form was sufficient (Pearson's $r>0.7$).

TABLE 1

Intensity Codes Physical Activity Questionnaire (Metabolic Equivalents)

Activity	METs	Activity	METs
Recreational walking	4.5	lawn tennis	6.0
Recreational bicycling	4.5	badminton	7.0
Volleyball	5.0	yoga	2.5
Gymnastics	4.5	tai chi	2.5
Dancing (folk)	5.5	speed skating	7.0
Swimming	6.0	skiing	7.0
Jogging	7.0	cross country skiing	7.0

Based on the total activity score, subjects were divided equally into three groups, least active, moderately active and most active, as shown in Table 2. The three groups differed considerably in activity levels, varying from 3.8 METs hours per week for the least active group to 35.0 METs hours per week for the most active group.

TABLE 2

Mean Age (years), Number, and Mean Level of Physical Activity (METs hours per week) of the Subjects in Each Activity Group

	Men	Women	Total
Least active	65.9	66.1	66.0
	43	112	155
	3.5	3.9	3.8
Moderately active	65.1	65.1	65.1
	59	97	156
	13.9	13.3	13.6
Most active	66.2	64.6	65.5
	87	68	155
	34.9	35.2	35.0

Measurements of Physical Fitness

Physical fitness was measured with the Groningen Fitness Test for the Elderly (Lemmink et al., 1991). The test consists of seven test items for the objective measurement of fitness.

1. Walking endurance. Participants walk on a rectangular course. The walking speed is increased by one km/h every three minutes, starting at a speed of four km/h, and ending at a speed of seven km/h. The participant must keep up the effort as long as possible. The score is adjusted to the highest speed sustained for three full minutes.

2. Flexibility of the hip joint and the spine (the "sit-and-reach" test). The participant sits on the floor, legs out-stretched, in front of a box (Lafayette, model 01285) and has to bend forward and push a slide over the table with the fingertips as far as possible. The shift of the slide is recorded. The best of three trials is taken as the obtained score.

3. Flexibility of the shoulder joint. In this item a cord is used, with a fixed handle on one end and a sliding handle on the other end. The participant holds the handles and passes the cord from in front of the body, over the head, to behind the body. The participant has to keep the arms straight and has to try to keep the arms as close together as possible. The shift of the sliding handle (s), combined with the length of the arm (l), is used to determine the score (score=arccos (s/2*l)). The score is the best trial of three.

4. Manual dexterity. The participant has to replace forty blocks from a full board to an empty board in a prescribed way as quickly as possible with his hand of preference. The time taken to complete the task is recorded.

5. Simple reaction time. The participant has to react to a visual signal by pushing a button. The score is the median out of fifteen trials.

6. Balance. The participant must try to keep a tilting platform in balance.

The total time during a thirty-second interval that the platform did not touch the floor is recorded. The score is the best trial of three.

7. Grip strength. The participant has to hold a handgrip dynamometer (Jamar, model 00105) in the preferred hand with arm at the side and must squeeze using maximum force. The score obtained is the best of three trials.

In addition, the Groningen Fitness Test for the Elderly includes a questionnaire for subjective evaluation of physical fitness. This questionnaire asks about experiences regarding the components of fitness compared to ten years ago (nine items) and compared to people of the same age (nine items). On both scales, the minimum score is nine points, where the participant thinks he is much less fit than ten years ago or than his peers, and the maximum score is forty-five points, where the participant believes himself to be much more fit. Also, participants have to give themselves a report-card mark on fitness between one (very poor) and ten (excellent).

Data Analysis

Data were analyzed using a 2 x 3 factorial covariance analysis for each of the seven test items for objective measurement of physical fitness and each of the three test items for subjective evaluation. The two independent variables were gender and physical activity (least, moderately, and most active). Age was used as a covariate. In addition, regression analysis was used to compare the rate of decline in fitness between the three activity groups. P-values less than five percent were considered to indicate statistical significance.

RESULTS

Objective Measurement of Physical Fitness

The means and standard deviations of the objective measurement of physical fitness are shown in Tables 3.1 and 3.2. Because of positive skewness of the dependent variables manual dexterity and simple reaction time, loglinear transformations were made before performing the analysis of variance.

The multivariate main effect of age was significant. (Wilk's $F(7,353)=20.73$, $p<.0005$). For all measures, the univariate main effect of age was significant (Table 4), with a decline in fitness with increasing age.

The multivariate main effect of physical activity was significant (Wilk's $F(14,708)=3.54$, $p<.0005$). The univariate main effects were significant for walking endurance, flexibility of the hip and spine, flexibility of the shoulder, and manual dexterity (Table 4). Comparing group means with Tukey correction for multiple comparisons (Tables 3.1 and 3.2) showed differences mainly between the least active groups on the one hand and the moderately active and most active groups on the other hand. Few differences were found between the moderately active and most active groups.

The multivariate age-activity interaction reached borderline significance [Wilk's $F(14,702)=1.70$, $p=.051$]. The univariate age-activity interaction was significant only for

TABLE 3.1

Means and Standard Deviations of Objective Measurement of Physical Fitness in Men, and the Results of Multiple Comparisons with Tukey Correction at 5 Percent Level

Test Item	Least Active	Moderately Active	Most Active
Walking endurance (km/h)	6.2 (0.8) [1] [2]	6.5 (0.8)	6.7 (0.6)
Flexibility hip (cm)	26.0 (10.9)	25.7 (9.9)	30.2 (10.0) [2]
Flexibility shoulders (°)	43.1 (5.8)	41.6 (5.4)	40.9 (5.2)
Manual dexterity (s)	46.7 (5.9) [2]	43.8 (4.2)	44.6 (4.9)
Simple reaction time (ms)	215 (37)	208 (25)	209 (35)
Balance (s)	25.0 (2.6)	25.1 (2.8)	25.2 (2.5)
Grip strength (N)	433 (76)	440 (85)	454 (64)

[1] = significantly different from most active
[2] = significantly different from moderately active

TABLE 3.2

Means and Standard Deviations of Objective Measurement of Physical Fitness in Women and the Results of Multiple Comparisons with Tukey Correction at 5 Percent Level

Test Item	Least Active	Moderately Active	Most Active
Walking endurance (km/h)	5.7 (0.9) [1] [2]	6.1 (0.8)	6.2 (0.8)
Flexibility hip (cm)	33.0 (8.5) [1]	35.0 (7.6)	36.3 (9.4)
Flexibility shoulders (°)	40.2 (5.9) [1] [2]	37.1 (7.4)	37.2 (6.3)
Manual dexterity (s)	44.9 (5.3) [1] [2]	42.6 (4.9)	41.8 (4.7)
Simple reaction time (ms)	221 (40)	214 (29)	212 (26)
Balance (s)	24.4 (2.6) [1]	25.0 (2.9)	25.5 (3.5)
Grip strength (N)	258 (57) [2]	278 (58)	266 (47)

[1] = significantly different from most active
[2] = significantly different from moderately active

TABLE 4

F-Ratios from Analysis of Covariance for Objective Measurement of Physical Fitness

	Source			
Test Item	Age	Gender	Activity	Age x Activity
Walking endurance	74.79***	53.14***	17.57***	3.37*
Flexibility hip	20.41***	67.35***	6.75**	3.44*
Flexibility shoulder	30.31***	34.94***	7.69**	0.69
Manual dexterity	77.46***	17.20***	12.02***	0.96
Simple reaction time	37.33***	4.24*	1.54	0.09
Balance	29.48***	65	2.18	0.30
Grip strength	63.71***	888.80***	1.92	2.65

* p<.05 ** p<.01 *** p<.001

TABLE 5

Slopes of Linear Regression Lines with Walking Endurance and Flexibility of the Hip and the Spine as Functions of Age

Test Item	Least Active	Moderately Active	Most Active
Walking endurance			
Men	-.036	-.070	-.042
Women	-.041	-.087	-.072
Flexibility hip			
Men	-.174	-.614	-.555
Women	-.108	-.322	-.665

walking endurance and flexibility of the hip and spine. For these test items, the slopes of the regression lines of the linear relationship with age are given in Table 5. For both variables the absolute value of the slopes are smaller for the least active groups compared to the moderately active and the most active groups, showing the performance differences due to physical activity decrease with age.

Subjective Evaluation of Physical Fitness

Tables 6.1 and 6.2 show the means and standard deviations of the test items concerning the subjective evaluation of physical fitness.

TABLE 6.1

Means and Standard Deviations of Subjective Evaluation of Physical Fitness in Men and the Results of Multiple Comparisons with Tukey Correction at 5 Percent Level

Test Item	Least Active	Moderately Active	Most Active
Compared to 10 years ago (pts)	21.1 (5.6) [1]	23.2 (4.9)	24.5 (4.4)
Compared to people of the same age (pts)	27.1 (4.7) [1 2]	30.1 (4.6)	30.6 (4.1)
Report card mark	6.4 (1.0) [1 2]	6.9 (1.0)	7.1 (0.9)

[1] = significantly different from most active
[2] = significantly different from moderately active

The multivariate main effect of age was statistically significant [Wilk's F(3,435)=7.34, p<.0005]. Two univariate main effects of age were significant: for fitness compared to ten years ago and the report card mark (Table 7). For these two items, the feelings regarding physical fitness became less positive with increasing age.

The multivariate main effect of physical activity was statistically significant [Wilk's F(6,870)=10.83, p<.0005]. The univariate main effects of activity were significant for all dependent variables (Table 7). Comparing group means with Tukey correction for multiple comparisons (Tables 6.1 and 6.2) showed differences mainly between the least active groups on the one hand and the moderately active and most active groups on the other hand. Few differences were found between the moderately active and the most active groups.

In none of the test items was the interaction effect Age x Activity significant (Table 7).

TABLE 6.2

Means and Standard Deviations of Subjective Evaluation of Physical Fitness in Women and the Results of Multiple Comparisons with Tukey Correction at 5 Percent Level

Test Item	Least Active	Moderately Active	Most Active
Compared to 10 years ago (pts)	20.5 (4.6) [1 2]	22.0 (3.4)	23.7 (4.3) [2]
Compared to people of the same age (pts)	25.9 (4.7) [1 2]	28.7 (4.4)	29.9 (4.0)
Report card mark	6.4 (1.0) [1 2]	6.8 (0.8)	7.1 (0.9)

[1] = significantly different from most active
[2] = significantly different from moderately active

DISCUSSION

Within the limitations of a cross-sectional design, which provides no evidence for a causal relationship, we can conclude that the results of this study provide no evidence for the assumption that physical activity can retard the age-dependent decline in physical fitness either in the objective measurement of physical fitness, or in the subjective evaluation. On the contrary, differences between active and inactive groups tend to decrease with age. This might indicate an age limitation for the effects of physical activity, which is consistent with the results of the studies of Kozma et al. (1991) and Suominen et al. (1980).

Buskirk and Hodgson (1987) assume that changes in endurance power (maximum oxygen uptake) may be curvilinear over the entire age range, with active individuals declining slowly as long as they maintain a regular exercise program, and sedentary individuals declining at a rapid rate during their 20's and 30's followed by a slower rate of decline as they further age. Therefore, from the age of 20, the differences between active and inactive may first increase, only to be followed by a decrease at a later age. In our study no curvilinear relation was found for either of the test items. As we investigated only subjects over 55 years of age, the assumption of a curvilinear relationship cannot be disproved by our study. Further research examining the entire age range is required.

Clarkson and Kroll (1978) suggest that the inter-individual variability in motor performance increases with age. This might violate the assumption of equality of variance required for the analysis of covariance. In this investigation, only the simple reaction time test showed violation of the assumption of equality of variance, even after the loglinear transformation, with increased variability in the subjects over 75 years of age. However, repetition of the analysis of covariance without the subjects over 75 years of age led to the same results.

TABLE 7

F-Ratios from Analysis of Covariance for Subjective Evaluation of Physical Fitness

	Source			
Test Item	**Age**	**Gender**	**Activity**	**Age x Activity**
Compared to 10 years ago	13.79***	5.52**	17.98***	1.26
Compared to people of the same age	0.09	6.03*	27.66***	0.41
Report card mark	7.69**	.32	22.24***	0.21

* p<.05 ** p<.01 *** p<.001

One problem with the assessment of the level of physical activity should be mentioned. A total activity score was obtained by weighing with intensity codes expressed as METs (Metabolic Equivalents). To determine the effect of physical activity on endurance, this is the correct procedure. On the other hand, if strength, flexibility, balance, reaction time or manual dexterity are considered as dependent variables, this method is not accurate. In these cases mechanic or cybernetic equivalents should be used. However, such methods of measurement are not available.

The subjects in this study were all relatively healthy and living independently. Therefore, generalizations can be made only to a population with these characteristics. Another problem is that, with increasing age, the sample will be less representative for the entire population of elderly, as most people aged 55 are fairly healthy and living independently, whereas only the strongest of those over 80 years of age are. Therefore, the effects of age will be underestimated. Furthermore, the cross-sectional design led to an underestimation of the effects of age because only the strongest reach very old age.

CONCLUSION

In this study, few differences were found between the moderately active and the most active groups for both objective measurement of physical fitness and subjective evaluation. The intensity level of the moderately active group appears to be sufficient to enhance physical fitness. This level corresponds to one hour of sports per week, for gymnastics or dancing, and two hours of walking or bicycling per week. The effect of physical activity was significant for the subjective evaluation of physical fitness. The age-activity interaction was significant only for walking endurance and flexibility of the hip and spine. For these test items, the score differences between the least active group and the moderately and most active groups decreased with age, which might indicate an age limitation for the effects of physical activity in old age.

REFERENCES

Agre JC, Pierce LE, Raab DM, McAdams M, Smith EL. Light resistance and stretching exercise in elderly women: effect upon strength. Arch Phys Med Rehabil 1988;69:273-6.

Badenhop DT, Cleary PA, Schaal SF, Fox EL, Bartels RL. Physiological adjustments to higher-or-lower-intensity exercise in elders. Med Sci Sports Exerc 1983;15:496-502.

Blumenthal JA, Emery CF, Madden DJ et al. Cardiovascular and behavioral effects of aerobic exercise training in healthy older men and women. J Gerontol 1989;44:M147-57.

Brown M, Holloszy JO. Effects of a low intensity exercise program on selected physical performance characteristics of 60-to-71-year olds. Aging 1991;3:129- 39.

Buskirk ER, Hodgson JL. Age and aerobic power: the rate of decline in men and women. Fed Proc 1987; 46:1824-9.

Clarkson PM, Kroll W. Practice effects on fractioned response time related to age and activity level. J Motor Behavior 1978;10:275-86.

Dehn MM, Bruce RA. Longitudinal variations in maximal oxygen intake with age and activity. J Appl Physiol 1972;33:805-7.

Ekdahl C, Jarnlo GB, Andersson SI. Standing balance in healthy subjects. Scand J Rehab Med 1989;21:187-95.

Gottsdanker R. Age and simple reaction time. J Gerontol 1982;37:342-8.

Haber P, Honiger B, Klicpera M, Niederberger M. Effect in elderly people 67-76 years of age of three-month endurance training on a bicycle ergometer. Eur Heart J 1984;5:37-9.

Hagberg JM, Graves JE, Limacher M et al. Cardiovascular responses of 70-to-79-year-old men and women to exercise training. J Appl Physiol 1989;66:2589-94.

Hopkins DR, Murrah B, Hoeger WWK, Rhodes RC. Effect of low-impact aerobic dance on the functional fitness of elderly women. Gerontologist 1990;30:189-192.

Kozma A, Stones MJ, Hannah TE. Age, activity, and physical performance: an evaluation of performance models. Psychol Aging 1991;6:43-9.

Lemmink KAPM, Brouwer WH, Bult P, van Heuvelen MJG, Rispens P. Fitheidstest voor Ouderen. Lichamelijke Opvoeding 1991;6:43-9.

Makrides L, Heigenhauser GJF, Jones NL. High-intensity endurance training in 20-to-30 and 60-to-70-year-old healthy men. J Appl Physiol 1990;69:1792-98.

Morey MC, Cowper PA, Feussner JR et al. Two-year trends in physical performance following supervised exercise among community-dwelling older veterans. J Am Geriatr Soc 1991;39:986-92.

Morey MC, Cowper PA, Feussner JR et al. Evaluation of a supervised exercise program in a geriatric population. J Am Geriatr Soc 1989;37:348-54.

Pearson MB, Bassey EJ, Bendall MJ. The effects of age on muscle strength and anthropometric indices within a group of elderly men and women. Age Ageing 1985;14:230-4.

Raab DM, Agre JC, McAdams M, Smith EL. Light resistance and stretching exercise in elderly women: effect upon flexibility. Arch Phys Med Rehabil 1988;69:268-72.

Rikli R, Busch S. Motor performance of women as a function of age and physical activity level. J Gerontol 1986;41:645-9.

Rogers MA. Effects of chronic, intense endurance exercise training on longitudinal changes in maximal oxygen uptake in older men. In: Harris S, Suominen H, Era P, Harris WH, eds. Physical Activity, Aging and Sports, Volume III: Toward Healthy Aging-International Perspectives-Part 1. Physiological and Biomedical Aspects. Albany, NY: Center for the Study of Aging, 1994:15-23.

Salthouse TA. Age and experience effects on the interpretation of orthographic drawings of three-dimensional objects. Psychol Aging 1991;6:426-33.

Seals DR, Hagberg JM, Hurley BF, Ehsani AA, Holloszy JO. Endurance training in older men and women I. Cardiovascular responses to exercise. J Appl Physiol 1984;57:1024-9.

Sherwood DE, Selder DJ. Cardiorespiratory health, reaction time and aging. Med Sci Sports 1979;11:186-9.

Sidney KH, Shephard RJ. Frequency and intensity of exercise training for elderly subjects. Med Sci Sports 1978;10:125-31.

Spirduso WW. Reaction and movement time as a function of age and physical activity level. J Gerontol 1975;30:435-40.

Spirduso WW, Clifford P. Replication of age and physical activity effects on reaction and movement time. J Gerontol 1978;33:26-30.

Steinhaus LA, Dustman RE, Ruhling RO et al. Aerobic capacity of older adults: a training study. J Sports Med Phys Fitness 1990;30:163-72.

Suominen H, Heikkinen E, Parkatti T, Forsberg S, Kiiskinen A. Effects of "lifelong" physical training on functional aging in men. Scand J Soc Med 1980;(Suppl. 14):225-40.

Taylor HL, Jacobs DR, Schucker B, Knudson J, Leon AS, Debacker G. A questionnaire for the assessment of leisure time physical activities. J Chron Dis 1978;31:741-55.

Wilkinson RT, Allison S. Age and simple reaction time: decade differences for 5,325 subjects. J Gerontol 1989;44:P29-35.

Physical Skills and Fitness of Groups from Different Environments

Halina Szwarc, M.D., F.A.

INTRODUCTION

The consequences of decreased activity in old age are a lower physical efficiency and increased progression of the aging process, as well as a higher incidence of diseases and biological disability. In geriatric prevention, gerontologists place most emphasis upon the necessity of regular physical activity.

Our previous papers showed that physical exercises of very low intensity can lead to an improvement of all respiratory parameters in people whose life was rather sedentary. The improvement was obtained after five to six weeks of exercise performance for 30 minutes five times a week (Szwarc, 1992).

The purpose of this investigation was to determine the physical skills, efficiency and general health status of senior students who were members of the Warsaw University of the Third Age (UTA) and of older persons from other environments.

METHODS

Eighty UTA students aged 60 to 87 years, who were divided into two groups, were examined before, during and after their participation in a recreation camp or on hiking tours. One group comprised 50 who participated in a recreation camp situated on the plain; the other group (hikers) was composed of 30 who were engaged in walking tours in the mountains 700 to 900 meters above sea level. The average age of the recreation campers was 71.6 years and of the hikers was 73 years.

The camp on the plain was designed for those who, because of their health or for other reasons, had a rather physically inactive way of life; they determined the time and distance of their daily walking tours themselves, usually walking four to six kilometers a day. The hikers participated in walking tours of 10 kilometers to 24 kilometers a day in the mountains.

All participants were examined at the Sport-Medicine Department of the Academy of Physical Education in Warsaw. After a complete medical examination, an electrocardiogram was taken before and after a step-up test. The height of step was 22 centimeters, and the number of ascents made as quickly as possible per 90 seconds was counted. Vital capacity and physical efficiency were tested.

The participants were obliged to make a daily brief report on their ailments or their well-being to a physician for the hikers and to a nurse for the recreational campers. The physician measured the heart rate and blood pressure of the hikers before and after the walking mountain tours.

In a separate study the physical skills of two groups were determined. One group was composed of 51 women who were UTA students; the second group comprised 44 other women who participated in practical exercises twice a week and whose average age was 70 years (range 55 to 89 years). They self-estimated their physical efficiency, health, and physical skills. Afterwards, the physical skills listed in the questionnaire were examined: knee bending, forward trunk bend, and balance - standing on one foot for 20 seconds.

RESULTS

Vital capacity of all participants was improved. This improvement was statistically significant by the t-test ($p<0.05$) for the participants of the recreation camp (Table 1).

TABLE 1

Vital Capacity
(Before and After Two-Week Camps)

Examined Group	1st examination (before the camp)	2nd examination (after the camp)
Recreation camp participants n=50, $\bar{x}$ age = 71.6	2,600 ml	2,900 ml*
Hikers n=30, $\bar{x}$ age=73	2,741 ml	2,880 ml

*$p<0.05$

The number of complaints by participants diminished (Table 2) and fitness increased. For example, 43 complaints of the motor apparatus were received before, but only 24 after, the intervention. The number of digestive system complaints decreased from 21 to 9. Out of 30 cases of sleep disturbances, 14 remained. Out of 20 cases of general weakness, only five remained.

Results of the step-up test indicated that fitness was improved: the number of steps climbed increased from two to seven ascents per 90 seconds. The stress electrocardiogram was positive in two recreation camp participants before the camp experience but became normal after the camp. The hikers had a lowering of resting pulse rate and systolic blood pressure as the daily mountain hikes increased from 10 to 24 kilometers (Table 3). The self-evaluation of health and physical efficiency was best for the hikers, less good for the UTA students, and worst for the general population aged 60 years and over (Table 4).

TABLE 2

Number of Complaints
(Before and After the Camp or Hiking Intervention)

Complaints	Recreation Camp Participants n=50 Number of complaints		Hikers n=30 Number of complaints	
	Before	After	Before	After
Circulatory system	35	6	14	8
Motor apparatus	27	12	16	12
Digestive system	15	4	6	5
Headache	11	2	7	3
Fears, excitement	11	0	7	1
Sleep disturbances	19	7	11	7
Apathy, depression status	10	2	2	0
General weakness	15	3	5	2
Summary of all complaints	143	36	68	38

Physical efficiency was self-evaluated as best by the hikers, with 63 percent "very good" and "good" efficiency and none "bad." In contrast, physical efficiency was estimated as "bad" in 10 percent of UTA students and in 29 percent of the general population (GUS, 1988). The general population, 60 years of age and over, estimated their own health as "bad" in 30 percent of instances, which is three times the percentage in the senior UTA students' group and five to six times more than in the hikers (Table 4, Figure 1).

In Poland, the General Office of Statistics has conducted country-wide examinations of the population with regard to various forms of physical and cultural recreation (GUS, 1982; GUS, 1985). Recent examinations were conducted in 1987 by GUS with collaboration of Lobozewicz (GUS, 1988; Lobozewicz, 1992). This author has applied the self-estimation method for the investigation of physical activity and some motor skills.

The aim of this second part of our investigation was to compare the motor skills as assessed first by self-evaluation (i.e., declared by the subject during an interview) with the results of subsequent actual examination of these motor skills. A group of 96 women - 51 UTA students and 45 others - was examined (Visan, 1992), with the results of physical efficiency in examined skills compared with the data previously declared by the women. The examinations took place in the gymnastic halls where the women exercised twice a week.

TABLE 3

Heart Rate and Blood Pressure
(before and after a daily hike)

Date	6 September	8 September	10 September	12 September
Distance	10 km	14 km	20 km	24 km
Before the hiking tour				
HR	63/min	64/min	62/min	61/min
BP	149/82 mm Hg	151/81 mm Hg	148/83 mm Hg	142/86 mm Hg
After the hiking tour				
HR	76/min	74/min	70/min	72/min
BP	152/83 mm Hg	152/83 mm Hg	158/84 mm Hg	149/84 mm Hg

TABLE 4

Self-Estimation of Physical Efficiency and Health by Group

	Very good and good Percent	Average Percent	Bad Percent
Physical Efficiency by Group			
Hikers N = 30	63	37	0
Recreation camp participants N=50	52	37	11
Senior students N=185	54	36	10
General population GUS N = 2641	33	38	29
Health by Group			
Hikers	37	58	5
Recreation camp participants	37	52	11
Senior students	18	71	11
General population GUS	17	54	30

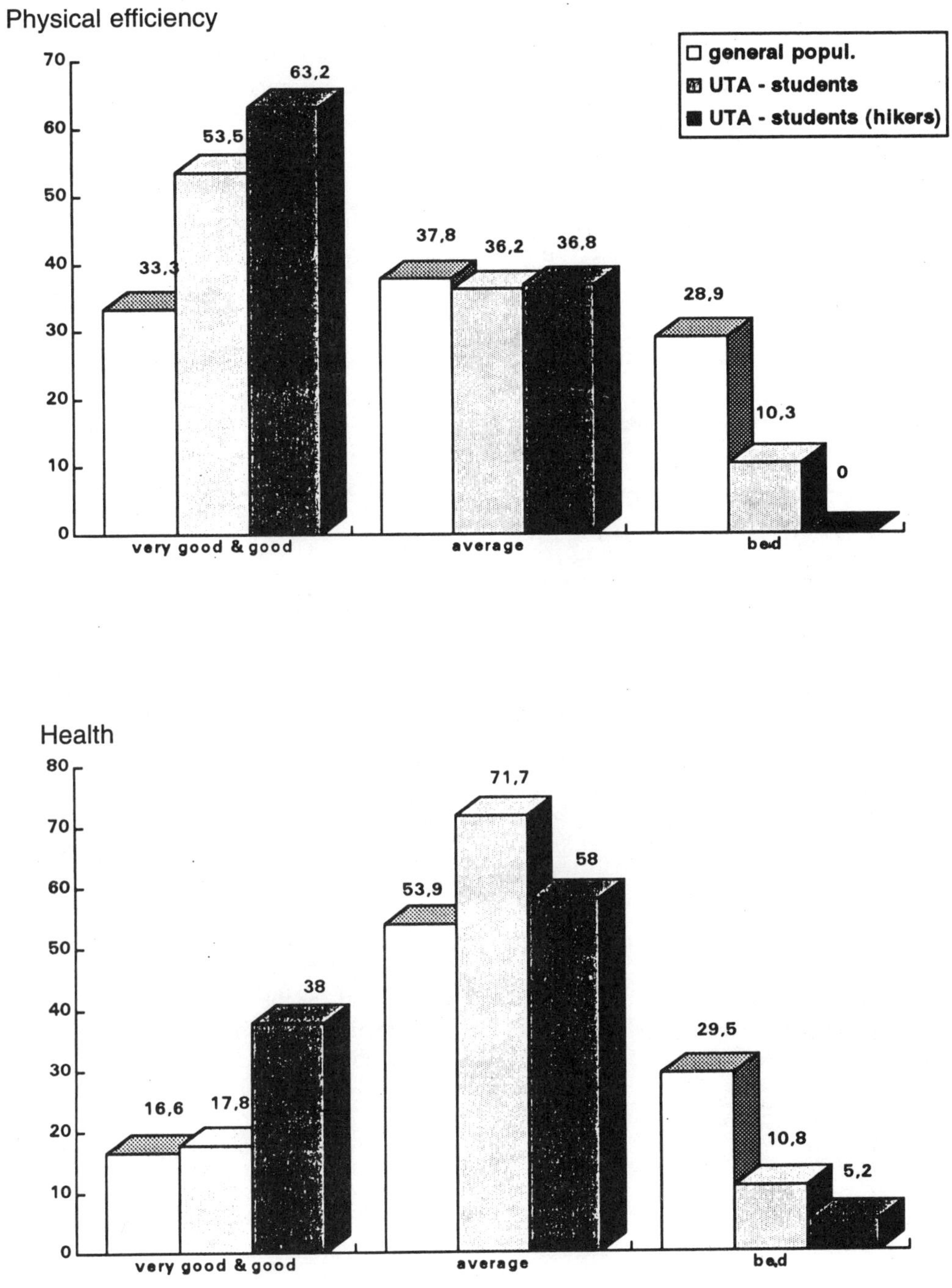

Figure 1. Self-estimation of Physical Efficiency and Health
(Age over 60)

The observed results of the efficiency parameters, knee bending, forward trunk bend, and 20 seconds standing on one foot, were better for the UTA students than for the other examined women. In addition, the difference between the self-estimation and investigated (actually observed) data was smaller in all investigated skills for the UTA students than the others (Table 5).

TABLE 5

Comparison of Obtained Results with the Data of Questionnaires (Self-Estimation)

Skills	Declared data Self-estimation		Performed		Error of estimation	
	Number	Percent	Number	Percent	Number	Percent
Forward trunk bend						
UTA students	48	94	44	86	4	8
Others	31	70	24	54	7	16
Knee bending						
UTA students	39	76.5	44	86	5	9.5
Others	24	54.5	27	61	3	6.5
Standing on one foot						
UTA students	42	82	29	57	13	25
Others	32	73	5	11	27	62

Table 5 shows that fewer faulty estimates were noted for the UTA students than for others. The errors of self-evaluation were in both directions, positive and negative. Most errors were in the declaration of the balance skill, standing on one foot.

CONCLUSION

According to our observations, low intensity training can increase the mobility of joints, eliminate joint aches (the most frequent complaint in old age), eliminate headaches and dizziness, improve coronary circulation and blood flow, and regulate arterial blood flow and systolic arterial blood pressure.

1. The physical activity of older people participating in the recreation camps or hiking groups improved vital capacity and physical fitness, especially in the hikers, and diminished the number of their complaints.

2. Results suggest that persons who are in better physical condition make fewer mistakes in the self-evaluation of their motor skills than do those who have lower physical efficiency.

3. The method of self-evaluation of motor functions is not correct, and the results obtained with it are not exact even for those who perform regular physical exercises in their leisure time.

4. The self-evaluation of physical skills and fitness cannot ensure results that are as valid as those obtained by the self-evaluation of health, which is a method widely applied in geriatric investigations.

REFERENCES

GUS. General Office of Statistics. Sytuacja zyciowa osob starszych. Warszawa, 1982, z. 127.

GUS. Sytuacja bytowa osob starszych w 1985 r. Warszawa 1985, z. 36.

GUS. Turystyka i rekreacja osob w starszym wieku. Warszawa 1988, z. 61.

Lobozewicz T. Stan. i uwarunkowania aktywnosci ruchowej ludzi w starszymwieku. Wydawnictwo AWF, Warszawa, 1992.

Szwarc H. Physical activity of older people and its influence on health, physical efficiency and fitness. In: Harris S, Harris R, Harris WS, eds. Physical Activity, Aging and Sports, Volume II: Practice, Program and Policy. Albany, NY: Center for the Study of Aging, 1992:262-71.

Visan J. Sprawnosc fizyczna starszych kobiet. Praca magisterska, AWFWarszawa, 1992.

Biomechanical Changes In Daily-Life Skills with Instruction and Practice in Women 60-75

Alberto Ayalon, Ph.D.
Yael Netz, Ph.D.

INTRODUCTION

The importance of biomechanical research in aging has been widely overlooked. Some anthropometric data provide limited information for elementary architectural needs, but a thorough understanding of the mechanical aspects of different activities in the aged is still nonexistent.

Adrian (1980) states that biomechanics of aging "refers then to the changes in the ability of the tissues and systems to create, attenuate, and tolerate forces, as well as the tissues' and the total body's ability to produce and regulate motion."

Of all the accidental deaths that occur among elderly people, those resulting from falls rank foremost. Thirty percent of people over 65 who live in the community fall each year. This rate increases to 40 percent in subjects over the age of 80 (Prudham and Evans, 1981; Campbell et al., 1981). Agate (1966) reported that, in persons over age 75, falls are the cause of more than two-thirds of accidental deaths, and constitute the only major accidental death classification in which women grossly outrank men.

An analysis of the possible causes of accidental falls seems to show manifestations of fundamental defects in elderly people as to the control of posture and physical ability (Tinetti et al., 1988; Stelmach et al., 1989). Murray et al. (1964) reported data on normal walking patterns of old men. Besides shorter steps by 3.1 cm., no differences were found in the measured mechanical variables as compared to young men.

Adrian (1980) summarizes an unpublished study by Klinger et al. In this study, twelve women aged 60 and older who participated in a regular exercise program were analyzed as to their ability in performing different daily-life exercise and sports skills. From the results, the subjects were divided into two levels of performance. Adrian reports that the women in the high level of performance "were characterized as moving faster, transferring body weight more easily, showing a greater range of motion, more erect trunk posture, and better coordination, evidenced by greater continuity of sequence of movements."

A comparison study of some mechanical variables from daily life activities in elderly and young people was done by Ayalon and Van Gueluwe (1975). Considerable differences were found between old people and young ones as to their mechanical behavior in activities of daily living. The results of this study also indicate that emphasis should be placed on training older people in the correct and safe ways of performing different tasks and that a physical training program by itself, without skills training, may not be enough to avoid faulty mechanics.

In relation to the prevention of falls Agate (1966) and Steinberg (1966) agree that a deep understanding of the mechanics of the falls will permit the proper design of facilities and of rehabilitation and education of the subjects.

The purpose of the present study was to analyze the biomechanical changes resulting from a program especially designed to improve six skills of daily living that can be considered potential hazards for falls.

METHODS

Ten healthy women 60 to 75 years of age (mean age 65.3 ± 5.3) were filmed at 32 fps. with a Bolex movie camera before and after a 10-session training program while performing the following skills:

1. Climbing stairs
2. Going down stairs
3. Walking
4. Lifting an object
5. Stepping over an obstacle
6. Sitting on a chair

The films were digitized, and selected biomechanical variables were analyzed and compared for each skill. The variables analyzed for each skill are presented in Table 1.

During the sessions, in addition to conventional fitness exercises, special emphasis was given to teaching and practice in performing the six skills described above.

The descriptive statistics for all the measured variables are presented in Table 2.

A Wilcoxon Matched-pairs Signed-ranks Test was used to evaluate the statistical differences among the pre- and post-tests and the levels of significance for the variables shown in Table 2.

RESULTS AND DISCUSSION

Climbing Stairs

In this skill, slower times were found in the post-test as compared to the pre-test. This change was statistically significant. Since control of movement was emphasized during practice, this result was expected.

The trunk inclination decreased significantly from pre- to post-tests. During practice, subjects were taught to climb stairs in two phases, as opposed to the findings of Ayalon and Van Gueluwe (1975) that elderly women tend to include a first phase where hip flexion is performed and the whole body is kept in balance on the supporting leg. This phase is considered dangerous and thus should be avoided. The improvement in this parameter, less verticality of the trunk, shows that learning took place.

TABLE 1

Variables Analyzed for Each Skill

SKILL	VARIABLE
Climbing stairs	Duration of one step. Angle of the trunk with the horizontal plane, hip and knee of forward leg at maximal hip flexion.
Going down stairs	Duration of one step. Angle of the trunk with the horizontal plane, hip and knee of forward leg at maximal hip flexion.
Gait	Stride length. Walking speed. Angle of the hip at maximal flexion. Angle of the knee at maximal flexion (recovery phase).
Lifting	Angles of trunk with horizontal plane, hip and knee at contact with the lifted object. Heel contact (y/n). Distance of forefoot from center of lifted object.
Stepping over obstacle	Clearing height. Angle of trunk with horizontal plane, hip and knee at maximal flexion. Angle of knee of back leg recovery at maximal flexion. Step length.
Sitting	Maximal trunk inclination with horizontal plane. Angles of thigh and shank at maximal trunk inclination. Maximal trunk inclination at buttocks contact with chair. Time to sit (to vertical position of trunk).

No changes were found at the hip joint at maximal hip flexion, but significant changes at the 0.05 level were found at the knee joint. The knee was more flexed at the post-test, meaning, probably, more awareness of the dangers of hitting the stairs while climbing.

Going Down Stairs

In this activity, as found in climbing stairs, the stepping times were significantly slower. As mentioned before, control of movement was emphasized and it was expected that elderly subjects should go down stairs more slowly in order to avoid falls.

Trunk inclination was found to decrease from 90 degrees in the post-test. This result was not positive, as a more vertical position (close to 90 degrees) should be considered for safety importance.

No differences were found in the hip and knee angles.

TABLE 2

Descriptive Statistics for Pre- and Post-Tests

		PRE-TEST		POST-TEST		
SKILL	VARIABLE	$\overline{X}$	SD	$\overline{X}$	SD	P
Climbing stairs	Step duration (s)	0.60	0.11	0.88	0.14	*
	Trunk angle (degrees)	98.00	5.96	78.41	8.89	*
	Hip angle (degrees)	102.71	8.71	105.39	10.38	
	Knee angle (degrees)	89.57	9.86	84.86	8.29	*
Going down stairs	Step duration (s)	0.51	0.22	0.72	0.08	*
	Trunk angle (degrees)	86.44	5.99	83.84	7.82	*
	Hip angle (degrees)	125.43	7.25	122.43	11.12	
	Knee angle (degrees)	98.73	13.14	95.07	14.03	
Gait	Stride length (m)	0.83	0.12	0.91	0.10	
	Walking speed (m/s)	0.80	0.16	0.84	0.14	
	Hip angle (degrees)	148.56	6.68	148.86	5.76	
	Knee angle (degrees)	121.14	4.67	120.43	3.74	
Lifting	Trunk angle (degrees)	12.29	10.52	30.19	1.60	*
	Hip angle (degrees)	52.31	3.38	53.76	13.55	
	Knee angle (degrees)	119.26	25.18	86.84	18.43	*
	Foot-object dist. (m)	0.19	0.05	0.16	0.19	
Stepping over obstacle	Clearing height (m)	0.23	0.08	0.13	0.03	*
	Trunk angle (degrees)	110.76	30.65	95.90	6.53	*
	Hip angle (degrees)	104.83	36.55	92.14	12.50	
	Knee angle (degrees)	88.54	8.00	90.34	16.43	
	Step length (degrees)	0.92	0.09	0.95	0.07	
Sitting	Trunk inclination I	74.29	36.28	65.89	19.99	
	Thigh angle (degrees)	59.70	13.99	44.59	2.84	*
	Shank angle (degrees)	97.89	6.50	104.19	7.75	
	Trunk inclination II	60.54	6.37	58.19	9.07	
	Time to sit (s)	0.75	0.21	1.06	0.28	*

*$p<0.05$

Gait

No statistically significant differences were found in the measured parameters for the gait analysis.

Lifting

Observable improvement was found in this skill. Subjects learned to incline the trunk less while bending the knees ($p<0.05$), as shown by the trunk inclination and by the smaller angles at the knee joint.

Although some positive but not significant changes were found, the distance from feet to lifted object was not improved. This is a key factor for correct lifting, and more emphasis is required in practice in order to achieve better results.

Stepping Over Obstacle

In this skill, two variables were found to be significantly different from pre- to post-tests.

The clearing height decreased as the result of training and the trunk inclination decreased.

The change can be explained as the result of practice and confidence on the control of the height of the foot.

The second difference, as in climbing stairs, was the result of the teaching and practice of the skill. A backwards tilt of the trunk can be dangerous. The trunk inclination angle should be even lower than that found in the post-test for correct performance of the activity.

Sitting

Keeping the trunk vertical was emphasized during practice but the results do not indicate that this principle was learned.

The time to sit was improved in the post-test. More controlled movements were recommended during practice sessions in order to avoid the danger of falling onto the chair which can result in a backwards movement and consequent fall.

CONCLUSION

Six skills of daily life (climbing stairs, etc.) that can be considered potential hazards for falls were analyzed biomechanically from digitized motion pictures in 10 subjects before and after they participated in 10 teaching and practice sessions aimed at improving these skills. After completion of this program of instruction and practice, certain biomechanical measurements during these subjects' performance of the skills were observed to have changed from the subjects' pre-intervention values.

REFERENCES

Adrian MS. Biomechanics and Aging. In: Cooper JM, Haven B, eds. Proceedings of the CIC Biomechanics Symposium. Indiana University. 1980:132-40.

Agate H. Accidents to older people in their homes. Brit Med J 1966;2:5517.

Ayalon A, Van Gueluwe B. A comparison study of some mechanical variables from daily life activities in elderly and young people. In: Simri U, ed. Physical Exercise and Activity for the Aging. Israel: Wingate Institute, 1975:209-20.

Campbell AJ, Reinken J, Allan BC, Martinez GS. Falls in old age: a study of frequency and related clinical factors. Age Ageing 1981;10:264-70.

Murray PM, Drought AB, Kory RC. Walking patterns of normal men. J Bone Joint Surg 1964;46:335-60.

Prudham D, Evans JG. Factors associated with falls in the elderly: a community study. Age Ageing 1981;10:141-46.

Steinberg FU. Gait disorders in old age. Genetics 1966;12:134.

Stelmach GE, Teasdale N, DiFabio RP, Phillips J. Age related decline in postural control mechanisms. Int J Aging Hum Dev 1989;29:205-23.

Tinetti ME, Speechley M, Ginter SF. Risk factors for falls among elderly persons living in the community. N Engl J Med 1988;319:1701-07.

An Age-Comparison of Circadian Rhythms in Physical Performance Measures

Greg Atkinson B.Sc.(Hon)
Adam Coldwells B.Sc.(Hon)
Thomas Reilly B.A., M.Sc., Ph.D.
James M. Waterhouse B.A., D.Phil.

INTRODUCTION

Physiological functions which oscillate once around the length of the solar day (24 hours) are termed circadian rhythms. Human circadian rhythms are well documented in many parameters ranging from whole-body activity to biochemical processes at the cellular level (Minors and Waterhouse, 1981). Many rhythms occur as a direct result of fluctuations in the environment (exogenous rhythms) but others persist when environmental conditions are kept constant (endogenous rhythms). The generation of endogenous rhythms is thought to involve areas of the brain in and around the suprachiasmatic nuclei (Moore, 1978). Circadian rhythms in humans comprise both endogenous and exogenous influences, and fluctuate "in phase" with the body temperature rhythm, peaking in the early evening. Circadian rhythms can be characterized by calculating the parameters of a best fitting cosine curve which are the mesor (24-hour mean), the acrophase (peak-time) and the amplitude (difference between mesor and peak values).

Research regarding the impact of aging upon circadian rhythms (reviewed by Brock, 1991) has focused predominantly on body temperature, hormonal secretions, hematological parameters and the urinary excretion of metabolites. The most consistent findings of this research are a reduction in the amplitudes or a "flattening" of the rhythms, as well as a rise with age in the variability of rhythm acrophases. Some studies have reported that rhythm acrophases of elderly subjects occur earlier than normal in the solar day (Czeisler et al., 1986; Sharma et al., 1989; Lieberman et al., 1989), in agreement with other observations of increased "morningness" (a preference for high levels of activity in the morning) in old age (Monk et al., 1991). These age-related changes in circadian parameters have been related to the documented susceptibility of elderly subjects to such rhythm disturbances as shift work (Reinberg et al., 1988) and transmeridian travel (Winget et al., 1984).

Recent research (reviewed by Reilly, 1990) has shown that circadian rhythms exist in many performance variables including strength (Coldwells et al., 1991), short-term high power output (Reilly and Down, 1986), prolonged exercise performance (Reilly et al., 1984) and the physiological responses to exercise (Reilly and Brooks, 1990). It has also been shown that the intensity of exercise that athletes are voluntarily prepared to sustain varies with time of day (Atkinson et al., 1992a). The peak work-rate chosen at 18:00 hours is not perceived to feel harder than the lower work-rates chosen at any other times of the day (Coldwells et al., 1993). These rhythms provide direct evidence that an individual's ability to exercise is at its lowest in the early hours of the morning. Circadian rhythms in performance have important implications for sport as well as for optimizing productivity and safety in industrial contexts. To date, there has been no systematic study of how circadian rhythms in short-term or prolonged human performance are affected by aging.

The present study was designed to compare circadian rhythms relevant to exercise performance between groups of aged and young individuals.

METHODS

Subjects

Fourteen male subjects volunteered for the study. All subjects were made fully aware of the experimental procedures and signed a subject consent form. This sample was divided into groups of young ($\bar{x} \pm$ SD age = 23.6 ± 3.4 years, 18-29 years, n=7) and old ($\bar{x} \pm$ SD = 50.7 ± 4.1 years, 47-60 years, n=7) subjects. All subjects were physically active, competing regularly in sport. The characteristics of the two groups are presented in Table 1.

TABLE 1

Mean ± SD Characteristics of the Young (n=7) and Old (n=7) Groups

Parameter	Young Group	Old Group
Age (years) ***	23.6 ± 3.4	50.7 ± 4.1
Body mass (kg)	72.4 ± 9.1	80.0 ± 6.0
Height (m)	1.76 ± 0.05	1.73 ± 0.09
Energy expenditure for activities in leisure time. (MJ day)	2.12 ± 1.37	1.25 ± 0.78

Energy expenditure in leisure time was estimated using a questionnaire (Lamb and Brodie, 1991).

*** denotes a significant difference between the groups (p<0.001)

Experimental Design

A test battery was administered to each subject at 02:00, 06:00, 10:00, 14:00, 18:00 and 22:00 hours in a counterbalanced sequence (six subjects in each group started the experiment at each of the six different time points; the additional seventh subject in each group performed his first test battery at 10:00 hours). At least eight hours separated each test session to allow for recovery. Subjects were kept awake for the 02:00 hours test time. For the tests at 06:00 hours, subjects were awakened at 05:00 hours after at least six hours sleep. A familiarization session with the equipment and test protocols was completed by the subjects prior to the experiment. Pre-test diet, physical activity and alcohol consumption were controlled for each subject according to Reilly and Brooks (1982). Room temperature in the laboratory was 18-22° C. over the period of testing. The relative humidity was 60-65 percent.

Experimental Procedure

At each time-point, arousal was measured by asking each subject to place a mark on a 10 cm horizontal line between extremes of "Alert" and "Drowsy" (Hoddes et al., 1973). Rectal temperature was then recorded using a digital clinical thermometer (Phillips). Resting pulse rate was also recorded by palpating the radial artery.

Right and left grip strengths were assessed using a Takei Kiki Kogyo (Tokyo) grip dynamometer. Leg strength and back strength were measured using a portable dynamometer (Takei Kiki Kogyo, Tokyo). The postures for measurement were standardized according to Coldwells et al. (1991). Flight time in a vertical jump was measured by asking the subjects to jump vertically as high as possible off a pressure-activated mat (Bosco et al., 1983). The best of three trials was recorded for all these performance measures.

Subjects were required to complete a self-chosen work-rate test (Atkinson et al., 1993a) at each time point. This psychophysiological test, designed to quantify the amount of work a subject is prepared to sustain, is similar in principle to the rating of acceptable lift tasks that have been used in industrial contexts. In brief, the test consisted of three minutes of exercise on a cycle ergometer (MONARK) at a work-rate that the subject could sustain for 30 minutes. Mean power production was calculated with a BBC computer from the ergometer braking resistance (set at four percent of body mass) and the chosen pedal frequency.

No more than two subjects at a time were administered the test battery. Competition between the subjects on the performance tests was discouraged by the use of screens to separate them from a knowledge of each other's results. Verbal motivation given by the experimenters during the strength and power tests was standardized.

Statistical analysis

Group data for each measure were subjected to cosinor analysis (Nelson et al., 1979). This involves a least-squares regression algorithm to determine the cosine wave that best fits the group data. A sinusoidiality test was employed to indicate whether a sine wave or a more complex model best described the data. The mesor, amplitude and acrophase were calculated together with the confidence intervals for each parameter. Students' t-tests were employed to compare these parameters between young and old groups. Group differences in the measures recorded at each time of day were also examined with Students' t-tests. The alpha level of significance used in the present study was five percent ($p<0.05$).

RESULTS

No significant differences were found between the groups with respect to the 24-hour means (mesors) of the parameters, except in flight time measured in the vertical jump. The mean flight time was 563.6 ms for the young group compared to 516.5 ms in the old group ($p<0.05$).

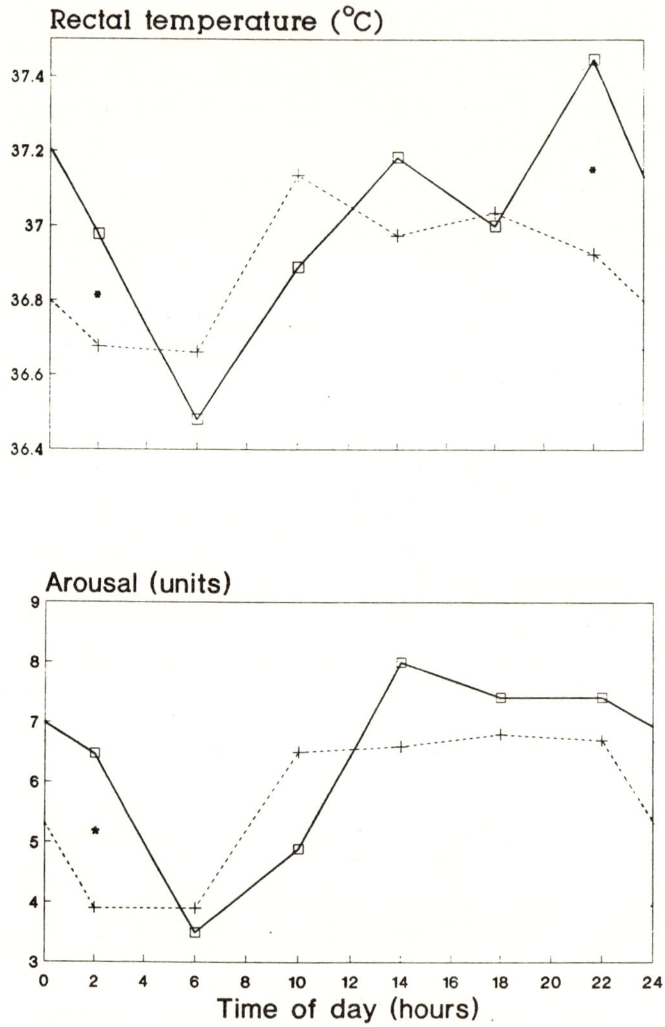

young □——□ old +-------+

* denotes a significant difference between the groups.

Figure 1. Circadian variation in rectal temperature and subjective arousal for the young and old groups.

It can be seen from Figure 1 that the circadian profiles of rectal temperature and arousal were different between the groups. Young subjects had significantly higher body temperature and arousal levels than aged subjects in the late evening and night (22:00 and 02:00 hours). The groups did not differ significantly in these parameters at the other times of day. Similar results were obtained when the scores for flight time in a vertical jump were compared between age-groups (Figure 2). The greatest difference between the groups was apparent

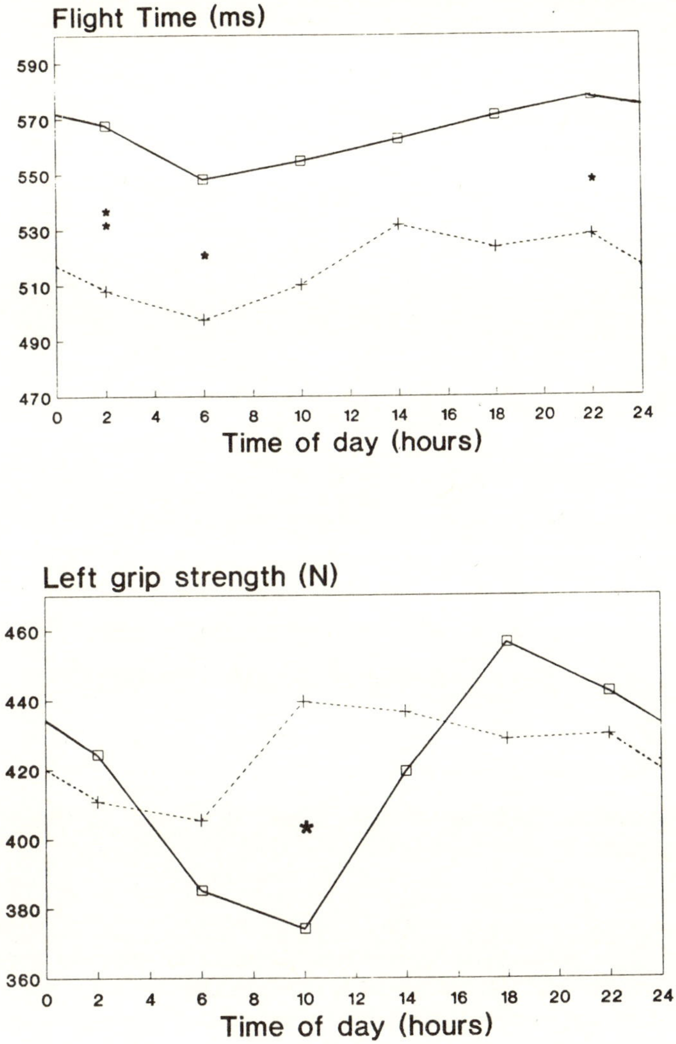

*(p<0.05) **(p<0.01) young □——□ old +------+

Figure 2. Circadian variation of flight time in a vertical jump and left grip strength for the young and old groups.

at 02:00 hours ($p<0.01$). For left grip strength (also Figure 2), the old subjects were actually significantly stronger than the young individuals but only at 10:00 hours ($p<0.05$). A similar trend was observed in the measure of self-chosen work-rate (Figure 3), although the group differences of 15 watts recorded at 10:00 and 14:00 hours did not reach statistical significance ($p>0.05$).

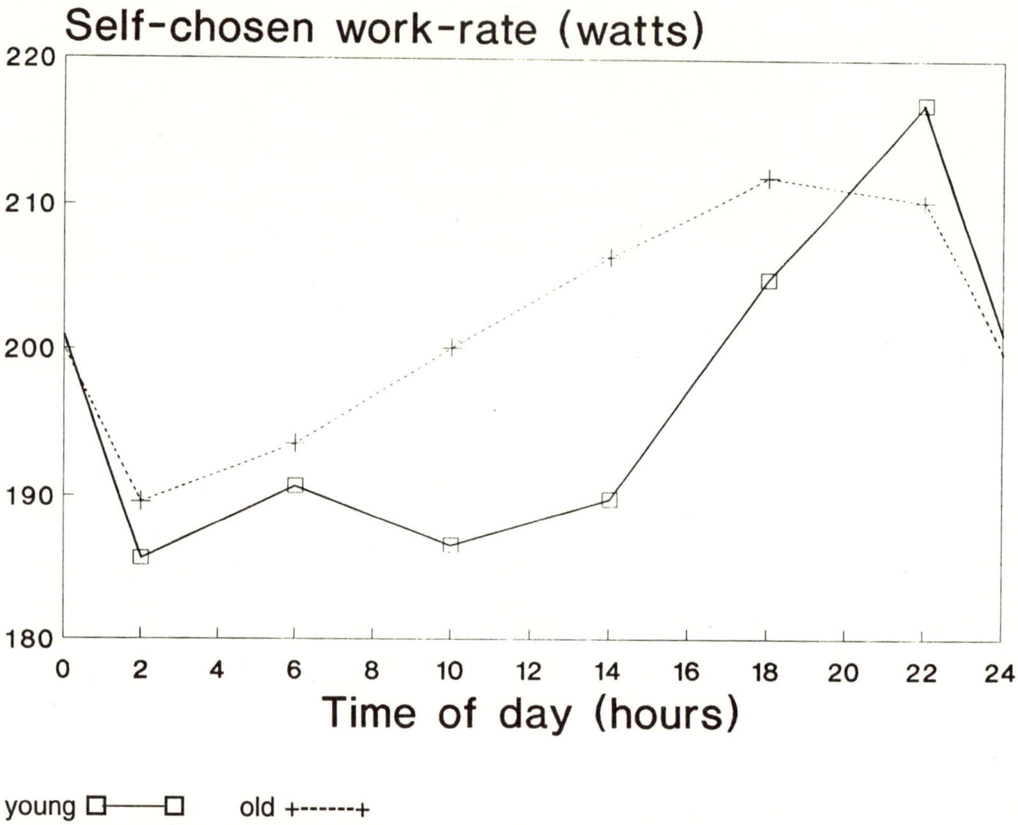

Figure 3. Circadian variation of self-chosen work-rate for the young and old groups.

Further analysis of the rhythm parameters, derived with the more powerful statistical technique of cosinor analysis, confirmed that the phasing of some circadian rhythms was different in elderly compared to young subjects (Figure 4). Significant circadian rhythmicity ($p<0.05$) was found for all measures in both groups except resting pulse rate in the old group. The sinusoidality test indicated that all significant rhythms were best described by a sine-wave ($p<0.05$), except those for back strength in both the young and the old groups. The circadian rhythm in back strength was characterized in both groups by a transient decline in performance in the afternoon. The fitted curves for rectal temperature and left grip strength peaked four to five hours earlier in the old group ($p<0.05$). Although rhythm acrophases in the other measures were not found to differ significantly when considered separately ($0.1>p>0.05$), the average acrophase for the six performance measures occurred 2.83 ± 1.48 hours earlier for the old group than for the young group ($p<0.01$).

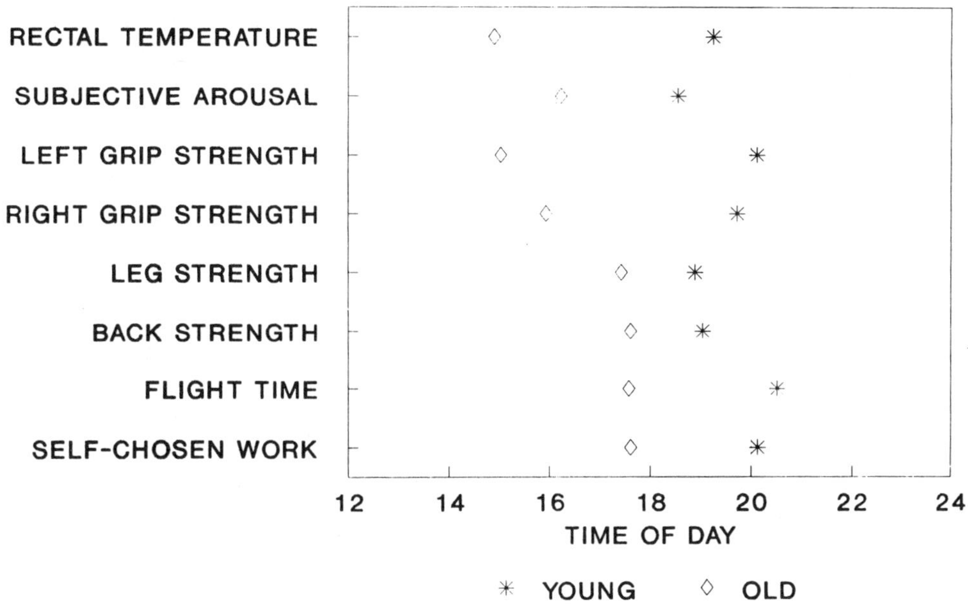

Figure 4. Rhythm acrophases (derived from cosinor analysis) for the measures in the young and old groups.

It can be seen in Figure 4 that some rhythm acrophases for the performance measures in the old group varied markedly from the acrophase of body temperature. This variance was used as a measure of "internal desynchronization." The mean phase deviation of the six performance measures from the body temperature rhythm was 2.0 hours in the old group compared to only 0.5 hours in the young group. A significant relation ($r=0.98$, $p<0.05$) was found in the old group between the deviation of each maximal performance measure from the body temperature rhythm and general performance of the old group (assessed by the comparison of the group 24-hour means in each performance measure). This relation is shown in Figure 5.

No effects of age were found on the rhythm amplitudes (Table 2), except for left grip strength and resting pulse rate (since this latter rhythm was found to be statistically significant in the young but not in the old group).

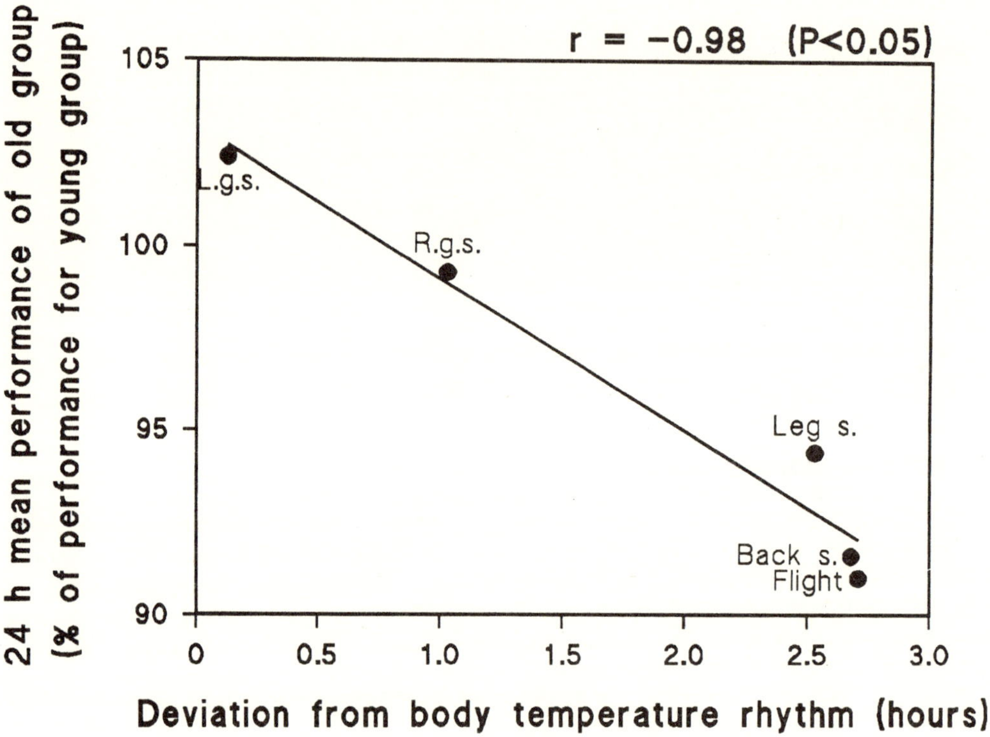

L.g.s. = left grip strength; R.g.s. = right grip strength; Leg s. = leg strength; Back s. = Back strength; Flight = Flight time in a vertical jump.

Figure 5. Relation between internal desynchronization and performance of the old group. Internal desynchronization is the time (in hours) the performance rhythm was out of phase with the body temperature rhythm. Performance of the old group is expressed as a percentage of the mesor for the young group. The mean performance of greater than 100 percent for L.g.s., for example, means that the old group performed better than the young group did over 24 hours.

TABLE 2

Mean Rhythm Amplitudes for the Young and Old Groups

Measure	Young Group	Old Group
Rectal Temp. (°C)	0.32	0.20
Arousal (units)	2.01	1.59
Pulse rate (% Mesor) *	5.86	NS**
Left grip (% Mesor) *	9.51	3.41
Right grip (% Mesor)	5.61	3.73
Leg strength (% Mesor)	7.27	7.86
Back strength (% Mesor)	6.82	7.02
Flight time (% Mesor)	2.36	3.02
S-C W-R (% Mesor)	6.05	5.03

The amplitudes of the rhythms in resting pulse rate and performance are expressed as percentages of the respective mesors.

* ($p<0.05$ for difference between the young and old groups)

** no significant rhythm found

DISCUSSION

The present study has confirmed with performance measures that there is a phase advance in the circadian rhythms of aged individuals. Monk et al. (1991) showed that increasing age is associated with earlier times of falling asleep and waking. This is manifested in age-related increases in "morningness" and earlier phasings of circadian rhythms in body temperature (Weitzman et al., 1982), cortisol secretion (Sharma et al., 1989) and arousal (Czeisler et al., 1986). These rhythms are believed to be most strongly related to physical and mental performance (Reilly, 1990). Lieberman et al (1989) monitored patterns of activity in a controlled environment with young and elderly subjects. In agreement with the present study, aged subjects reported less sleepiness in the morning and the acrophase of the activity rhythm peaked two hours earlier than for the young individuals. Van Gool and Mirmiran (1986) maintained that it is difficult to attribute these results to an aging effect on the endogenous circadian time-keeping system. It was argued that age-related changes in the sleep-wake cycle may be a reflection of a reduced social pressure to maintain a diurnal existence (i.e., retirement from work). However, several studies have reported changes in the sleep-wake cycle of elderly subjects even when the social environments of young and old subjects are identical (Weitzman et al., 1982; Czeisler et al., 1986).

Although the exact causes of age-related changes in the phasing of circadian rhythms are unclear, it is likely that the results of the present study have implications for the timing of veteran sports events and fitness tests as well as for the designing of shift work regimes for aged employees. Since the circadian rhythms of aged athletes are phase advanced, age differences in athletic performance may be reduced in the morning but exacerbated in the late evening (Figures 1-3). In addition, it could be argued that older shift workers would be most effectively employed on earlier shifts (e.g., morning) than younger workers. The results of studies involving animal models (Rosenberg et al., 1989; Buresova et al., 1990) may be relevant to this argument. Older animals required a significantly shorter time than young animals for their rhythms to adjust to an eight-hour phase advance of the light-dark cycle. Although this protocol was analogous to changing from an afternoon to a morning shift in human shift workers, further research is needed to confirm these results in humans.

There is evidence that the phasing of different circadian rhythms within individuals changes with age (Brock, 1991). It is postulated that an "uncoupling" of initially mutually coupled rhythms can occur more readily in aged subjects, resulting in a state termed "internal desynchronization." Research with young adults has established that most rhythms relevant to human performance are "coupled" to the body temperature rhythm (Reilly, 1990). In the present study, the acrophases of some performance rhythms in the old group were found to differ markedly (2.5 hours) from that of body temperature. Monk (1989) believed that such internal desynchronization could contribute to the deterioration in performance that is a characteristic of aging. This is supported by the fact that those athletes competing at the Los Angeles Olympics who had internally synchronized rhythms were more successful than athletes evidencing internal desynchronization (Reinberg et al., 1985). The negative relation between internal desynchronization and performance found in the present study meant that age differences in performance were greatest in those measures that were most inappropriately phased from body temperature (flight time, leg strength, back strength). This relation, however, may be restricted to measures of maximal performance since self-chosen work-rate on a cycle ergometer peaked 2.5 hours later than body temperature in the old group without affecting general performance.

The amplitudes of rhythms in physical performance seemed to be largely unaffected by age in the athletic subjects examined in this study. This is in contrast to the results of other circadian rhythm studies which have treated age as an independent variable (Weizman et al., 1982; Scheving et al., 1974). One of the most consistent findings in these studies is a decrease in amplitude of the body temperature rhythm, an observation which has also been found to be associated with poor tolerance to shift work in older workers (Reinberg et al., 1988). In the present study, some rhythm amplitudes were markedly lower in the old group compared to the young group (e.g., body temperature, arousal), but only the group differences in resting pulse rate and left grip strength reached statistical significance. Although this was probably due to the use of small sample sizes, it is possible that the results were influenced by the fact that the older subjects were athletes. Harma et al., (1982) and Atkinson et al. (1993b) reported that rhythm amplitudes are greater in subjects who carry out high levels of habitual physical activity and are physically fit. The athletic old group examined in the present study showed rhythm amplitudes in some measures that were higher than those of an inactive, unfit young group examined in the study by Atkinson et al., (1993b). This may indicate another benefit of maintaining physical activity in old age, that of prolonging efficient circadian rhythm control. Future research should confirm if physical fitness can reduce the age-related decline in circadian rhythm control.

CONCLUSION

Age differences in physical performance were found not to be consistent over the course of a day. This has implications for the scheduling of sports events, fitness tests and work shifts to veteran athletes.

REFERENCES

Atkinson G, Coldwells A, Reilly T, Waterhouse J. Circadian rhythmicity in self-chosen work-rate. In: Gutenbruner C, Hilderbrandt G, Moog R (eds). Chronobiology and Chronomedicine. Frankfurt: Peter Lang 1993a:478.

Atkinson G, Coldwells A, Reilly T, Waterhouse J. A comparison of circadian rhythms in work performance between physically active and inactive subjects. Ergonomics, 1993b;36:273-81.

Bosco CP, Luhtanen P, Komi P. A simple method for the measurement of power in jumping. Eur J Appl Physiol 1983;50:273-82.

Brock MA. Chronobiology and aging. J Am Geriatr Soc 1991;39:74-9.

Buresova M, Benesova O, Illnerova H. Aging alters resynchronisation of the circadian system in rats after a shift of the light-dark cycle. Eperientia 1990;46:75.

Coldwells A, Atkinson G, Reilly T. The validity and reliability of back and leg dynamometry. J Sports Sci 1991;9:334.

Coldwells A, Atkinson G, Reilly T, Waterhouse J. Self-chosen work-rate determines day-night differences in work capacity (abstr). Ergonomics 1993;36:313.

Czeisler CA, Rios CD, Sanchez R et al. Phase advance and reduction in amplitude of the endogenous circadian oscillator correspond with systematic changes in sleep-wake habits and daytime functioning in the elderly. Sleep Res 1986;15:268.

Harma MI, Ilmarinen J, Yletyinen I. Circadian variation of physiological functions in physically average and very fit dayworkers. J Human Ergol 1982;11(Suppl):33-46.

Hoddes E, Zarcone V, Smythe HR, Dement WC. Quantification of sleepiness: a new approach. Psychophysiol 1973;10:431-6.

Lamb, KR, Brodie DA. Leisure time physical activity as an estimate of physical fitness: a validation study. J Clin Epidemiol 1991;44:41-52.

Lieberman HR, Wurtman JJ, Teicher MH. Circadian rhythms of activity in healthy young and elderly humans. Neurobiol Aging 1989;10:59-265.

Minors D, Waterhouse J. Circadian Rhythms and the Human. London: Wright, PSG, 1981.

Monk TH. Circadian rhythm. Clin Geriatr Med 1989;5:331-46.

Monk TH, Reynolds III CF, Buysse DJ et al. Circadian characteristics of healthy 80-year-olds and their relationship to objectively recorded sleep. J Gerontol 1991;46:M171-5.

Moore RY. Central neural control of circadian rhythms. In Ganong WF, Martini L, eds. Frontiers in Neuroendocrinology, Vol 5. New York: Raven Press, 1978;185-206.

Nelson W, Tong TL, Lee J-K, Halberg F. Methods for cosinor-rhythmometry. Chronobiologia 1979;6:305-23.

Reilly T. Human circadian rhythms and exercise. Crit Rev in Biomed Eng 1990; 18:165-80.

Reilly T, Brooks G. Investigation of circadian rhythms in metabolic responses to exercise. Ergonomics 1982;25:1093.

Reilly T, Brooks G. Selective persistence of circadian rhythms in physiological responses to exercise. Chronobiol Internat 1990;7:59.

Reilly T, Down A. Time of day and performance on all-out arm ergometry. In: Reilly T, Watkins J and Borms J, eds. Kinanthropometry III. London: E and FN Spon 1986:296.

Reilly T, Robinson G, Minors DS. Some circulatory responses to exercise at different times of day. Med Sci Sports Exerc 1984;16:477.

Reinberg A, Proux S, Bartal J et al. Circadian rhythms in competitive sabre fencers: internal desynchronisation and performance. Chronobiol Internat 1985;2:195.

Reinberg A, Motohashi Y, Bourdeleau P et al. Alteration of period and amplitude of circadian rhythms in shift workers. Eur J Appl Physiol 1983;57:15-25.

Rosenberg RS, Zee PC, Turek FW. Age-related changes of hamster circadian rhythms. Sleep Res 1989;18:525.

Scheving, LE, Harrison WH, Gordan P Pauly JE. Circadian variation in residents of a senior citizens home. In: Scheving L, Halberg F, Pauly J, eds. Chronobiology. Tokyo: Igaku Shoin, 1974:353.

Sharma M, Palacios-bois J, Schwartz G et al. Circadian rhythms of melatonin and cortisol in aging. Biol Psychiatry 1989;25:305-9.

Van Gool, WA, Mirmiran M. Aging and circadian rhythms. Prog Brain Research 1986;70:255-77.

Weitzman, ED, Moline, ML, Czeisler CA, Zimmerman, JC. Chronobiology of ageing: temperature, sleep-wake rhythms and entrainment. Neurobiol Aging 1982;3:299-309.

Winget CM, DeRoshia CW, Markley CL et al. A review of physiological and performance changes associated with desynchronosis of biological rhythms. Aviat Space Environ Med 1984;55:1085-1096.

Section 3

Therapeutic Exercise and Practice

Prognostic Indicators of Rehabilitation in the Frail Elderly

Jaakko Valvanne, M.D., Ph.D., Elina Saloheimo, M.D.
Tuula Nurminen, Dr.P.H., Marjatta Ahonen, P.T. , Seija Salovaara, R.N.

INTRODUCTION

The ultimate goal of geriatric rehabilitation is to restore independence in activities of daily living often lost due to a medical or surgical event, so that patients can eventually return to home and family. The recovery from acute illnesses is often time consuming in the elderly because of multiple diseases and social dependence.

To avoid using scarce rehabilitative resources for patients unlikely to benefit from geriatric intervention, effective targeting strategies are needed. Criteria for targeting most commonly include age, physical disease, geriatric conditions, functional impairment, and social problems (Winograd, 1991).

The aims of this study were to identify those elderly patients who would benefit from active rehabilitation, improve the assessment of elderly patients in a general hospital, and call positive attention to a problematic patient group.

SUBJECTS

Subjects studied were 50 consecutive elderly, aged 65 years or more, admitted to the rehabilitation ward of Malmi City Hospital between November 1989 and May 1990. Patients were referred from acute medical wards of the same district hospital mainly because of stroke, multiple joint disease and mental incapacity. Either they needed a special rehabilitation program or their recovery from acute illness was slow and discharge to home seemed unlikely.

Of the study sample, 28 subjects were eventually discharged home, fourteen were permanently institutionalized, seven were referred to acute care because of worsening condition, and one patient died.

METHODS

The assessments were carried out within two days after admission to the rehabilitation ward. The physical disability was estimated with Barthel's ADL (Activities of Daily Living) index (Mahoney and Barthel, 1965, modified by Collin et al., 1988). The observers were trained nurses. The self-selected walking speed of those able to walk independently (with or without aids) was recorded. The apparatus used to measure walking speed consisted of a pair of infrared beams with photosensors mounted 2.0 m apart and 1.2 m above floor level, as recommended by Friedman et al., 1988 (Figure 1). The patients were asked to rate their health by using a ten centimeter continuum. Depression was assessed by a physician according to DSM III-criteria (American Psychiatric Association, 1980).

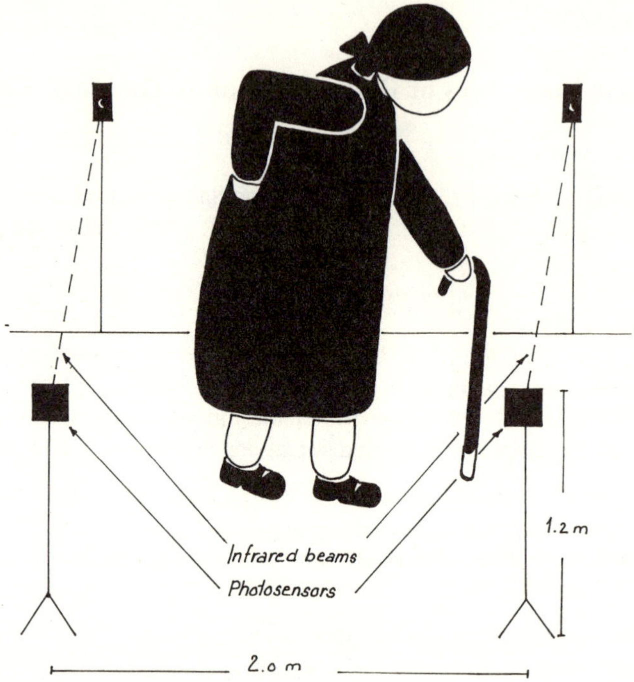

Figure 1. Measurement of self-selected gait speed

The estimates and confidence limits for the differences in discharge percentage were calculated according to the chi-square function procedure (Miettinen and Nurminen, 1985). To test for trend in the percentages according to the level of Barthel's index and gait speed, the chi-square statistic of Armitage was used (Armitage, 1955).

RESULTS

The results of the study are shown in Table 1. Age, sex or subjective health did not distinguish those discharged to home. In contrast, Barthel's scores and ability to walk were predictive of good outcome. The other indicators - primary diagnosis, gait speed and depressive state - were not statistically significant. The patients with locomotor disease had the highest discharge rate, but the differences in discharge between the main diagnosis groups were not statistically significant. Two-thirds of the patients could walk independently on admission, and 70 percent of those fastest in walking (> 0.6 m/s) were discharged home. However, walking speed's ability to predict the outcome did not reach statistical significance. The crude assessment of walking ability was more predictive: two-thirds of those able to walk independently were discharged home as compared with one third of those who were unable to walk without help.

TABLE 1

Prognostic Value of Different Indicators in Elderly Patients Admitted to Rehabilitation Ward

Indicator	N	Discharged home N	Discharged home %	Difference in discharge percentage[c]
Age (years)				
65 - 79	27	16	59	7 (-20, 34)
80 +	23	12	52	
Sex				
male	14	9	64	12 (-19, 38)
female	36	19	53	
Main diagnosis				
locomotor disease	8	6	75	28 (-15, 60)
cerebrovascular accident	19	11	58	11 (-22, 42)
mental deterioration	8	4	50	3 (-37, 43)
other	15	7	47	
Barthel's index				
17-20	15	12	80[d]	40 (4, 67)
9-16	20	10	50	10 (-23, 41)
0-8	15	6	40	
Ambulation				
able	35	23	66	32 (2, 57)
unable	15	5	33	
Gait speed (m/s)				
≥ 0.6	10	7	70[e]	29 (-11, 59)
≥ 0.4 - < 0.6	14	9	64	23 (-13, 53)
> 0.0 - < 0.4	9	5	56	14 (-25, 50)
0[a]	17	7	41	
Subjective health[b]				
poor	15	9	60	7 (-27,39)
fair	18	10	56	3 (-29, 34)
good	17	9	53	
Major depression				
no assessment	11	7	64	35 (-13, 69)
no	32	19	59	31 (-10, 59)
yes	7	2	29	

[a]unable to walk, [b]using a ten centimeter continuum: good <4.7 cm, fair from ≥4.7 cm to <7.6 cm, poor ≥7.6 cm, [c]95% confidence interval in parenthesis, [d]test for trend in percentages: χ^2 = 4.8, P = 0.03, [e]test for trend in percentages: χ^2 = 2.6, P = 0.11.

The better the physical functioning, the better the outcome. Discharge to home was twice as common in the group with high scores (from 17 to 20) of Barthel's ADL index as in the group that scored eight points or less. Subjective health was not associated with discharge home, but the patients with depression had low discharge rates. However, because the number of patients with the diagnosis of major depression was only seven, the study was inconclusive when discharge of this group was considered.

DISCUSSION

The major aim of the study was to find simple measurements that could help identify elderly patients who would benefit from active rehabilitation after acute medical conditions. In agreement with previous studies (Isaacs, 1965; Stewart, 1980), the results suggest that good physical functioning in daily activities is of prognostic value.

Age of the patients is one of the most important determinants of outcome in stroke rehabilitation, the difference being most obvious between age groups under and over 65 years (Isaacs and Marks, 1973). In this study, older age itself did not have prognostic significance among patients above 65 years.

Although cognitive disturbance worsens prognosis according to some studies (Isaacs, 1965; Isaacs and Marks, 1973), mental deterioration did not affect the outcome of the subjects in this study. Similarly, the prognosis in the other main diagnostic groups did not differ from each other convincingly.

Gait speed is an objective but inexpensive method of monitoring gait rehabilitation in the elderly. It is a valid measure of mobility, correlates closely with any aid being used (Wade et al., 1987), and relates to the frequency of falls (Wolfson et al., 1990). Serial recordings showing improvement in walking speed have proved useful in predicting eventual independent mobility of poorly mobile subjects, and walking speed at discharge clearly separates those requiring long-term hospital care from those sufficiently mobile to be discharged home (Friedman et al., 1988).

In this study, the association of discharge home with gait speed on admission was not statistically significant in trend analysis. Serial records might be more informative. The crude assessment of ambulation ability was more predictive.

Subjective health has been considered a useful prognostic indicator of predicting future changes in daily functioning (Grand et al., 1988; Mor et al., 1989), but in this study it did not predict those elderly patients who would benefit from comprehensive rehabilitation.

Nearly one-third of those patients who were properly assessed for mood had major depression, in agreement with the previous finding in a rehabilitation hospital that 28 percent of the patients were clinically depressed (Gans, 1981). In the present study, the frequency of being discharged to home was reduced by half in the depressive group, but this difference did not reach statistical significance. Of course, diagnosing and treating depression in the slowly recovering frail elderly is of crucial importance.

No single instrument seems to be sensitive enough for the identification of those elderly who would benefit from intensive rehabilitation. Functional assessment is important in predicting the future outcome. Although the prognosis of those elderly who have lost their independence during an acute episode seems to be poor, some of them recover eventually.

REFERENCES

American Psychiatric Association: Diagnostic and Statistical Manual of Mental Disorders, 3rd ed. Washington, DC: American Psychiatric Association, 1980.

Armitage P. Tests for linear trends in proportions and frequencies. Biometrics 1955;11:375-86.

Collin C, Wade DT, Davies S, Horne V. The Barthel ADL index: a reliability study. Int Disabil Studies 1988; 10:61-3.

Friedman PJ, Richmond DE, Baskett JJ. A prospective trial of serial gait speed as a measure of rehabilitation in the elderly. Age Ageing 1988;17:227-35.

Gans JS. Depression diagnosis in a rehabilitation hospital. Arch Phys Med Rehabil 1981;62:386-9.

Grand A, Grosclaude P, Bocquet H, Pous J, Albarede JL. Predictive value of life events, psychosocial factors and self-rated health on disability in an elderly rural French population. Soc Sci Med 1988;27:1337-42.

Isaacs B. Prognostic factors in elderly patients in a geriatric institution. Gerontol Clin 1965;7:202-15.

Isaacs B, Marks R. Determinants of outcome of stroke rehabilitation. Age Ageing 1973;2:139-49.

Mahoney FL, Barthel DW. Functional evaluation: the Barthel Index. Maryland State Med J 1965;14:61-5.

Miettinen O, Nurminen M. Comparative analysis of two rates. Stat Med 1985; 4:213-26.

Mor V, Murphy J, Masterson-Allen S et al. Risk of functional decline among well elders. J Clin Epidemiol 1989;42:895-904.

Stewart CPU. A prediction score for geriatric rehabilitation prospects. Rheumatol Rehabil 1980;19:239-45.

Wade DT, Wood VA, Heller A, Maggs J, Hewer RL. Walking after stroke. Scand J Rehab Med 1987;19:25-30.

Winograd CH. Targeting strategies: an overview of criteria and outcomes. J Am Geriatr Soc 1991;39:25S-35S.

Wolfson L, Whipple R, Amerman P, Tobin JN. Gait assessment in the elderly: a gait abnormality rating scale and its relation to falls. J. Gerontol 1990; 45:M12-19.

Predictors of Declining Mobility

Jaakko Valvanne, M.D., Ph.D.
Timo Erkinjuntti, M.D., Ph.D.
Reijo Tilvis, M.D.

INTRODUCTION

Disability is a serious threat to independent living, and its prevention is a major task for geriatricians and health professionals. In the eighties and early nineties, several studies were published on the risks of changes in the functional status of the aged (Palmore et al., 1985; Pinsky et al., 1987; Lichtenstein and Thomas, 1987; Colvez et al., 1987; Grand et al., 1988; Manton, 1988; Guralnik and Kaplan 1989; Harris et al., 1989; Jagger et al., 1989; Lammi et al., 1989; Mor et al., 1989; Jette and Branch, 1990; Reuben et al., 1990). However, predictors of declining mobility are less well established.

In the Helsinki Aging Study, the data from a random sample of the aged population were analyzed in order to determine whether health, well-being and functional capacity are predictive of changes in mobility. Special attention was paid to different diseases and symptoms.

SUBJECTS

The study involved a random sample of persons born in 1904, 1909 and 1914 and registered in Helsinki city. The random sample consisted of 795 subjects, of whom 651 (82 percent) attended a clinical examination (Table 1). Five hundred and fifty-four (554) of them were not bedridden at entry (including wheelchair-bounds) and were reexamined one year later.

METHODS

The comprehensive assessment consisted of a structured interview by public health nurses and a clinical examination by general practitioners.

The assessment of mobility was carried out by the examining physician in the basic study and by the nurse at follow-up. The five hierarchical stages of mobility were:

1. No difficulties: independently without any aid.
2. Minor difficulties: independently with a cane.
3. Moderate difficulties: able to move independently only with assistance of other aids (e.g., crutches, walker or wheel chair).
4. Major difficulties: needs assistance by one person (includes being wheeled by one person).
5. Unable: bedridden.

TABLE 1

Subjects Studied

Age (years)	Gender	Random sample	Subjects studied originally	Non-Bedridden subjects followed for one year
75	Men	84	73	61
	Women	190	166	151
80	Men	74	59	52
	Women	192	153	130
85	Men	54	44	34
	Women	201	156	126
Total		795	651	554

Objective health, need of care and intellectual functioning were assessed by the physician at entry, according to following ratings:

1. objective health: healthy, fairly healthy, sick, very sick.
2. need of care: independent, needing help in heavy duties, needing help in light duties, needing help in basic activities of daily living (ADL's).
3. dementia: healthy (CDR 0), questionable dementia (CDR 0.5), mild dementia (CDR 1), moderate dementia (CDR 2), severe dementia (CDR 3) (Hughes, 1982).

Statistical analyses were performed using standard BMDP software (Dixon 1988). The frequencies were compared using Chi-square test (BMDP 4F), and the independent associations of the main correlates with declining mobility were analyzed using stepwise logistic regression analysis (BMDP LR). The 95 percent confidence intervals for the population values of odds ratios and relative risks were calculated (Morris and Gardner, 1989). The standardization of rates of declining mobility was carried out by the indirect method (Armitage, 1971).

RESULTS

The percentage of the 651 participants living in institutions, i.e., in homes for the elderly, in nursing homes or in hospitals, was eight, 17 and 31 percent of the 651 subjects, respectively, in the age groups of 75, 80 and 85 years.

According to the cross-sectional data, the percentage of physically disabled doubled with every five years of age of the subjects (Table 2). Nearly 90 percent of the 75-year-olds walked independently without cane or other aid, whereas only one of two of the 85-year-olds could walk without aids, and one of ten among them was bedridden. Sex differences were insignificant.

TABLE 2

Mobility Distribution (Percent) in Random Age Cohorts in Helsinki in 1989

	Age (years)		
Mobility	**75**	**80**	**85**
No difficulties	87	75	49
Minor difficulties	7	13	24
Moderate difficulties	4	5	13
Major difficulties	<1	3	6
Bedridden	2	4	9

Statistical significance between age-groups: $p<0.001$

Of the 144 drop-outs, 95 percent were known to live at home, the rest in institutions. The mobility of 58 refusers was determined by a telephone interview carried out by one of the authors(JV). No significant differences in mobility distribution between them and the study participants was found.

The capability of moving remained unchanged in the majority of the subjects within one year (Figure 1). One of ten of the 75-year-olds and one of five among the older groups deteriorated. In a minority the mobility even improved. These changes were equally frequent in both genders.

Table 3 shows that declining locomotion was associated with some sociodemographic factors (i.e., institutionalization and need of home care), poor quality of life and symptoms such as dizziness and tendency to fall.

Figure 2 demonstrates that both the initial need of care and initial objective health correlated with changes in the capability of moving. Thus, in less than 10 percent of the healthiest the mobility deteriorated, whereas the respective figure was about 30 percent in the group of the very sick and ADL-dependent. The same tendency was obvious concerning the number of regular drugs, difficulties in daily duties and disabling diseases (Figure 3). Only a few of the subjects free of disabling diseases declined, compared to one-third of the subjects with many disabling diseases.

According to the logistic regression analysis, three clinical observations (abnormal gait, dyspnea on exertion and kyphosis) were major independent risk factors for deteriorating mobility (Table 4). Of the diagnosed diseases, peripheral arterial diseases, heart failure, and dementia were the most important predictors of deteriorating mobility.

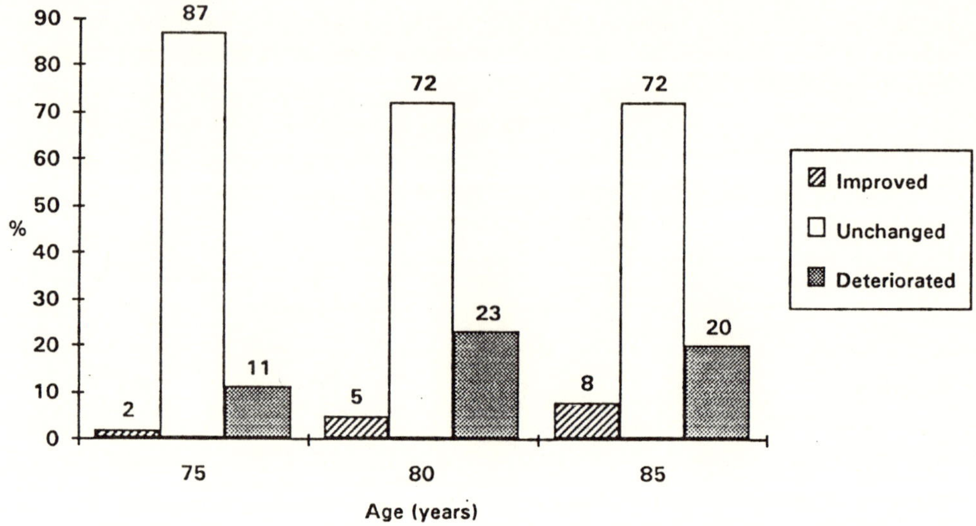

Figure 1. Changes in mobility (percent) in ambulatory subjects within one year by age

Age and sex were also included in both logistic regression analyses, but they were non-significant.

Interestingly, slight abnormalities at base-line examination clearly predicted deterioration of mobility within one year (Table 5). That was evident, e.g., for abnormalities in walking, kneeling and posture. Presence of slight difficulties were associated with doubling the risk of decreased mobility.

DISCUSSION

The study was performed in a random sample of 75, 80 and 85-year-old people living both at home and in institutions. It was characterized by a relatively low number of drop-outs (18 percent), who did not differ markedly from the study participants. Thus, this study reveals quite accurately the prevalence of locomotor difficulties in an elderly urban population.

According to the present data, mobility remained fairly stable during one-year follow-up. In one of five (11 to 23 percent) it declined and in one of twenty (two to eight percent) it improved within one year, which is in agreement with two comparable studies. Reuben et al. (1990) followed elderly (65+) Medicare beneficiaries for one year and found that 20 percent of the subjects declined in their advanced activities of daily living (AADL) level, 63 percent showed no change and 17 percent improved their exercise level. Similarly, when the stability of instrumental and basic activities (IADL and BADL) of another group of Medicare beneficiaries was followed for one year, 14 percent of both 75 to 84 and 85+-year-olds improved, whereas 17 percent and 23 percent deteriorated, respectively (Lichtenstein et al., 1987).

TABLE 3

Significant Odds Ratios of Variables Associated with Deteriorating Mobility within One Year

Variable	Odds Ratio	95 Percent Confidence Interval
Sociodemographic factors:		
Institutionalization	2.1	(1.2 - 3.7)
Need of home care*	2.2	(1.0 - 4.6)
Quality of life:		
Poor subjective health*	1.8	(1.1 - 2.9)
Feeling of uselessness*	2.2	(1.3 - 3.6)
Use of analgetics*	1.9	(1.1 - 3.1)
Symptoms:		
Dizziness*	1.8	(1.1 - 3.0)
Falling tendency*	1.6	(1.0 - 2.7)
Clinical signs:		
Abnormal gait	3.3	(2.1 - 5.2)
Difficulties in undressing	1.9	(1.1 - 3.3)
Dyspnea on slight exertion	2.8	(1.5 - 5.2)
Kyphosis	2.8	(1.8 - 4.4)
Poor vision	2.2	(1.3 - 3.8)
Diagnoses:		
Myocardial infarction	1.7	(1.0 - 3.0)
Heart failure	2.0	(1.3 - 3.0)
Peripheral arterial disease	2.5	(1.6 - 3.9)
Transient ischemic attack	1.9	(1.0 - 3.4)
Stroke	2.0	(1.0 - 4.1)
Dementia	2.0	(1.2 - 3.6)
Urinary incontinence	2.5	(1.5 - 4.2)

The following factors were also tested by X^2 test: gender, marital status, social class, depressive mood, smoking and drinking habits, use of hypnotics, headache, arthralgias, nausea, auscultation of heart and lungs, blood pressure, hearing, diabetes mellitus, angina pectoris, atrial fibrillation, hypertension, chronic obstructive pulmonary diseases, Parkinson's disease, major depression and malignant diseases. They did not show any statistically significant association with declining mobility.

* refers to non-institutionalized subjects.

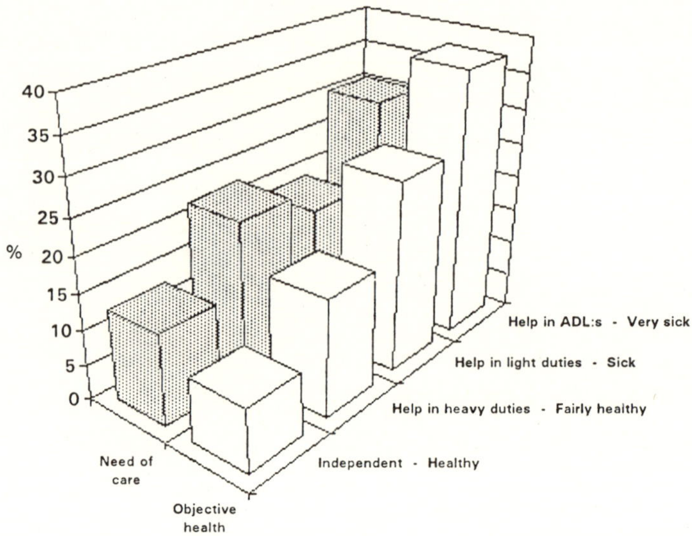

Figure 2. Age adjusted rates (percent) of declining mobility according to the need of care and objective health

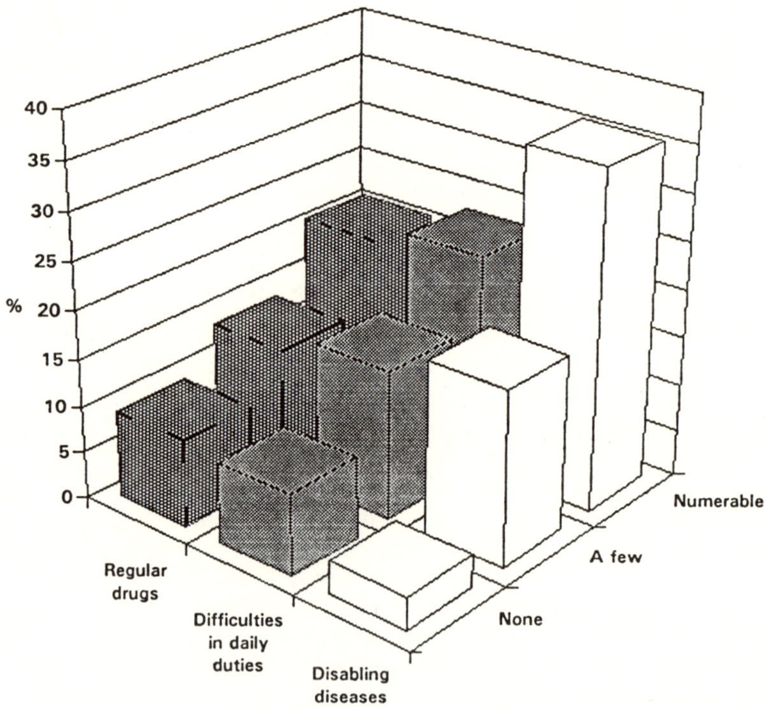

Figure 3. Age-adjusted rates (percent) of deteriorating mobility according to the number of drugs, difficulties in daily duties and disabling diseases

TABLE 4

Clinical Findings and Diagnoses as Independent Risk Factors for Deteriorating Mobility

Variable	Risk Ratio	95 Percent Confidence Interval
Clinical finding		
Abnormal gait	1.8	(1.4 - 2.5)
Dyspnea on slight exertion	1.5	(1.1 - 2.1)
Kyphosis	1.3	(1.0 - 1.7)
Disease		
Peripheral arterial disease	1.4	(1.1 - 1.8)
Heart failure	1.3	(1.0 - 1.6)
Dementia	1.3	(1.0 - 1.6)

In the present study general health and well-being were closely associated with changes in mobility. In previous studies, subjective health (Grand et al., 1988; Mor et al., 1989), feelings of uselessness (Grand et al., 1988) and falling tendency (Mor et al., 1989) have been associated with declining functional ability. In keeping with these observations, the associations of global ratings, i.e., objective health and need of care, with declining mobility are also clear after adjusting for age.

This study showed that cognitive impairment, heart failure and peripheral vascular diseases are serious medical threats to independence. The previous results concerning the importance of heart and circulatory diseases and dementia have been contradictory. Their association with declining mobility has been demonstrated in several studies (Palmore et al., 1985; Colvez et al., 1987; Harris et al. 1989; Grand et al., 1988; Lammi et al., 1989), although some studies have failed to reveal any relationship (Colvez et al., 1987; Guralnik and Kaplan, 1989; Mor et al., 1989).

The most important observation of the present study was the clinical significance of mild disturbances. Minor impairments, regardless of their causes and sites, seemed to predict a progressive decline in physical functioning. The importance of slight difficulties as an indicator of further decline has also been highlighted in two recent studies (Manton, 1988; Harris et al., 1989).

According to these results, more attention should possibly be paid to those individuals who initially have only mild manifestations of their disability. Whether this progressive decline can be prevented or postponed by exercise or by other therapeutic measures should be studied.

TABLE 5

Percent of Subjects with Deteriorating Mobility within One Year by Degree of Disability at Entry

	Age (years)		
Clinical finding	**75**	**80**	**85**
Walking			
normal	7	15	15
slightly abnormal	25	43	26
obviously abnormal	24**	38***	26
Kneeling			
normal	8	13	9
slightly abnormal	13	29	22
obviously abnormal	19	35**	30*
Standing up from a chair			
normal	8	20	22
slightly abnormal	26	36	17
obviously abnormal	27***	27	26
Undressing			
normal	8	23	21
slightly abnormal	40	19	15
obviously abnormal	38***	40	41
Posture			
normal	9	18	15
slight kyphosis	25	32	23
moderate/severe kyphosis	22*	44*	44*

Statistical significance between groups: $^*p<0.05$, $^{**}p<0.01$, $^{***}p<0.001$

REFERENCES

Armitage P. Statistical Methods in Medical Research. Oxford: Blackwell Scientific Publications, 1971:384-91.

Colvez A, Robine JM, Jouan-Flahault CH. Risk and risk factors of disability in the elderly. Rev Epidemiol Sante Publique 1987;35:257-69.

Dixon WJ (Ed.). BMDP Statistical Software Manual. Berkeley: University of California Press, 1988.

Grand A, Grosclaude P, Bocquet H, Pous J, Albarede JL. Predictive value of life events, psychosocial factors and self-rated health on disability in an elderly rural French population. Soc Sci Med 1988;27:1337-42.

Guralnik JM, Kaplan GA. Predictors of healthy aging: prospective evidence from the Alameda Study. Longitudinal study of physical ability in the oldest-old. Am J Public Health 1989;79:703-8.

Harris T, Kovar MG, Suzman R, Kleinman JC, Feldman JJ. Longitudinal study of physical ability in the oldest-old. Am J Public Health 1989;79:698-702.

Hughes CP, Berg L, Danziger WL, Coben LA, Martin RL. A new clinical scale for the staging of dementia. Brit J Psychiat 1982;140:566-72.

Jagger C, Clarke M, Cook AJ. Mental and physical health of elderly people: five-year follow-up of a total population. Age Ageing 1989;18:77-82.

Jette AM, Branch LG, Berlin J. Musculoskeletal impairments and physical disablement among the aged. J Gerontol 1990;45:M203-208.

Lammi U-K, Kivela S-L, Nissinen A, Punsar S, Puska P, Karvonen M. Predictors of disability in elderly Finnish men - a longitudinal study. J Clin Epidemiol 1989;42:1215-25.

Lichtenstein RL, Thomas JW. A comparison of self-reported measures of perceived health and functional health in an elderly population. J Community Health 1987;42:213-30.

Manton KG. A longitudinal study of functional change and mortality in the United States. J Gerontol 1988;43:S153-61.

Mor V, Murphy J, Masterson-Allen S et al. Risk of functional decline among well elders. J Clin Epidemiol 1989;42:895-904.

Morris JA, Gardner MJ. Calculating confidence intervals for relative risks, odds ratios, and standardised ratios and rates. In: Gardner MJ, Altman DG, eds. Statistics with confidence. Confidence intervals and statistical guidelines. Br Med J, 1989:50-63.

Palmore EB, Nowling JB, Wang HS. Predictors of function among the old-old: a 10-year follow-up. J Gerontol 1985;40:244-50.

Pinsky JL, Leaverton PE, Stokes J. Predictors of good function: the Framingham study. J Chron Dis 1987;40:159-67S.

Reuben DB, Laliberte L, Hiris J, Mor V. A hierarchical exercise scale to measure function at the advanced activities of daily living (AADL) level. J Am Geriatr Soc 1990;38:855-61.

Aerobic Exercise Lowers Biological Age of Patients with Coronary Heart Disease or Hypertension

Kiyoji Tanaka, Ph.D., Masaki Takeda, M.S., Yoko Hayakawa, M.S.
Katsumi Asano, Ph.D., Yoshiyuki Matsuura, Ph.D., Yutaka Watanabe, M.D.
Teruo Hiyama, M.D.

INTRODUCTION

Aging might be defined as the loss of an individual's ability to adapt to his/her environment (Smith, 1980). Shock et al. (1984) defines it as more the result of an interaction among many specific characteristics within an individual than of a single process. Even though aging is inevitable, it is clear that by maintaining moderate to high levels of physical conditioning the individual can have the functional capacity of the average person who is 20 or more years younger (Tanaka et al., 1990a). In this context, the authors of the present study have recently developed a useful equation for estimating vital age or the so-called biological age (sometimes referred to as functional age or physiological age) of Japanese people (Tanaka et al., 1990b, 1991a, 1991b). The difference between vital age and commonly used biological age is that the former is predicted through the assessment of various factors measured not only under resting conditions but also under exercise conditions.

Blair et al. (1989) found, from the review of 10 longitudinal studies reported in the literature, an inverse relationship between physical work capacity, maximal oxygen uptake, or heart rate during submaximal exercise and future risk of coronary heart disease. There is an accumulated body of evidence that moderate exercise can produce higher levels of physical fitness which may protect against early mortality (Blair et al., 1989; Ekelund et al., 1988; Leon et al., 1987; Paffenbarger et al., 1986; Pekkanen et al., 1987). The hypothesis is that the initiation of an appropriate exercise program can slow the rate of mortality or aging and partially reverse the effects of a sedentary lifestyle even in middle-aged and older persons. The purpose of this study was to evaluate the effects of a six-month exercise program on vital age in patients with coronary heart disease or essential hypertension.

TABLE 1

Equations for Calculating Vital Age of Japanese Women

$$VA = 8.90\ VAS + 49.0 + Z$$

$$VAS = .016X_1 + .011X_2 + .004X_3 + .004X_4 + .004X_5 + .034X_6 -064X_7 -12X_8 -.037X_9 -.005X_{10} -.367X_{11} -1.035,$$

$$Z = .33X_{12} -16.17 \text{ (for age correction)};$$

where X_1 = abdominal girth (cm), X_2= systolic blood pressure (mm Hg), X_3= cholesterol (mg/dl), X_4 = low-density lipoprotein cholesterol (mg/dl), X_5 = triglycerides (mg/dl), X_6= hematocrit (%).
X_7 = oxygen uptake corresponding to lactate threshold (ml/kg/min)
X_8 = heart rate corresponding to lactate threshold (b/min)
X_9= side step, X_{10} = single leg balance with eyes closed (s)
X_{11} = forced expiratory volume for one second (1), and
X_{12} = chronological age.

VA: vital age, VAS: vital age score, Z: correction factor

SUBJECTS

Twenty-four female patients with coronary heart disease (52.6 ± 7.6 yr, n=12) or essential hypertension (51.0 ± 9.7 yr, n=12) who were between the ages of 40 and 69 years, served as subjects. The cardiac patients had either stable angina pectoris, coronary artery spasm, well-documented previous myocardial infarction, or a coronary artery bypass grafting operation within the prior two years. Most of these patients had angiographically confirmed coronary artery disease but were considered to be in New York Heart Association functional class I or II. Only two patients experienced slight ischemic pain (claudication) during exercise. The hypertensive patients had a clinical history of mild/moderate hypertension and were classified as WHO stages I-II. All the 24 subjects were non-smokers. The study design was reviewed and approved by the Tsukuba Health/Fitness Study Committee Review Board for the Use of Human Subjects. Informed consent was obtained from both patient and her spouse before any patient was allowed to participate in the study.

Most patients were taking one or more medications for management of their cardiovascular and/or other medical conditions. Those medications included beta-adrenergic blocking agents (n=5), vasodilators (n=4), digitalis (n=1), antiarrhythmic agents (n=3), hyperlipidemia agents (n=2), calcium channel blockers (n=13), etc. No alteration in the medication regimen occurred throughout the entire study period with the exception of one patient in each group. The control group (n=11) consisted of six patients with coronary heart disease and five patients with essential hypertension, aged from 44 to 69 years (53.2 ± 8.5), and were prescribed medications similar to those for the experimental groups.

METHODS

Exercise Program and Other Interventions

Table 2 illustrates a medically supervised, exercise-based rehabilitation program, designed with the belief that the initiation of physical conditioning can slow the rate of decline in functional capacity and improve prognosis of cardiac disease or hypertension (Tanaka et al., 1986, 1989). The subjects participated in the exercise conditioning program two sessions per week, 90 to 120 minutes each session, for a period of six months, and also an unsupervised exercise conditioning program 2.4 ± 0.6 days per week, 30-40 minutes each session, throughout the entire study.

Each conditioning session was supervised by at least two of the authors and/or experienced exercise instructors. The unsupervised, self-controlled program consisted of calisthenics, walking or jogging, non-device muscular exercise, and stretching. The intensity of exercise was set, on the average, at an individually determined work rate corresponding to lactate threshold (Tanaka et al., 1986, 1989). Goals of the program were individualized to meet the needs of each patient (ACSM, 1991). The contents of both supervised and unsupervised programs appeared to be equivalent in the two groups.

TABLE 2

In-Hospital Supervised Exercise Program

1.	Warm-up: calisthenics, stretching	15-20 min
2.	Leg cycling or walking at a work rate corresponding to lactate threshold	30-40 min
3.	Non-device muscle exercises and flexibility exercises	20-30 min
4.	Cool-down: stretching	10 min

Perceived exertion (12 to 14 in Borg's 15-grade scale ranging from 6 to 20), work rate, heart rate, breathing pattern, and/or blood pressure were periodically monitored as a training clue in all patients. Continuous electrocardiographic (ECG) monitoring during the exercise program was also done in patients judged to be at increased cardiac risk.

Measurement of Lactate Threshold

The test began with a two-minute period of warm-up cycling at 60 revolutions per minute without load and then for one minute at 15 watts. The test continued by increasing the work load by 15 watts every minute until symptoms limited further exercise or the authors terminated the exercise. Only three of the 24 patients were controlled with antiarrhythmics or digitalis at the time of testing. The oxygen uptake ($\dot{V}O_2$), work rate, and heart rate corresponding to lactate threshold were measured during the cycling exercise test. All metabolic measurements of expiratory gases were determined by standard techniques of open-circuit spirometry with Fukuda Sangyo IS-5000 System.

Multiple samples of venous blood (1 ml each) were drawn from the antecubital vein every minute during exercise. The lactate threshold was defined as the point in exercise of increasing intensity at which lactate (La) concentration abruptly increased in a non-linear fashion. For discerning the point, the log [$\dot{V}O_2$]-log{La} transformation method was used.

Computation of vital age

The rationale behind the concept and computation of vital age has been described in detail by Tanaka et al. (1990b, 1991a, 1991b), and is very similar to that summarized by others (Clark 1960; Hofecker et al., 1980; Nakamura et al. 1988, 1990) for biological age. A total of 34 physiological and anthropometric variables was selected as a representative subset of the very large number of characteristic changes of aging. The correlation matrix among the selected 11 variables was factored by principal component analysis. The criterion for selection was that the variables had a positive or negative linear trend with chronological age in cross-sectional and longitudinal data (Borkan and Norris, 1980). The first principal component was used as an overall index of age-related changes in various physiological variables on the assumption that healthy individuals would be biologically more youthful than diseased individuals. As shown in Table 1, vital age (VA) of each patient was estimated from the equations for determining vital age score (VAS) and correction factor (Z) (Tanaka et al., 1990b, 1991a). The distortion of VA at the regression edges as a function of chronological age was corrected by calculating Z (Dubina et al., 1984).

RESULTS

At the onset of the study, no statistically significant difference existed in either vital or chronological age between the two groups. Mean vital age was found to be significantly higher than mean chronological age in both groups (Figure 1). However, the vital age for both groups decreased significantly following the six-month aerobic exercise program. Among the 11 variables that constitute the vital age prediction equation, the oxygen uptake corresponding to lactate threshold increased significantly by approximately 29 percent and 23 percent on the average for Groups Coronary and Hypertensive, respectively.

After the completion of the study, mean vital age of each group decreased significantly (50.5 ± 8.9 yr and 52.1 ± 9.1 yr, respectively) and approximated the mean chronological age. Although cholesterol and low-density lipoprotein cholesterol remained unchanged, high-density lipoprotein cholesterol tended to increase on the average. Mean vital age of a usual-care control group remained essentially unchanged. Remarkable reductions in vital age were due to significant increases in lactate threshold and some other physical fitness elements and significant decreases in systolic blood pressure, triglycerides, and abdominal girth, all of which were factors in the vital age prediction equation (Table 3).

When data for the two exercise groups were pooled and analyzed, side step and single leg balance with eyes closed were found to increase by 13 percent ($p<0.05$) and 28 percent ($p<0.05$), respectively; significant decreases were observed in body weight (two percent),

TABLE 3

Descriptive Studies (Mean ± SD) for Selected Variables Measured Before and After the Supervised Exercise Conditioning Program in Two Exercise Groups

	CHD		Hypertension	
	Pre	Post	Pre	Post
Stature, cm	151.0 ± 4.8	151.0 ± 4.7	151.5 ± 5.0	151.6 ± 5.0
Body Mass, kg	56.1 ± 12.0	54.2 ± 10.8*	56.9 ± 10.5	55.3 ± 9.7*
BMI	24.6 ± 5.4	23.9 ± 5.0*	24.8 ± 5.2	24.1 ± 5.1*
Body Fat, %	32.7 ± 11.5	29.3 ± 8.4*	32.3 ± 8.5	30.1 ± 8.3*
Body Fat, kg	18.3 ± 12.5	15.9 ± 8.8*	18.4 ± 9.7	16.7 ± 8.2
FFM, kg	37.8 ± 3.0	38.3 ± 3.8	38.5 ± 3.4	38.6 ± 3.6
Chest Girth, cm	89.0 ± 11.1	88.0 ± 10.7	90.1 ± 9.7	88.5 ± 10.0
Abdominal Girth (max), cm	86.5 ± 14.7	85.3 ± 14.6	87.2 ± 10.1	85.3 ± 9.2*
Abdominal Girth (min), cm	82.0 ± 16.9	81.0 ± 16.0	82.5 ± 9.4	81.6 ± 9.5
Triceps Skinfold, mm	21.8 ± 6.9	19.1 ± 4.8*	22.2 ± 7.5	19.5 ± 6.4*
Subscapular Skinfold, mm	28.1 ± 12.7	25.2 ± 10.3*	27.0 ± 9.8	24.4 ± 8.5*
Abdominal Skinfold, mm	35.6 ± 12.6	30.2 ± 9.8*	33.9 ± 10.7	29.8 ± 8.9*
Suprailiac Skinfold, mm	25.8 ± 14.5	21.8 ± 11.7*	25.1 ± 12.9	22.6 ± 10.2*
FVC, l	2.61 ± 0.36	2.65 ± 0.34	2.57 ± 0.54	2.67 ± 0.55
$FEV_{1.}$ l	2.15 ± 0.33	2.27 ± 0.30*	2.13 ± 0.55	2.23 ± 0.47*
$FEV_{1.}$ %	82.4 ± 4.2	85.7 ± 4.3	82.9 ± 4.5	83.6 ± 4.4
SBP, mm Hg	145.6 ± 12.8	136.9 ± 15.3*	151.7 ± 13.0	143.0 ± 14.1*
Total Cholesterol, mg/dl	204.3 ± 48.9	201.5 ± 37.8	200.3 ± 35.5	198.1 ± 32.4
HDL Cholesterol, mg/dl	43.5 ± 12.7	44.5 ± 14.9	41.5 ± 12.3	44.2 ± 11.9
LDL Cholesterol, mg/dl	131 ± 38.9	132.3 ± 42.2	131.5 ± 39.2	130.8 ± 40.8
Triglyceride, mg/dl	148.4 ± 91.6	124.0 ± 75.5*	136.3 ± 80.0	115.7 ± 69.3*
Hemoglobin, g/dl	13.4 ± 1.3	13.5 ± 0.9	13.7 ± 1.2	13.6 ± 1.1
Hematocrit, %	40.1 ± 3.8	40.0 ± 2.3	41.4 ± 3.6	40.4 ± 3.7
$\dot{V}O_2$@LT, ml/kg/min	13.2 ± 2.8	16.8 ± 3.1*	13.4 ± 2.5	16.6 ± 2.7*
HR@LT, b/min	114.5 ± 19.5	114.6 ± 18.0	116.3 ± 17.2	117.4 ± 15.4
Peak $\dot{V}O_2$, ml/kg/min	17.6 ± 4.1	24.6 ± 6.0*	18.5 ± 3.9	24.2 ± 4.5*
Peak HR, b/min	138.3 ± 30.3	147.3 ± 23.2	144.3 ± 31.0	153.4 ± 20.7
Side Step	26.3 ± 6.2	30.1 ± 5.1*	26.1 ± 6.5	28.7 ± 6.0*
One-Foot Balance, s	11.5 ± 11.4	14.4 ± 14.0*	14.6 ± 14.0	17.8 ± 9.4*
Trunk Extension, cm	32.7 ± 8.3	37.8 ± 8.7	38.8 ± 10.4	40.2 ± 9.0
Trunk Flexion, cm	11.5 ± 5.0	16.4 ± 5.7*	11.9 ± 6.3	16.3 ± 5.5*
Vertical jump, cm	24.0 ± 8.5	25.4 ± 7.0	25.4 ± 8.6	26.8 ± 8.0
Grip Strength, kg	25.2 ± 6.0	27.2 ± 5.3	27.3 ± 6.3	29.4 ± 6.3

* $p<0.05$

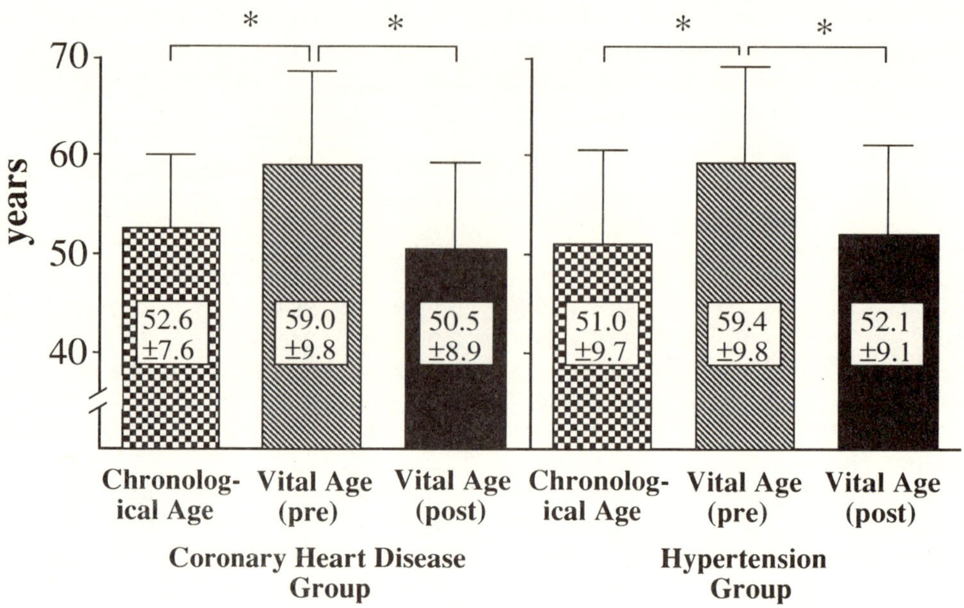

Figure 1. The effects of exercise program on vital age of patients with coronary heart disease or hypertension

abdominal girth (two percent), skinfold thickness at various sites, systolic blood pressure (nine percent), and triglycerides (20 percent). Forced expiratory volume for one second increased by three percent ($p<0.05$). In addition, significant improvements were observed for both groups in the flexibility of the hamstrings muscle group and the lower back, the sit-ups, and the push-ups with the knees on the floor.

In the control group (n=11) no change occurred in any of the body composition, cardiorespiratory, blood pressure, blood lipid, and physical fitness measures; and, therefore, the vital age of this group, which was significantly higher than their mean chronological age, remained unchanged (Figure 2).

DISCUSSION

It is not unusual to find that some individuals in middle and late adulthood who practiced a good life style are in much better physical and mental health than those who failed to do so. There are many individuals who do not look their age. During the last two decades several investigators (Borkan and Norris, 1980; Furukawa et al., 1975, Heikkinen et al., 1974; Hollingsworth et al., 1965; Nakamura et al., 1988, 1990; Tanaka et al., 1990b) have attempted to measure biological age, which, hypothetically, is the objective measure of a person's physical health or aging status. However, there is still no universally accepted standard for measuring it (Dean, 1988). Sensitivity of vital age as an index of physical health or aging status needs to be confirmed from the longitudinal standpoint.

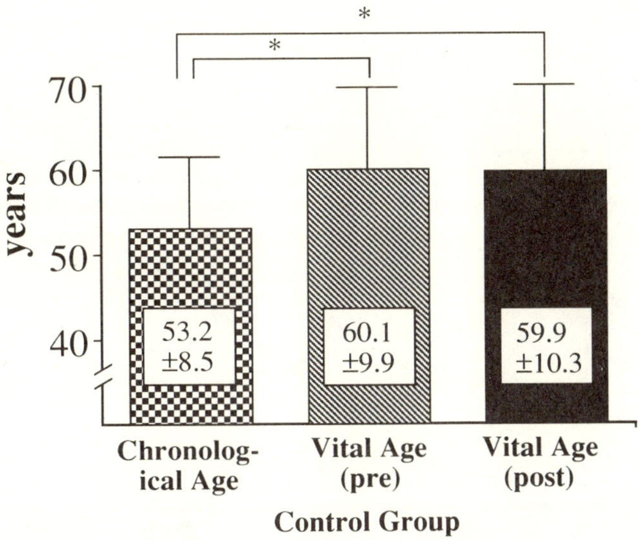

Figure 2. Vital age and chronological age in a usual-care control group

Based on the belief that assessing functional status is likely to be a much more rational basis for categorizing an individual's age than is chronological age, the present study was undertaken to determine the effects on vital age of aerobic exercise in patients with coronary heart disease or hypertension. Another interest was the comparison of exercise trainability between two groups.

Figure 1 indicates that patients diagnosed with either coronary heart disease or hypertension, with a regular exercise program, show almost the same vital age as their chronological age, indicating the positive effects of exercise. This is consistent with the cross-sectional study of Tanaka et al. (1991a), which demonstrated that significantly high vital ages resulted in the groups with coronary heart disease, hypertension, and obesity, while the vital ages in the hypertensive or obese subjects who had been extensively trained tended to approximate their chronological ages. The finding that, after the completion of the study, mean vital age of each group (50.5± 8.9 yr and 52.1 ± 9.1 yr, respectively) approximated the mean chronological age is not surprising, since patients without complications may achieve physical work capacity levels comparable to those of healthy sedentary people (Wohl et al., 1977; DeBusk et al., 1979). Although greater biological youthfulness may be suggested for the trained patients, extrapolating the conclusion that aerobic exercise itself retards the rate of aging is perilous (Borkan and Norris, 1980).

The upper panel in Figure 3 shows that in the Coronary Group a significantly high correlation existed between vital age obtained at the beginning of the study and vital age obtained immediately after the exercise program. As shown in the lower panel, similar results were obtained in the Hypertension Group. The slope of the regression line was almost parallel to that of the identity line, that is 1.0 in both groups, indicating that the

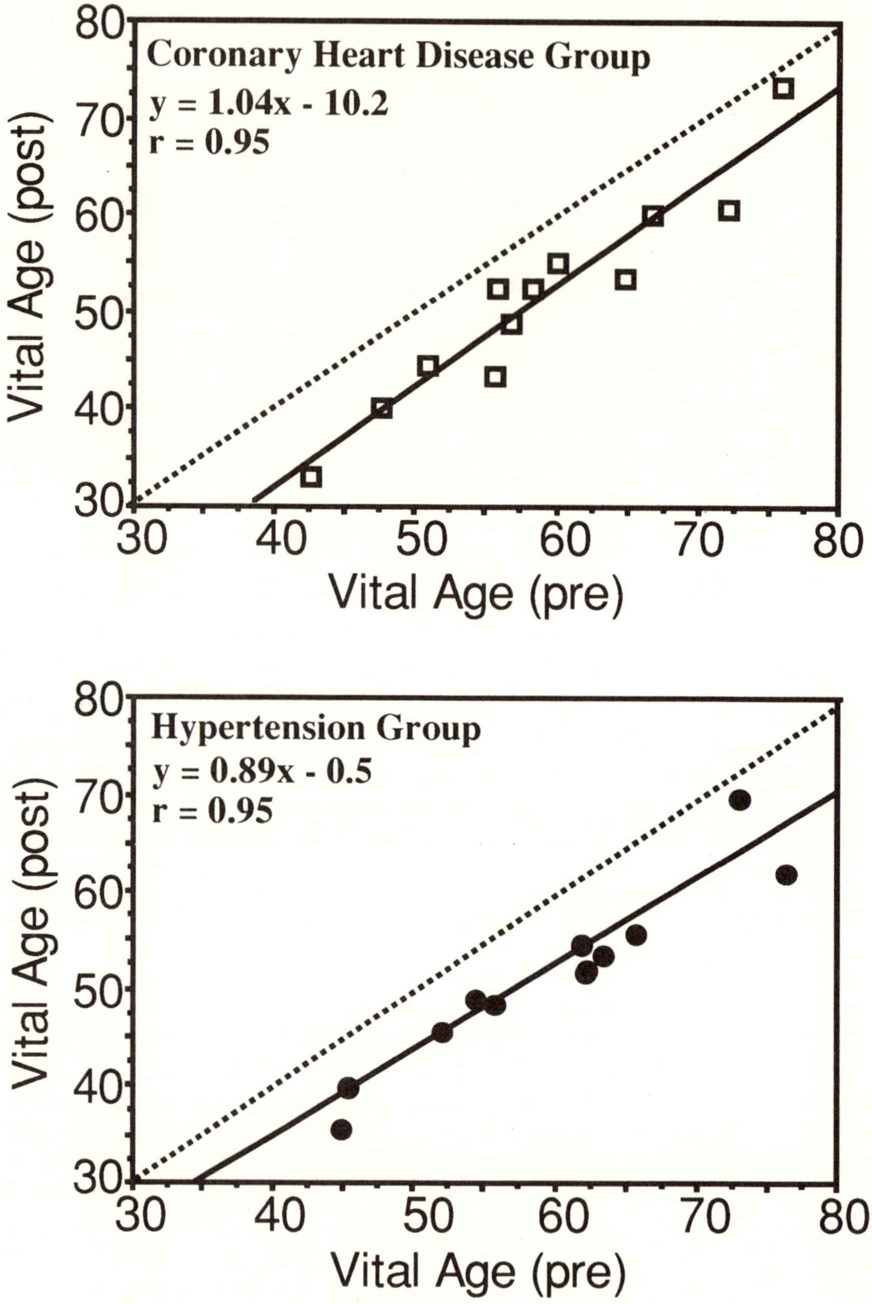

Figure 3. Scatter diagram between vital age assessed prior to exercise program for X-axis and vital age assessed following exercise program for Y-axis in patients with coronary heart disease (upper panel) or hypertension (lower panel).

effects of exercise can be seen throughout a wide range of age. Remarkable reductions in vital age were due to (1) significant increases in lactate threshold and some other physical fitness elements, and (2) significant decreases in systolic blood pressure, triglycerides, and abdominal girth, all of which were predictors in the equation of vital age.

Significant increases in oxygen uptake at lactate threshold and peak oxygen uptake may be attributed to skeletal muscle adaptations to six months of endurance-type exercise training. Major adaptations in skeletal muscle include alterations in fiber subtype distribution (i.e., conversion of type II b fibers into type II a, an increase in fiber size, an increase in capillarization, a decrease in the activity of some glycolytic enzyme activities, and an increase in mitochondrial respiratory enzyme activities (Coggan et al., 1992). These adaptations to physical training seem to play a major role in the decreased reliance on carbohydrate during submaximal exercise, thereby increasing endurance performance (Holloszy and Coyle, 1984).

Chronic physical activity of an endurance nature appears to result in moderate reductions (about 10 mm Hg) in both systolic and diastolic blood pressures of hypertensive individuals (Seals and Hagberg, 1984; Hagberg and Seals, 1986). The significant decrease in blood pressure following exercise conditioning in hypertensive persons is consistent with the results of several studies (Bonanno and Lies, 1974; Boyer and Kasch, 1970; Cade et al., 1984; Choquette and Ferguson, 1973; Duncan et al., 1985; Kiyonaga et al., 1985). Furthermore, it is worth noting that the number of premature ventricular depolarizations per minute of exercise and per day decreased remarkably in some subjects following the physical conditioning.

CONCLUSION

The results indicate that aerobic exercise may alter overall physiologic profiles of patients with coronary heart disease or essential hypertension and rejuvenate them.

Greater biological youthfulness or slower biological aging can be seen for the trained state. Elderly persons who finished a supervised exercise program should continue a three-to-five-days per week controlled exercise program. Studies are continuing to determine the amount of exercise needed and the duration for which the rejuvenation in vital age is maintained.

ACKNOWLEDGEMENT

This work was supported, in part, by Grant-in-Aid for General Scientific Research by The Ministry of Education, Science and Culture, and by a grant from the University Research Project Board, University of Tsukuba.

REFERENCES

American College of Sports Medicine: Guidelines for Exercise Testing and Prescription. Philadelphia: Lea & Febiger, 1991:187-99.

Blair SN, Kohl HW III, Paffenbarger RS Jr., Clark DG, Cooper KH, Gibbons LW. Physical fitness and all-cause mortality: a prospective study of healthy men and women. JAMA 1989;262:2395-2401.

Borkan GA, Norris AH. Assessment of biological age using a profile of physical parameters. J Gerontol 1980;35:177-84.

Bonanno JA, Lies JE. Effects of physical training on coronary risk factors. Am J Cardiol 1974;33:760-83.

Boyer JL, Kasch FW. Exercise therapy in hypertensive men. JAMA 1970;211: 668-71.

Cade R, Mars D, Wagemaker H et al. Effect of aerobic exercise training on patients with systemic arterial hypertension. Am J Med 1984;77:785-90.

Choquette G, Ferguson RJ. Blood pressure reduction on borderline hypertensives following physical training. Can Med Assoc J 1973;108:699-703.

Clark JW. The aging dimension: a factorial analysis of individual differences with age on psychological and physiological measurements. J Gerontol 1960;15:183-7.

Coggan AR, Spina RJ, King DS et al. Skeletal muscle adaptations to endurance training in 60- to 70-yr-old men and women. J Appl Physiol 1992;72:1780-6.

DeBusk RF, Houston N, Haskell W, Fry G, Parker M. Exercise training soon after myocardial infarction. Am J Cardiol 1979;44:1223-9.

Dean W. Biological Aging Measurement. Los Angeles: The Center for Bio-Gerontology, 1988:3-31.

Dubina TL, Mints AY, Zhuk EV. Biological age and its estimation. II. Introduction to a correction to the multiple regression model of biological age and assessment of biological age in cross-sectional and longitudinal studies. Exp Gerontol 1984;19:133-43.

Duncan JJ, Farr JE, Upton J, Hagan D, Oglesby ME, Blair SN. The effects of aerobic exercise on plasma catecholamines and blood pressure in patients with mild essential hypertension. JAMA 1985;254:2609-13.

Ekelund LD, Haskell WL, Johnson JL, Whaley FS, Criqui MH, Sheps DS. Physical fitness as a predictor of cardiovascular mortality in asymptomatic North American men: the Lipid Research Clinics Mortality Follow-up Study. N Engl J Med 1988;319:1379-84.

Furukawa T, Inoue M, Kajiya F et al. Assessment of biological age by multiple regression analysis. J Gerontol 1975;30:422-34.

Hagberg JM, Seals DR. Exercise training and hypertension. Acta Med Scand (Suppl) 1986;711:131-6.

Heikkinen E, Kiiskinen A, Kähty B, Rimpelä M, Vuori I. Assessment of biological age: methodological study in two Finnish populations. Gerontologia 1974;20:33-43.

Hofecker G, Skalicky M, Kment A, Niedermullar H. Models of the biological age of the rat. I. A factor model of age parameters. Mech Ageing Dev 1980;14:345-59.

Hollingsworth JW, Hashizume A, Jablon S. Correlations between tests of aging in Hiroshima subjects - an attempt to define "Physiologic Age". Yale J Biol Med 1965;38:11-26.

Holloszy JO, Coyle EF. Adaptations of skeletal muscle to endurance exercise and their metabolic consequences. J Appl Physiol 1984;56:831-8.

Kiyonaga A, Arakawa K, Tanaka H, Shindo M. Blood pressure and hormonal responses to aerobic exercise. Hypertension 1985;7:125-31.

Leon AS, Connett J, Jacobs DR Jr, Rauramaa R. Leisure-time physical activity levels and risk of coronary heart disease and death. JAMA 1987;258:2388-95.

Nakamura E, Miyao K, Ozeki T. Assessment of biological age by principal component analysis. Mech Ageing Dev 1988;46:1-18.

Nakamura E, Moritani T, Kanetaka A. Biological age versus physical fitness age in women. Eur J Appl Physiol 1990;61:202-8.

Paffenbarger RS Jr, Hyde RT, Wing AL, Hsieh CC. Physical activity, all-cause mortality and longevity of college alumni. N Engl J Med 1986;314:605-13.

Pekkanen J, Marti B, Nissinen A, Tuomilchto J, Pusar S, Karvonen MJ. Reduction of premature mortality by high physical activity: a 20-year follow-up of middle-aged Finnish men. Lancet 1987;1:1473-7.

Seals DR, Hagberg JM. The effect of exercise training on human hypertension: a review. Med Sci Sports Exerc 1984;16:207-15.

Shock NW, Geulich RC, Andres R et al. Normal human aging. The Baltimore longitudinal study of aging (NIH Publication No. 84-2450). Washington, DC: U.S. Government Printing Office, 1984.

Smith EL. Age: the interaction of nature and nurture. In: Smith EL, Serfass RC, eds. Exercise and Aging. New Jersey: Enslow, 1980:11-7.

Tanaka K, Yoshimura T, Okuda T et al. Physiological alterations in obese women: the effects of caloric restriction plus physical training at an intensity corresponding to or above anaerobic threshold. Bull Phys Fitness Res Inst 1986;62(Suppl):26-40.

Tanaka K, Kim HS, Wakita M, Nakadomo F,Hasama T, Maeda K. Effects of aerobic conditioning plus caloric restriction in obese middle-aged women. Jpn J Appl Physiol 1989;19:495-504.

Tanaka K, Takeshima N, Kato T, Niihata S, Ueda K. Critical determinants of endurance performance in middle-aged and elderly endurance runners with heterogeneous training habits. Eur J Appl Physiol 1990a;59:443-9.

Tanaka K, Matsuura Y, Nakadomo F, Nakamura E. Assessment of vital age of Japanese women by principal component analysis. Jpn J Phys Educ 1990b;35:121-31.

Tanaka K, Yoshimura T, Maeda K et al. Validity of CHD risk factor-dependent "vital age" as an index of health and aging status. J Jpn Atheroschler Soc 1991a;19:303-10.

Tanaka K, Nakadomo F, Takeshima N, Nakamura E, Matsuura Y. Longitudinal alterations in vital age of obese middle-aged women following a supervised aerobic conditioning plus caloric restriction program. Bull Phys Fitness Res Inst 1991b;77:73-81.

Wohl AJ, Lewis HR, Campbell W et al. Cardiovascular function during early recovery from acute myocardial infarction. Circulation 1977;56:931-7.

Benefits of Habitual Walking on Coronary Artery Disease Risk Factors in Middle-Aged and Older Males

Yasuo Kimura, Ed.D.
Minoru Kubota, B.L.
Shoichi Yamazaki, Ph.D.

INTRODUCTION

Recent research suggests that regular physical activities and leisure-time activities are associated with a decreased incidence of coronary artery disease and increased longevity (Blair et al., 1989; Slattery et al., 1989), probably by altering plasma lipid and lipoprotein levels. In the past decade, walking has become one of the most popular activities for fitness. The popularity of walking is due to the fact that it is simple, inexpensive, and can be performed by individuals of all ages and abilities with very little risk of injury. Previous studies suggest that brisk or vigorous walking exercise improves aerobic power (Jette et al., 1988; Pollock et al., 1971) and cardiovascular health (Blair 1985; LaPorte et al., 1985), reduces body mass and fat (Pollock et al., 1971; Porcari et al., 1989; White et al., 1984), decreases depression and anxiety (Porcari et al., 1988), and decreases total blood cholesterol and increases high-density lipoprotein cholesterol (Cook et al., 1986). However, little information is available regarding the effects of daily mild aerobic exercise, such as walking, on the major risk factors for coronary artery disease (Kimura et al., 1991; Oja et al., 1991).

The purpose of this study, therefore, was to compare the beneficial effects of habitual walking exercise on selected coronary artery disease risk factors of middle-aged and older walkers with those of age-matched sedentary men.

METHODS

Subjects

Forty-nine male volunteers participated in this study. The subjects were assigned to four groups: older walkers (N=14, aged 58 ± 7 years, mean ± SD), older sedentary males (N = 11, 56 ± 6 years), middle-aged walkers (N = 13, 47 ± 6 years), and middle-aged sedentary males (N = 11, 44 ± 9 years). Those who took a daily walk of 30 minutes or more were referred to as walkers (trained group) and those who walked less than this were referred to as non-walkers (untrained group). Consecutive years of walking exercise in the older and middle-aged walkers averaged 15 and eight years, respectively. Walking distances and frequency in the last year were 8 ± 2 km per day and 5 ± 1 days per week, respectively, for both walkers' groups. Each subject completed a medical history questionnaire and was examined prior to his participation in this study. All subjects were healthy, free from coronary artery disease and not taking any medications. Each subject was fully informed regarding the design and risks of this project prior to giving a written informed consent.

Measurements

Resting heart rate, resting blood pressure, height, body weight, and skinfold thickness measurements were taken on all subjects. Resting heart rate and blood pressure were measured after each subject sat quietly for at least 15 minutes. Resting heart rate was measured by counting the radial pulse for 60 seconds. Resting blood pressure was measured in a sitting position on the right arm by auscultation of the first and fourth of Korotkoff's sounds, using a calibrated standard sphygmomanometer and stethoscope.

Skinfold thickness measurements were made with an Eiken skinfold caliper (made by the National Nutrition Research Institute, Tokyo) at two sites (triceps and subscapular) by the same technician through accepted procedures. The sum of the two skinfolds measured was converted to body density by Nagamine and Suzuki's (1964) equation for Japanese adults, and the body density was converted to the percentage of body fat (percent body fat) by Brozeck et al.'s (1963) equation. Body mass index was calculated as weight (mass, kg)/ height ($m^{2)}$.

Maximal oxygen uptake was estimated during graded treadmill walking by a modified Balke protocol (Balke and Ware, 1959). Oxygen consumption and ventilation were measured every 30 seconds with an automated analyzer (AEROBIC PROCESSERE R1500A, SAN-EI, Tokyo).

Following an overnight fast of 12 to 14 hours and free from any vigorous exercise for 24 hours, approximately 10 ml of blood was drawn from an anticubital vein. Plasma was immediately separated by centrifugation. Total cholesterol was determined by the Wako Cholesterol B test kit, and triglycerides were analyzed by an enzymatic method. High-density lipoprotein cholesterol was determined by a heparin-Mn++ precipitation procedure. Low-density lipoprotein cholesterol was estimated by the indirect method of Friedewald et al. (1972).

To estimate the intensity of habitual walking exercise, heart rate during walking was measured using a pocket-size electrocardiographic recorder (HEART RATE MEMORY, Vine, Tokyo). The number of steps was determined by a pedometer (MANPO METER EC-500, Yamasa, Tokyo). The Yamasa MANPO METER is also designed to estimate caloric expenditure roughly from the number of steps on the bases of age, sex, and body weight of each subject.

Statistics

Statistical analyses were made by analysis of variance to evaluate overall differences among the groups. Student's t-test was used for paired data of groups, if the overall multivariate F was significant ($p<0.05$). All data are expressed as mean ± standard deviation (SD).

RESULTS

Characteristics of the Habitual Walkers

On the average, both walkers' groups had an exercise heart rate of 121 ± 11 beats per minute which was measured immediately after an exercise session, 67 percent of maximal heart rate reserve or 52 percent of maximal oxygen uptake for exercise intensity according to the individual heart rate-oxygen consumption regression in the laboratory test. The number of steps counted were from 12800 to 20000 (mean 16500 steps) and the estimated caloric expenditure by walking ranged from 350 to 500 Kcal (mean 440 Kcal).

Anthropometric Data

As shown in Table 1, there were marked differences in body weight, sum of skinfolds, estimated content of body fat, and body mass index between the trained and untrained males in both older and middle-aged groups. Percent fat was significantly lower in both older and middle-aged walkers than in their age-matched untrained controls (13 vs. 16 percent and 13 vs. 17 percent).

TABLE 1

Anthropometric Profiles of the Four Subject Groups

	n	Body Weight (kg)	Sum of skinfolds[a] (mm)	Relative body fat (%)	Body mass index (kg/m^2)
Older Group					
Walkers	14	55.2 ± 5.0	16.4 ± 4.2	12.5 ± 2.2	21.2 ± 1.2
Non-walkers	11	59.3 ± 8.6*	25.3 ± 8.0*	15.7 ± 3.6*	23.0 ± 2.0*
Middle-aged					
Walkers	13	58.7 ± 5.6*	17.3 ± 4.1†	12.7 ± 2.4†	21.6 ± 1.1
Non-walkers	11	62.7 ± 8.1*#	26.6 ± 6.9*#	16.9 ± 3.1*#	22.8 ± 1.4*

Values are mean ± SD
[a] Triceps + subscapular
* $p<0.05$ for difference from older walkers
† $p<0.05$ for difference from older non-walkers
# $p<0.05$ for difference from middle-aged walkers.

Heart Rates and Blood Pressure

Both groups of walkers had significantly lower heart rates at rest than either group of untrained subjects (Table 2). No significant differences among the four groups were found in resting diastolic blood pressure and resting systolic blood pressure.

TABLE 2

Cardiovascular Measurements in the Four Subject Groups

	n	Resting heart rate (bpm)	Systolic BP (mm Hg)	Diastolic BP (mm Hg)	Maximal O_2 uptake (ml/kg/min)
Older Group					
Walkers	14	66 ± 9	132 ± 19	82 ± 11	42.6 ± 5.5
Non-walkers	11	73 ± 10*	135 ± 19	84 ± 12	35.5 ± 6.3*
Middle-aged					
Walkers	13	70 ± 14†	130 ± 16	80 ± 14	45.2 ± 5.1†
Non-walkers	11	74 ± 11*#	132 ± 18	82 ± 12	38.4 ± 6.7*#

Values are mean ± SD
bpm:beats per minute
BP: blood pressure
* $p<0.05$ for difference from older walkers
† $p<0.05$ for difference from older non-walkers
# $p<0.05$ for difference from middle-aged walkers.

Maximal Oxygen Uptake

As shown in Table 2, maximal oxygen uptake capacity (43 ± 6 ml/kg/min for older walkers; 45 ± 5 ml/kg/min for middle-aged subjects) was approximately 7 ml/kg/min, or 18 to 20 percent, higher in both trained groups than in the untrained respective groups but six percent lower in the older walkers than in middle-aged walkers.

Plasma Lipid and Lipoprotein Evaluation

As shown in Table 3, total cholesterol was slightly higher (six to eight percent) in the older trained group (216 mg/dl) than in the other three groups. Low-density lipoprotein cholesterol level in the older walkers' group was similar to that in the untrained peers (122 vs. 126 mg/dl), whereas the middle-aged walkers had a significantly lower concentration of low-density lipoprotein cholesterol than the untrained peers. High-density lipoprotein cholesterol concentration of older walkers was markedly higher than that of non-walkers (67 vs. 53 mg/dl) but not significantly different from that of middle-aged walkers. As a result, the ratios of low-density lipoprotein cholesterol to high-density lipoprotein cholesterol and total cholesterol to high-density lipoprotein cholesterol were significantly lower in the older trained group than in both untrained age-groups, but the older trained had 10 percent and 3 percent higher ratios, respectively, although these differences were not statistically significant, than the middle-aged trained group had. Similarly, both trained groups had a lower concentration of triglycerides compared to the untrained males in both age-matched untrained groups.

TABLE 3

Plasma Lipid and Lipoprotein Data for Four Subject Groups

	n	Total cholesterol (mg/dl)	HDL cholesterol (mg/dl)	LDL cholesterol (mg/dl)	Triglyceride (mg/dl)	LDL cholesterol/ HDL cholesterol (Unit)	Total cholesterol/ HDL cholesterol (Unit)
Older group							
Walkers	14	216 ± 33	67 ± 16	122 ± 30	87 ± 26	1.86 ± 0.47	3.09 ± 0.87
Non-walkers	11	200 ± 35†	53 ± 16*	126 ± 32	128 ± 52*	2.30 ± 0.70*	3.63 ± 1.15*
Middle-aged							
Walkers	13	204 ± 28	79 ± 13†	114 ± 26	87 ± 27†	1.67 ± 0.58†	2.98 ± 0.92†
Non-walkers	11	204 ± 27	54 ± 13#	129 ± 24#	116 ± 41*#	2.15 ± 0.87*#	3.78 ± 1.13*#

Values are mean ± SD.
HDL: high density lipoprotein
LDL: low density lipoprotein
* $p<0.05$ for difference from older walkers
† $p<0.05$ for difference from older non-walkers
# $p<0.05$ for difference from middle-aged walkers.

DISCUSSION

Habitual Walking and Cardiovascular Health

Recent epidemiological evidence suggests an association between an individual's level of physical activity and the risk of developing coronary artery disease (Leon et al., 1987; Paffenbarger et al., 1986). A recent review reveals that physical inactivity does seem to be causally associated with coronary artery disease (Powell et al., 1987). Blair (1985) and LaPorte et al. (1985) suggested that increasing physical activity by walking 2.4 to 3.2 km per day (about 30 minutes) and/or moderate levels of energy expenditure (approximately 200 to 500 Kcal per day) utilized during exercise and leisure time activities will dramatically reduce the incidence of coronary artery disease in the general population. Casperson (1987) also stated that, after analysis of the research literature about the relationship between physical inactivity and coronary heart disease, physical inactivity is a far more important risk factor than elevated serum cholesterol, smoking, and hypertension, the three major risk factors. In other words, a sedentary person is 1.9 times more likely to develop coronary artery disease than the more active person. Leaf et al. (1989) suggest that the protective effect of leisure time physical activity on coronary artery disease occurs through mechanisms involving favorable changes in plasma lipoprotein. Higher levels of energy expenditure resulted in only slightly greater reduction in risk. Åstrand (1960) states that one should train at approximately 50 percent of maximal oxygen intake. The cross-sectional nature of the present study may explain some differences in results, when they occur, between it and some of the other (longitudinal) training studies described below.

Resting Heart Rate and Blood Pressure

Most studies show a reduction in heart rate to the mid to low 60's (Pollock, 1973). In this study both trained groups' resting heart rates were significantly lower than the age-matched untrained group's rates, although it is not clear whether this difference was due to genetic factors, training or both. These findings reflect an increased efficiency of the heart as well as a decreased myocardial oxygen demand and agree with others indicating that aerobically trained individuals tend to have lower resting heart rates than untrained individuals (Fox et al., 1988; Franklin et al., 1978; Pollock et al., 1973). The intensity of exercise has been suggested to be one of the most important factors when physical training is used to reduce blood pressure (Kiyonaga et al., 1985).

Hagberg (1990) suggests that an exercise intensity corresponding to that of brisk walking may be sufficient to lower blood pressure at rest. In the present study, the blood pressure measurements failed to yield significant group differences. These findings agreed with other reports of no resting blood pressure changes in normals with physical training (Luria and Koepke, 1975; Pollock, 1973). The mean resting blood pressure of the untrained groups exceeded that of the trained group, as would be expected (Fox et al., 1988).

Body Composition

In the present study, the measured and estimated anthropometric profiles of the walkers were better than those of the non-walkers. Both walkers' groups had a significantly lower total body weight, sum of skinfolds, percent body fat, and body mass index than both age-matched non-walkers. This finding agrees with the literature indicating that trained men have a lower body fat content than untrained individuals (Fox et al., 1988; Holloszy, 1974; Pollock et al., 1971, 1975; Porcari et al., 1989). Losses in body mass are related to total caloric expenditure. In order to achieve significant alterations in lean and fat weights effectively, the threshold stimulus has been reported to be at the minimal amount of energy expenditure of 200 to 300 Kcal per exercise session when frequency of exercise is three to four days per week (Pollock et al., 1975). In this study, habitual walking in both walkers' groups was performed five to six days per week, expending approximately 350 to 500 Kcal per exercise session. Although the intensity of exercise in this study was lower (about 50 percent of maximal oxygen uptake) than that reported previously in several of the running regimens, the increased frequency and duration of exercise added to its total kilocaloric expenditure.

Effects on Aerobic Power

Studies investigating the aerobic training benefits of walking have reported improvements in maximal oxygen uptake comparable with other forms of training, such as cycling, running and graded treadmill walking, in sedentary middle-aged men when intensity (85 to 90 percent of maximal heart rate reserve) is maintained at similar levels (Pollock et al., 1975). In a study by Jette et al. (1988), 35-to-53-year-old men and women walked three times per week for 12 weeks at speeds eliciting 60 percent of maximal oxygen uptake. Improvements in maximal oxygen uptake were significant for both men (9.7 percent) and women (17.3 percent). As estimated from the recorded heart rates, the intensity of habitual walking was slightly over 50 percent of the maximal oxygen uptake. Although the American College of Sports Medicine (1986) recommends exercise intensities in excess of 50 percent of maximal oxygen uptake to improve aerobic power, the minimal threshold may be below this value. This finding is consistent with the suggestion that for submaximal endurance training the total training time as the product of session time and frequency is more important than the training intensity (Wenger and Bell, 1986). In an investigation by Seals et al. (1984b), subjects walked during exercise sessions that require approximately 40 percent of maximal heart rate reserve (107 ± 6 beats per minute) and were conducted over a six-month period. Maximal oxygen uptake increased by 11 percent. This may be partially explained by the fact that the lower training heart rate (intensity) values for walkers, compared to the values found in joggers, were offset by an increased duration and frequency of participation.

Plasma Lipids and Lipoprotein Evaluation

Cross-sectional and training studies show clearly that adequate aerobic exercise is liable to lead to changes in plasma lipoproteins. These include elevations in plasma high-density lipoprotein cholesterol, particularly the high-density lipoprotein 2 cholesterol subfraction, which has been particularly associated with low risk of coronary artery disease (Gordon et al., 1977), and elevations in apolipoprotein A-1, the principal peptide of high-density lipoprotein. Also the very low-density lipoprotein cholesterol concentrations in highly active people who have exercised consistently over a long period of time are impressively low (Wood et al., 1984). A threshold amount of exercise, therefore, seems to be necessary in order to see a statistically significant effect on lipoprotein (Haskell, 1986; Williams et al., 1982).

There are numerous studies which suggest that blood triglycerides and low-density lipoprotein cholesterol significantly decreased and high-density lipoprotein cholesterol significantly increased following endurance exercise training at an intensity of 70 to 80 percent of maximal oxygen uptake (Dufaux et al., 1982; Farrell and Barboriak, 1980; Holloszy et al., 1964). However, only a few have focused on the effects of low-intensity exercise, such as walking, on blood high-density lipoprotein cholesterol. In addition, the existing data are conflicting. Cook et al. (1986) observed that high-density lipoprotein cholesterol levels for postal carriers, who have walked about 25 miles per week over a duration of 15 to 28 years, were significantly higher than those of industrial workers in blue collar occupations. In contrast, the report by Gaesser and Rich (1984) showed no significant increases of serum high-density lipoprotein cholesterol in 18 weeks of the low (45 percent of maximal oxygen uptake) intensity physical training with a cycle ergometer. Weltman et al. (1980) also failed to demonstrate any significant changes in plasma high-density lipoprotein cholesterol in the 10 weeks of brisk walking training performed at 45 minutes per session four days per week. Seals et al. (1984a) observed increased high-density lipoprotein cholesterol following high-intensity (80 to 90 percent of maximal heart rate) endurance training of older men and women, but changes were not significant in their low-intensity (60 percent maximal heart rate) group.

Although the middle-aged walkers tended to have lower levels of low-density lipoprotein cholesterol than their sedentary counterparts, in the older group the walkers had similar low-density lipoprotein cholesterol to those of the sedentary males. The higher levels of total cholesterol and low density lipoprotein cholesterol in the older walkers in contrast to the middle-aged walkers appear to be solely attributable to the difference in age, because there were no differences in other factors, such as body composition or level of exercise training, that influence lipid/lipoprotein profile. The fact that the older walkers had a significantly lower triglyceride concentration, similar to those of middle-aged walkers, than the sedentary males in both age groups suggests the favorable effect of exercise training on the prevention of coronary artery disease in older males (Aberg et al., 1985).

High-density lipoprotein cholesterol is generally thought to increase only with vigorous physical activity - the equivalent of 10 miles jogging every week for nine months (Thompson et al., 1988). Walking, however, has been shown to elevate high-density lipoprotein cholesterol levels. It has been suggested that high-density lipoprotein cholesterol has an inverse effect on the development of coronary artery disease (Cook et al., 1986; Gordon et al., 1977; Manninen et al., 1988; Ward et al., 1989).

The lower value of atherogenic index of low-density lipoprotein cholesterol/high-density lipoprotein cholesterol ratio in the older walkers compared to the sedentary individuals in both untrained groups was mainly induced by the elevation of high-density lipoprotein cholesterol level. However, when compared with the middle-aged walkers, the older walkers had slightly higher atherogenic indexes. The total cholesterol/high-density lipoprotein cholesterol ratio has been suggested as a more important indicator of coronary artery disease risk than total cholesterol or high-density lipoprotein cholesterol alone because it combines two coronary artery disease risk factors (Gordon et al., 1977).

There were only occasional complaints of leg fatigue, and none of the subjects suffered from musculoskeletal problems in this study. The present study points to the importance of the total amount of work (energy cost) accomplished as the important criterion for cardiovascular health, body composition, and blood lipid improvement. Thus, results of this study could indicate a decreased risk of coronary artery disease.

CONCLUSION

Habitual exercise by mild walking proved safe and effective. It favorably modified the plasma lipid profile, altered body composition and improved cardiovascular function, and may reduce the risk of coronary artery disease occuring in middle-aged and older males.

ACKNOWLEDGMENTS

Part of this study was presented at The 3rd International Conference on Physical Activity, Aging and Sports (University of Jyväskylä, Jyväskylä, Finland, 1992). The authors express thanks to all the subjects who offered their time and efforts, to Mr. Toshinobu Ban, MT for his technical assistance for the analyses of blood, and Professor Michio Kuzumaki for checking the English in this manuscript.

REFERENCES

Aberg H, Lithell H, Selinus I, Hedstrand H. Serum triglycerides are a risk factor for myocardial infarction but not for angina pectoris. Results from 10-year follow-up of Uppsala primary preventive study. Atherosclerosis 1985;54:89-97.

American College of Sports Medicine. Guidelines for Exercise Testing and Prescription, 3rd ed. Philadelphia: Lea & Febiger, 1986:134-9.

Åstrand I. Aerobic work capacity in men and women with special reference to age. Acta Physiol Scand 1960;49(Suppl 169):211-7.

Balke B, Ware RW. Experimental study of physical fitness of Air Force personnel. US Armed Forces J 1959;10:667-71.

Blair SN. Physical activity leads to fitness and pays off. Physician Sportsmed 1985;13:153-7.

Blair SN, Kohl HV III, Paffenbarger RS Jr. et al. Physical fitness and all-cause mortality. A prospective study of healthy men and women. JAMA 1989;262:2395-401.

Brozeck J, Grande F, Anderson JT, Keys A. Densitometric analysis of body composition: revision of some quantitative assumptions. Ann NY Acad Sci 1963;110:113-40.

Caspersen CJ. Physical inactivity and coronary heart disease. Physician Sportsmed 1987;15:43-4.

Cook TC, LaPorte RE, Washburn RA, Traven ND, Slemenda CW, Metz KF. Chronic low level physical activity as a determinant of high-density lipoprotein cholesterol and subfractions. Med Sci Sports Exerc 1986;18: 653-7.

Dufaux B, Assmann G, Hollmann W. Plasma lipoproteins and physical activity: a review. Int J Sports Med 1982;3:123-36.

Farrell PA, Barboriak J. The time course of alterations in plasma lipid and lipoprotein concentrations during eight weeks of endurance training. Atherosclerosis 1980;37:231-8.

Fox EL, Bower RW, Foss ML. The Physiological Basis of Physical Education and Athletics, 4th ed. Philadelphia: W.B. Saunders Co., 1988.

Franklin BA, Besseghini I, Golden LH. Low intensity physical conditioning: effects on patients with coronary heart disease. Arch Phys Med Rehabil 1978;59:276-80.

Friedewald WT, Levy RI, Frederickson DS. Estimation of the concentration of low-density lipoprotein cholesterol in plasma without use of the preparative ultracentrifuge. Clin Chem 1972;18:499-502.

Gaesser GA, Rich RG. Effects of high- and low-intensity exercise training on aerobic capacity and blood lipids. Med Sci Sports Exerc 1984;16:269-74.

Gordon T, Castelli WP, Hjortland MC, Kannel WB, Dawber TB. High density lipoprotein as a protective factor against coronary heart disease. The Framingham study. Am J Med 1977;62:707-14.

Hagberg KM. Exercise, fitness, and hypertension. In: Bouchard C, Shephard RJ, Stephens T, Sutton JR, McPherson BD, eds. Exercise, Fitness, and Health. Champaign, IL: Human Kinetics Books, 1990:455-66.

Haskell WL. The influence of exercise training on plasma lipids and lipoproteins in health and disease. Acta Med Scand 1986;711(Suppl):25-37.

Holloszy JO, Skinner JS, Toro G, Cureton TK. Effects of a six month program of endurance exercise in the serum lipids of middle-aged men. Am J Cardiol 1964;14:753-60.

Holloszy JO. The effects of endurance exercise on body composition. In: Vague J, Boyer J, eds. The Regulation of the Adipose Tissue Mass. New York: American Elsevier, 1974:254-8.

Jette M, Sidney K, Campbell J. Effects of a twelve-week walking program on maximal and submaximal work output indices in sedentary middle-aged men and women. J Sports Med Phys Fitness 1988;28:59-66.

Kimura Y, Kubota M, Yamazaki S. Effects of habitual walking on geriatric disease (in Japanese, abstract). Jpn J Phys Fitness Sports Med 1991;40:610.

Kiyonaga A, Arakawa K, Tanaka H, Shido M. Blood pressure and hormonal responses to aerobic exercise. Hypertension 1985;7:125-31.

LaPorte RE, Dearwater S, Cauley JA, Slemenda C, Cook T. Cardiovascular fitness: is it really necessary? Physician Sportsmed 1985;13:145-50.

Leaf DA, Parker DL, McAfee SR. The relationship of leisure time activity to plasma lipids, lipoproteins, blood pressure, and percent body fat. J Cardiopulmonary Rehabil 1989;9:497-504.

Leon AS, Connett J, Jacobs DR, Rauramaa R. Leisure-time physical activity levels and risk of coronary heart disease and death: the multiple risk factor intervention trial. JAMA 1987;258:2388-95.

Luria MH, Koepke, KR. The physical conditioning effects of walking. J Sports Med Phys Fitness 1975;15: 272-4.

Manninen V, Elo MO, Frick MH et al. Lipid alterations and decline in the incidence of coronary heart disease in the Helsinki Heart Study. JAMA 1988; 260:641-51.

Nagamine S, Suzuki S. Anthropometry and body composition of Japanese young men and women. Hum Biol 1964;36:8-15.

Oja P, Manttari A, Heinonen A et al. Physiological effects of walking and cycling to work. Scand J Med Sci Sports 1991;1:151-7.

Paffenbarger RS Jr., Hyde RT, Wing AL et al. Physical activity, all-cause mortality, and longevity of college alumni. N Engl J Med 1986;314:605-13.

Pollock ML. The quantification of endurance training programs. In: Wilmore JH, ed. Exercise and Sports Sciences Reviews. New York: Academic Press, 1973:155-88.

Pollock ML, Miller HS, Jr., Janeway R, Linnerud AC, Robertson B, Valentino R. Effects of walking on body composition and cardiovascular function of middle-aged men. J Appl Physiol 1971;30:126-30.

Pollock ML, Dimmick J, Miller HS Jr., Kendrick Z, Linnerud AC. Effects of mode of training on cardiovascular function and body composition of middle-aged men. Med Sci Sports 1975;7:139-45.

Porcari JP, Ward A, Morris D et al. Comparison of weight loss in males and females after 16 weeks of fitness walking and/or diet. Med Sci Sports Exerc(abstract) 1989;21:S102.

Porcari JP, Ward A, Morgan W et al. Effect of walking on state of anxiety and blood pressure. Med Sci Sports Exerc(abstract) 1988;20:S85.

Powell KE, Thompson PD, Casperson CJ, Kendrick, JS. Physical activity and the incidence of coronary heart disease. Ann Rev Public Health 1978;8:253-87.

Seals DR, Hagberg JM, Hurley BF, Ehsani AA, Holloszy JO. Effects of endurance training on glucose tolerance and plasma lipids in older men and women. JAMA 1984a;252:645-9.

Seals DR, Hagberg JM, Hurley BF, Ehsani AA, Holloszy JO. Endurance training in older men and women. I. Cardiovascular responses to exercise. J Appl Physiol 1984b;57:1024-9.

Slattery ML, Jacobs DR Jr., Nichaman MZ. Leisure time physical activity and coronary heart disease death. The US Railroad Study. Circulation 1989;79:304-11.

Thompson PD, Cullinane EM, Sady SP et al. Modest changes in high-density lipoprotein concentration and metabolism with prolonged exercise training. Circulation 1988;78:25-34.

Ward A, Morris D, Porcari J et al. Effects of walking and/or low fat diet on total cholesterol and HDL cholesterol and risk ratio (abstract). Circulation 1989;80:509-14.

Weltman A, Matter S, Stamford A. Caloric restriction and/or mild exercise: effects on serum lipids and body composition. Am J Clin Nutr 1980;33:1002-9.

Wenger HA, Bell CJ. The interactions of intensity, frequency and duration of exercise training in altering cardiorespiratory fitness. Sports Med 1986;3:346-56.

White MK, Yeater RA, Martin RB et al. Effects of aerobic dancing and walking on cardiovascular function and muscular strength in postmenopausal women. J Sports Med Phys Fitness 1984;24:159-66.

Williams PT, Wood PD, Haskell WL et al. The effects of running mileage and duration on plasma lipoprotein levels. JAMA 1982;247:2674-9.

Wood PD, Williams PT, Haskell WL. Physical activity and high-density lipoproteins. In Miller NE, Miller GJ, eds. Clinical and Metabolic Aspect of High-Density Lipoprotein. Elsevier: Amsterdam 1984:131-65.

Effects of Lactate Threshold Level Training in Patients with Coronary Heart Disease

Masaki Takeda, M.S., Kiyoji Tanaka, Ph.D., Katsumi Asano, Ph.D.
Hyun Soo Kim, Ph.D., Yasuhito Kumazaki, M.S.
Yutaka Watanabe, M.D., Teruo Hiyama, M.D.

INTRODUCTION

The most difficult problem in designing exercise programs is the prescription of the appropriate exercise intensity (ACSM, 1991), since the safe and optimal intensity required for improving the aerobic capacity of patients with coronary heart disease is not known. Usually, target heart rate, oxygen uptake adjusted for the desired relative intensity, metabolic requirements or rating of perceived exertion have been used to determine exercise intensity not only for middle-aged persons but also for older persons or patients with chronic disease. The percentage of functional capacity and maximal heart rate which a given individual is able to sustain for a specified period varies with each individual. Marathon runners are able to maintain 80 percent of their maximal oxygen uptake for over two hours, but poorly conditioned individuals exercising at 80 percent of maximal oxygen uptake are fatigued in a few minutes. This variance may be explained in part by differences in the relative intensity of the exercise at which blood lactate increases. These differences in the ability to sustain a given exercise intensity must be taken into consideration in developing the exercise prescription (ACSM, 1991).

When exercise intensity increases above lactate threshold, an excess load is imposed on cardiorespiratory function (Rousseau et al., 1973; Coyle et al., 1983; Hagberg et al., 1984; Tanaka et al., 1986). Tanaka et al. (1986) have demonstrated (1) that stroke volume peaks at a higher heart rate for the trained than the untrained, as does lactate threshold and (2) that stroke volume for the untrained is diminished when the work rate exceeds that corresponding to the lactate threshold. The oxygen uptake at lactate threshold varies largely from 40 percent to 80 percent of maximal oxygen uptake in sedentary persons whether asymptomatic or symptomatic. One can hypothesize, therefore, that lactate threshold is an optimal exercise intensity.

Prescribing exercise at the lactate threshold level is more important from the viewpoint of safety for patients with coronary heart disease than for persons without heart disease. It has not been ascertained, however, whether the intensity of exercise at the lactate threshold level is appropriate and effective for patients with coronary heart disease. The purposes of this study were to determine if lactate threshold is an optimal intensity of exercise in patients with coronary heart disease, and to evaluate the effect of 12 months of lactate threshold level training on aerobic capacity.

METHODS

Subjects

Nine patients (two males and seven females), aged 46 to 69 (56.6 ± 8.3) participated in this study. The body weight and stature of these patients averaged 54.4 ± 7.4 kg and 152.1 ± 8.6 cm, respectively. Of the nine subjects, seven were patients with stable angina pectoris (one male and six female) and two (one male and one female) with a well-documented previous myocardial infarction. Seven patients with angina pectoris had abnormal ST-segment depression during treadmill exercise test. Two patients (one male and one female) had angiographically proven coronary heart disease, including one major vessel with ≥75 percent stenosis. All patients were taking medications such as calcium antagonists (seven patients), beta-adrenergic blocking agents (three patients), nitrate (one patient), and diuretics (one patient) before the initiation of this study, but the dosages were identical during the entire study period. None of the subjects had smoking and exercise habits before the initiation of this study. Informed consent was obtained from each patient.

Assessment of Lactate Threshold and Peak Oxygen Uptake

Submaximal and near maximal aerobic capacity of the patients were evaluated by the oxygen uptake at lactate threshold and peak oxygen uptake. Both were measured by a symptom-limited maximal cycling exercise test on a Monark cycle ergometer. Following two to four minutes of unloaded warm-up cycling at 60 revolutions per minute, a workload of 15 watts was administered and thereafter increased by 15 watts every minute (Tanaka et al., 1989, 1990). All metabolic measurements of expiratory gases were determined by standard techniques of open circuit spirometry with Fukuda Sangyo IS-5000 system. For determination of lactate threshold, a series of blood samples were drawn from the antecubital vein every minute during exercise. Lactate threshold was detected as the point during exercise of increasing intensity at which lactate increased in a nonlinear fashion, utilizing the log-log transformation method (Beaver et al., 1985). Lactate concentration was measured by the electrochemical enzymatic method with a Yellow Institute lactate analyzer (Model 23). Aerobic capacity of each patient was tested before training and three, six, and 12 months after the initiation of training.

Lactate Threshold Level Training

The patients participated in an in-hospital supervised exercise training program two days per week, 90 and 120 minutes each session, for a period of 12 months, and also a self-controlled exercise training program two to three days per week, 30 to 40 minutes each session, throughout the entire study period. The supervised program included a 15-minute warm-up period of calisthenics and stretching exercises; 15 to 30 minutes of continuous cycling at the intensity corresponding to lactate threshold; 30 to 40 minutes of aerobic dancing or ground walking; 10 to 15 minutes of non-device muscle exercise; and 10-minute cool-down. The intensity of exercise was maintained at lactate threshold level throughout the study period. The absolute intensity in terms of work rate was, however, increased since most patients showed a remarkable increase in oxygen uptake at lactate threshold at three-month and six-month follow-up tests. Each training session was supervised by at least two of the authors. In the self-controlled training program, patients were instructed to do exercise at a work rate, heart rate or rating of perceived exertion corresponding to lactate threshold as exactly as possible.

Statistical analyses

The significance of the differences between four sets of data (i.e., before training and three, six, and 12 months after training) was tested with a repeated-measures ANOVA design. Scheffe F-test was used for the variables which were found to be significant after ANOVA. Pearson product-moment correlation technique was applied to test the correlation between variables. Statistical significance was accepted only when p values were less than 0.05 in all analyses. Values are shown in mean ± standard deviation (M ± SD).

RESULTS

Aerobic capacity measured on four exercise test occasions are presented in Table 1. Oxygen uptake at lactate threshold and peak oxygen uptake averaged 13.8 ± 2.3 and 19.7 ± 3.7 ml/kg/min respectively before training (Figure 1). Oxygen uptake at lactate threshold corresponded to 71.3 percent of peak oxygen (Figure 2). The lactate threshold relative to peak oxygen uptake was 10 to 20 percent higher than the relative exercise intensity recommended by the American College of Sports Medicine (ACSM, 1991) for coronary heart disease patients at the initial stage of the program (Figure 2). The absolute value of oxygen uptake at lactate threshold highly correlated (R = 0.89) with peak oxygen uptake (Figure 3). Relatively large individual differences (57.0 to 85.5 percent) were seen in lactate threshold relative to peak oxygen uptake before training (Figure 4).

TABLE 1

Aerobic Capacity Measured on Four Exercise Test Occasions

Variables	Before	3 mo	6 mo	12 mo
Oxygen uptake at lactate threshold (ml/kg/min)	13.8 ± 2.3	18.0 ± 2.7*	18.6 ± 2.9*	18.8 ± 1.6*
change (%)		31.7 ± 16.4	36.9 ± 25.4	39.0 ± 25.2
Peak oxygen uptake (ml/kg/min)	19.7 ± 3.7	26.5 ± 4.4*	27.9 ± 4.5*	27.1 ± 3.4*
change (%)		39.9 ± 39.2	47.4 ± 41.1	43.4 ± 38.1
Lactate threshold relative to peak oxygen uptake (%)	71.3 ± 8.4	68.7 ± 7.4	66.8 ± 3.3	69.9 ± 5.9

* Significantly different from the pre-training mean value

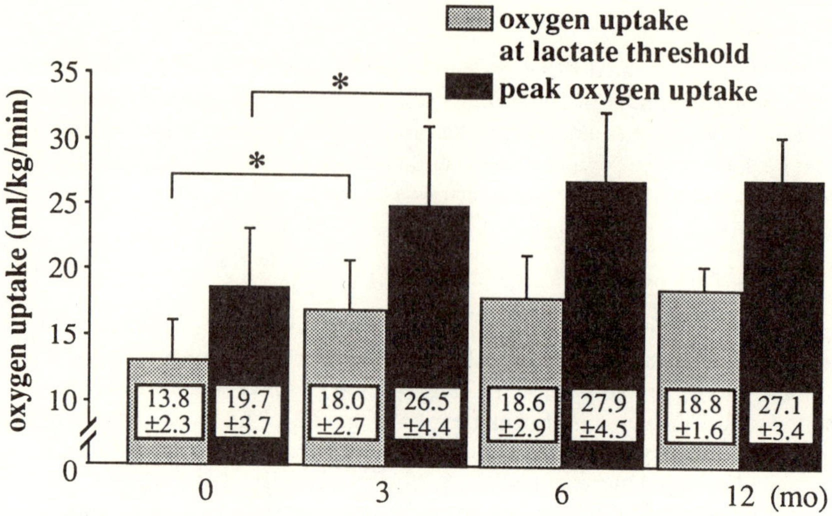

Figure 1. Changes in oxygen uptake at lactate threshold and peak oxygen uptake during program

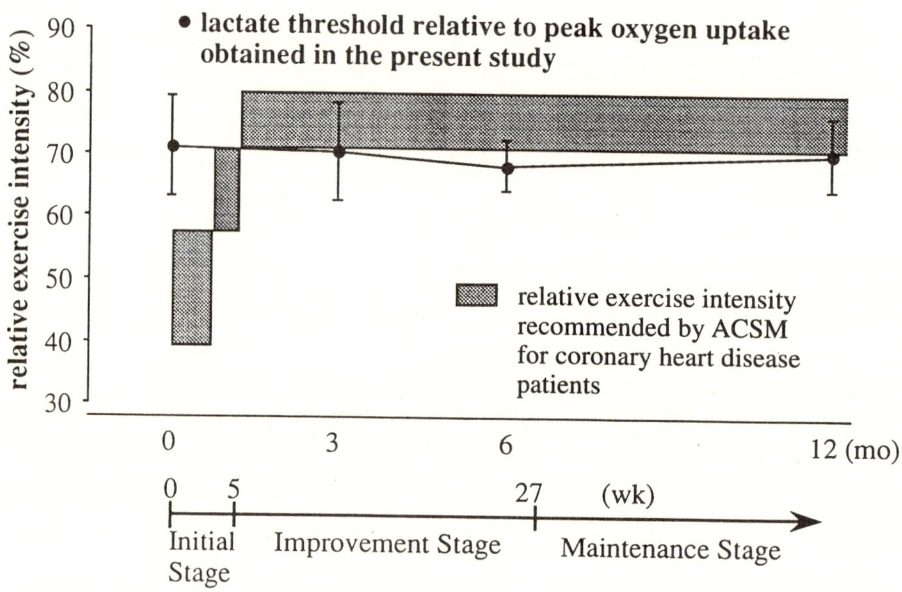

Figure 2. Training intensity prescribed in the present study (ACSM: American College of Sports Medicine)

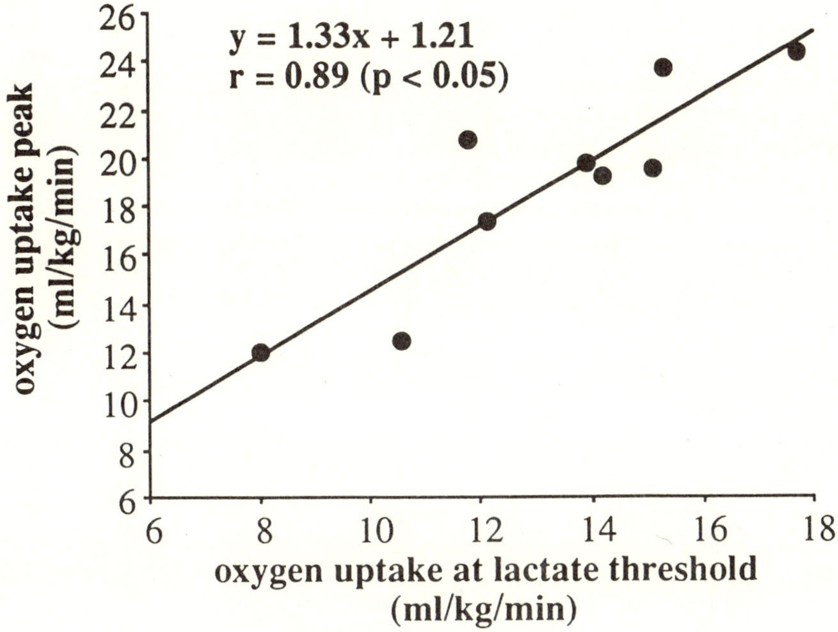

Figure 3. Relationship between oxygen uptake at lactate threshold and peak oxygen uptake before training

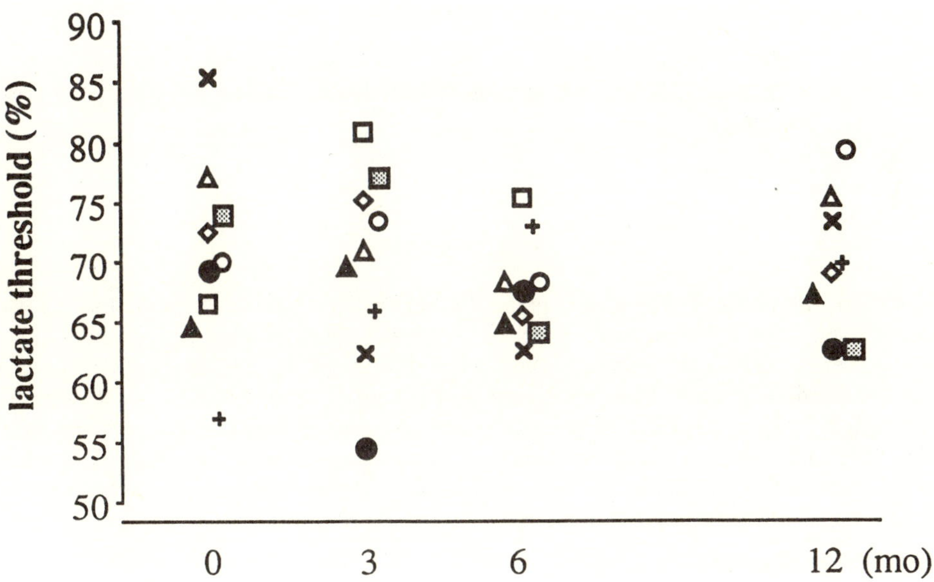

Figure 4. Distribution of lactate threshold relative to peak oxygen uptake for each patient on four exercise test occasions

With training, there were significant increases of 31.7 percent in oxygen uptake at lactate threshold and of 39.9 percent in peak oxygen uptake after three months of training, but thereafter both remained essentially unchanged (Table 1 and Figure 1). The absolute amount of change in peak oxygen uptake during the first three months correlated significantly with the change in oxygen uptake at lactate threshold (Figure 5).

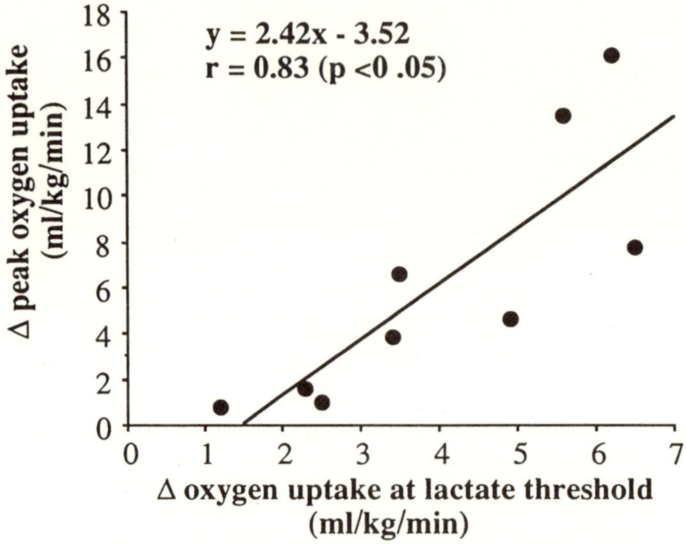

Figure 5. Relationship between change (Δ) oxygen uptake at lactate threshold and peak (Δ) oxygen uptake observed during the first three months of training

DISCUSSION

Various techniques can be used to prescribe and monitor exercise intensity. In the present study, lactate threshold level was used as an exercise intensity for cardiac patients, most of whom were middle-aged women, in the belief that lactate threshold is safe and enables them to continue exercise for a relatively long period of time. Whether lactate threshold level might be an optimal and effective intensity for coronary heart disease patients has not been adequately studied. The present study attempted to determine the effects of 12 months of exercise training at the lactate threshold level on the aerobic capacity of patients with stable angina pectoris and/or a previous myocardial infarction.

Initial Level of Aerobic Capacity

Oxygen uptake at lactate threshold (13.8 ml/kg/min) corresponded to 71.3 percent of peak oxygen uptake (19.7 ml/kg/min), which is similar to the results of Coyle et al. (1983).

They reported that lactate threshold of untrained patients occurred at 67 percent of maximal oxygen uptake during treadmill exercise test. It appears that these figures are somewhat higher than those of normals. This may be due to a lower peak oxygen uptake as a result of impaired cardiac function such as a decrease in stroke volume (Coyle et al., 1983).

Although the lactate threshold relative to peak oxygen uptake was 10 to 20 percent higher during the initial stage of the program (Figure 2) than the relative intensity recommended by the American College of Sports Medicine for coronary heart disease patients, the level might be low enough not to impair cardiac function during exercise and recovery. In fact, no patients experienced cardiac complications during exercise. While the oxygen uptake at lactate threshold correlated highly ($R = 0.89$) with peak oxygen uptake (Figure 3), relatively large individual differences (57.0-85.5 percent) were seen in lactate threshold relative to peak oxygen uptake before training (Figure 4). This means that, if a given relative intensity (e.g., 70 percent of peak oxygen uptake) is prescribed for all patients, intensity may become considerably higher or lower than lactate threshold for some patients. From this point of view, a lactate threshold that is from 40 percent to 80 percent of peak (or maximal) oxygen uptake appears to be a suitable exercise intensity.

Changes in Aerobic Capacity with Exercise Training

Many positive circulatory effects during submaximal or angina threshold exercise have been reported after several months of exercise training (Clausen and Trap-Jensen, 1970; Detry et al., 1971; Redwood et al., 1972; Rousseau et al., 1973; Ferguson et al., 1974; Clausen, 1976; Greenberg et al., 1979; Verani et al., 1981; May et al., 1984; Sullivan et al., 1985). In the present study, oxygen uptake at lactate threshold (31.7 percent) and peak oxygen uptake (39.9 percent) improved largely in a relatively short period, but thereafter both attained to plateau (Figure 1). Due to the considerably low initial level of aerobic capacity as usually found in cardiac patients, the post-training value of aerobic capacity was average for the same group (Clausen, 1976), even after aerobic capacity improved largely. However, it is worthwhile for those patients to improve their aerobic capacity to the same level as normals.

The significant correlation between the change in oxygen uptake at lactate threshold and the change in peak oxygen uptake (Figure 5) observed during the first three months agrees with the results of Sullivan et al. (1985), who has obtained an $R = 0.45$ between the change in ventilatory threshold and the change in peak oxygen uptake after 12 months of training. Lactate threshold correlates well with muscle respiratory capacity (Ivy et al., 1980; Hagberg, 1984), while maximal oxygen uptake appears to be more closely related to cardiovascular factors such as cardiac output (Hagberg, 1984). The fact that exercise training at lactate threshold level improved not only submaximal but also maximal aerobic capacity indicates that both peripheral and central adaptations may have occurred with training.

The most important finding is that no significant improvements occurred in oxygen uptake at lactate threshold and peak oxygen uptake from month three to the end of the study, although absolute exercise intensity was increased at months three and/or six. These data indicate that lactate threshold level may not always be of sufficient intensity to induce further improvement in aerobic capacity of patients after several months of exercise training. Hurley et al. (1984) have shown that normal men have to exercise at a higher percent of blood lactate concentration. However, Saltin et al. (1969) found that blood lactate concentration at the same relative intensity of exercise did not change in 42 men after a training program that induced an 18 percent increase in maximal oxygen uptake. The data obtained in the present study support the results of Saltin et al. (1969). Hurley et al. (1984) attributed the discrepancy between studies to differences in training frequency and intensity. Recent studies (Ehsani et al., 1981, 1982; Hagberg et al., 1983, 1991) have shown that high-intensity and prolonged endurance exercise training can, in selected patients, result in a higher double product at the onset of significant ST-segment depression (>0.1 mV) and a direct cardiac benefit such as the improvement in stroke volume. These results do not imply that all patients should initiate such an intense training program, but rather indicate that, in selected patients undergoing a training stimulus well in excess of that conventionally prescribed for coronary patients, the training-induced adaptations may be substantially greater than previously believed (Hagberg, 1991). On the basis of these studies, there may be more room to increase aerobic capacity for coronary patients. However, concerning the safety of high intensity training, the American Association of Cardiovascular and Pulmonary Rehabilitation (1991) proposes that unconventionally vigorous exercise (>85 percent of functional capacity) should be avoided by patients with coronary artery disease. In the present study, almost all patients could exercise over 12 months at a heart rate or work rate at lactate threshold, which corresponded to below 85 percent of peak uptake. In this context, lactate threshold would be a safe exercise intensity and be consistent with or just below the intensity recommended by the American College of Sports Medicine for patients at the maintenance stage. It should be further examined whether an exercise intensity higher than lactate threshold is safe and tolerable for most coronary heart disease patients, whether similar training effects could be obtained at an exercise intensity lower than lactate threshold, or whether it is necessary to further improve aerobic capacity in these patients.

CONCLUSION

Despite the inherent limitation of this study of two males and seven females, lactate threshold may be a suitable exercise intensity for coronary heart disease patients with a variety of lactate thresholds relative to peak oxygen uptake. Although lactate threshold level training significantly improves aerobic capacity of coronary heart disease patients in a relatively short period, this capacity seems to remain unchanged after that. Another approach may be necessary for further improving the aerobic capacity of most coronary heart disease patients whose aerobic capacities have reached a plateau.

ACKNOWLEDGEMENTS

We express our sincere appreciation to Akira Kudo and Kazunobu Arima for their technical assistance. Appreciation is also extended to all the patients who served as subjects.

REFERENCES

American Association of Cardiovascular and Pulmonary Rehabilitation, Guidelines for Cardiac Rehabilitation Programs. Champaign: Human Kinetics, 1991:9-15.

American College of Sports Medicine. Guidelines for Exercise Testing and Prescription. Fourth Edition. Philadelphia: Lea & Febiger, 1991:93-119.

Beaver WL, Wasserman K, Whipp BJ. Improved detection of lactate threshold during exercise using a log-log transformation. J Appl Physiol 1985;59:1936-40.

Clausen JP, Trap-Jensen J. Effects of training on the distribution of cardiac output in patients with coronary heart disease. Circulation 1970;42:611-24.

Clausen JP. Circulatory adjustments to dynamic exercise and effects of physical training in normal subjects and in patients with coronary heart disease. Prog Cardiovasc Dis 1976;18:459-95.

Coyle EF, Martin WH, Ehsani AA et al. Blood lactate threshold in some well-trained ischemic heart disease patients. J Appl Physiol 1983;54:18-23.

Detry JMR, Roussau M, Vandenbroucke G, Kusumi F, Brasseur L, Bruce RA. Increased arteriovenous oxygen difference after physical training in coronary heart disease. Circulation 1971;44:109-18.

Ehsani AA, Heath GW, Hagberg JM, Sobel BE, Holloszy JO. Effects of 12 months of intense exercise training on ischemic ST-segment depression in patients with coronary heart disease. Circulation 1981;64:1116-24.

Ehsani AA, Martin WH, Heath GW, Coyle EF. Cardiac effects of prolonged and intense exercise training in patients with coronary artery disease. Am J Cardiol 1982;50:246-54.

Ferguson RJ, Petitclerc R, Choquette G et al. Effects of physical training on treadmill exercise capacity, collateral circulation and progression of coronary disease. Am J Cardiol 1974;34:764-9.

Greenberg MA, Arbeit S, Rubin IL. The role of physical training in patients with coronary heart disease. Am Heart J 1979;97:527-34.

Hagberg JM, Ehsani AA, Holloszy JO. Effects of 12 months of intense exercise training on stroke volume in patients with coronary artery disease. Circulation 1983;67:1194-9.

Hagberg JM. Physiological implications of the lactate threshold. Int J Sports Med 1984;5:107-9.

Hagberg JM. Physiologic adaptations to prolonged high-intensity exercise training in patients with coronary artery disease. Med Sci Sports Exerc 1991;23:661-7.

Hurley BF, Hagberg JM, Allen WK, Seals DR, Young JC, Cuddihee RW, Holloszy JO. Effect of training on blood lactate levels during submaximal exercise. J Appl Physiol 1984;56:1260-4.

Ivy JL, Withers RT, Van Handel PJ, Elger DH, Costill DL. Muscle respiratory capacity and fiber type as determinants of lactate threshold. J Appl Physiol 1980;48:523-7.

May GA, Nagle FJ. Changes in rate-pressure product with physical training of individuals with coronary heart disease. Phys Ther 1984;64:1361-7.

Redwood DR, Rosing DR, Epstein SE. Circulatory and symptomatic effects of physical training in patients with coronary-artery disease and angina pectoris. N Engl J Med 1972;286:959-65.

Rousseau MF, Brasseur LA, Detry JM. Hemodynamic determinants of maximal oxygen intake in patients with healed myocardial infarction: influence of physical training. Circulation 1973;48:943-9.

Saltin BL, Hartley LH, Kilbom Å, Åstrand I. Physical training in sedentary middle-aged and older men. Scand J Clin Lab Invest 1969;24:323-34.

Sullivan M, Ahnve S, Froelicher VF, Meyers J. The influence of physical training on the ventilatory threshold of the patients with coronary heart disease. Am Heart J 1985;109:458-63.

Tanaka K, Yoshimura T, Sumida S et al. Transient responses in cardiac function below, at, and above anaerobic threshold. Eur J Appl Physiol 1986;55:356-61.

Tanaka K, Kim HS, Wakita M, Nakadomo F, Hazama T, Maeda K. Effects of aerobic conditioning plus caloric restriction in obese middle-aged women. Jpn J Appl Physiol 1989;19:495-504.

Tanaka K, Takeshima N, Kato T, Niihata S, Ueda K. Critical determinants of endurance performance in middle-aged and elderly endurance runners with heterogeneous training habits. Eur J Appl Physiol 1990;59:443-9.

Verani MS, Hartung GH, Hoepfel-Harris J, Welton D, Pratt CM, Millar RR. Effects of exercise training on left ventricular performance and myocardial perfusion in patients with coronary heart disease. Am J Cardiol 1981;47:797-803.

Physical Activity and Hip Fracture: Comparison of Leisure Physical Activity and Autonomy Levels of Women 60 Years and Over, Half with No History of Fracture and Half Prior to a Hip Fracture

Andrée Imbach, Ph.D., Daniel Picard, M.D., M.Sc., F.R.P.C.(C)
François Lessard, M.D., F.R.P.C.(C), Pierre Sabouret, M.D.
Lesly Germain M.D., F.R.C.S.(C), Colette Lortie, P.Dt.
Maryse Boulard, P.Dt., M.Sc.

INTRODUCTION

A previous study on the nutritional status of 137 elderly women living in Montreal (Delvin et al., 1988) found an inadequate daily intake of calcium in 84 percent of the sample and a similarly poor intake of dietary vitamin D, which correlated with low serum values of 25-hydroxyvitamin D, in 70 percent of the sample. The suspicion of a high risk of osteoporosis in these women together with the high incidence of hip fracture in the Quebec population, 4.5 per 1000 inhabitants over 65 years of age (Government of Quebec, 1988), prompted a broader study of the etiology of hip fracture in the context of postmenopausal osteoporosis. The principal objectives of this study were to identify the characteristics of a population of autonomous women over 60 years of age, living independently, who sustain a hip fracture and to compare them with a group having no history of fracture. Since regular exercise may help to maintain bone density and prevent falls and thus reduce the risk of osteoporotic fractures (Cummings et al., 1985), physical activity past and present was assessed and is reported here.

SUBJECTS

The subjects were 64 French-Canadian women between 60 and 84 years of age (mean 70.6 years). Thirty-two women were being admitted to the hospital for a hip fracture (subcapital or intertrochanteric) sustained after little or no trauma. These were paired by age with 32 women having no history of fracture and no established diagnosis of osteoporosis. Control subjects were recruited through a radio information program for senior citizens, bulletin boards in church halls and apartment buildings for seniors or were relatives of university employees. All subjects were living independently in the community, were lucid and normally physically active for their age. They had no previous history of neoplasms, steroid therapy, abnormal thyroid function or alcoholism. The research protocol was reviewed and approved by the Ethics Committee of each participating hospital. Participants gave informed written consent after the nature, purpose, risks and benefits of the study were explained.

METHODS

Assessment Methods

For the functional assessment of the subjects, "mobility" was scored on a scale of 12 according to their ability to move around the house and outside, a perfect score indicating that the subject had no physical difficulty with walking, managing stairs or getting around in normal or bad weather. The level of "autonomy" was scored on a scale of 6, according to the amount of help needed (in hours/week) to perform the necessary home duties, like cleaning, shopping, cooking, washing and whether help from the family or community services was unnecessary, occasional, habitual or essential. Subjects were questioned on the frequency of their outings, whether every day, few times a week or seldom.

To find out how active these women had been during their lifetime, a questionnaire on sports and other leisure physical activities was administered. It started with the time of the study for control subjects, and just prior to their hip fracture for the hospitalized group, then went back in time to their adult life (before menopause), and then to adolescence and childhood. Each type of physical activity practiced was allocated an intensity level in METS metabolic equivalents according to the values published by Taylor et al. (1978). For each subject the average intensity level of that physical activity was then converted to a score from 0 to 6 as described in Table 1, a method modified from Blair (1984) to allow for a better discrimination of subjects.

For childhood, adolescence and adult life, because the duration and frequency of leisure physical activity could not be assessed, only intensity levels of activities were considered. However, for the time of the study or prior to the hip fracture, the time duration each week

TABLE 1

MET Values Of Intensity Levels of Activity and Corresponding Scores

Level of Physical Activity	Number of METS	Score
Sedentary	< - 1.0	0
Light activity	1.1 - 2.9	1
Moderate activity	3.0 - 3.9	2
	4.0 - 4.9	3
Hard activity	5.0 - 5.9	4
	6.0 - 6.9	5
Very hard activity	> - 7.0	6

of leisure physical activity was recorded as well as the frequency of its practice, which was scored from 1 to 4, dependent on whether practice was once or less than once per week, a few times a week, every day less than one hour, or one hour or more every day. The time spent each week for each activity was noted, allowing for the calculation of an average intensity per week (METS/week). This value multiplied by the weight in kg gave for each subject the average energy expenditure attributable to physical activity in kJ per week or day.

Statistical Analysis

Data on physical activity were of two types: estimations of past activity based on an ordinal scale of response and multiple of resting metabolism (METS), measured on an interval scale. To take into account the level of measurement of these variables as much as the paired condition of the two samples to be compared, estimations of past activity were analyzed using Wilcoxon matched-pairs rank test, and data related to METS were submitted to a paired t-test. All analyses were conducted at an alpha level of .05.

RESULTS

Mobility and autonomy

The women admitted to hospital with a hip fracture were, prior to their fracture, as mobile as their control counterparts. On a maximum score of 12 for mobility, fractured women scored 11.5 ± 1.1, while the control group scored 11.9 ± 0.7 (NS). However, as shown in Figure 1, 20 percent of the women who sustained a hip fracture were already significantly less autonomous before the fracture than the control women who all scored "perfectly autonomous" (p=0.04). Asked whether they were going out every day, few times/week or seldom, 87 percent of control women answered every day, as compared to 62 percent of the women with a hip fracture; this difference was significant (p = 0.02).

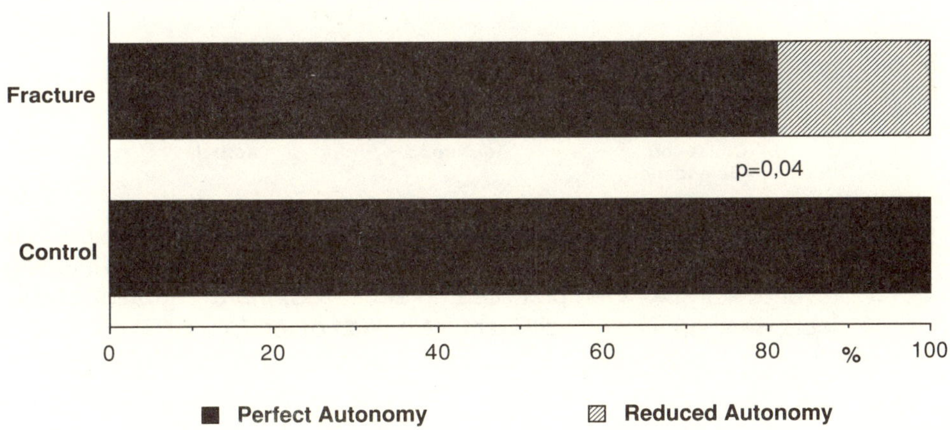

Figure 1. Assessment of autonomy level as expressed in percent of subjects with perfect autonomy scores (maximum of 6) and those with reduced autonomy (less than 6). Significantly different: (p = 0.04).

Lifelong Physical Activity Level

Figure 2 presents the average intensity of leisure physical activities practiced at different times of life. Scores refer to intensities in METS as shown in Table 1. Both groups of women were very similar in childhood and adolescence, practicing the usual sports and games: swimming, skipping rope, bicycling, skating, skiing, playing tennis and team sports like volleyball.

The difference in physical activity level appears in adulthood, the control group remaining significantly more active than the women who will later fracture a hip ($p = 0.05$). In addition to walking more, they dance, do gymnastics, work in the garden, bicycle and play tennis. At the time of the study (actual), the involvement of both groups in leisure physical activities had markedly decreased (NS), but more so in the fracture group. The most popular activity is walking, while some are still involved in gymnastics. The sum of the three scores for the time periods assessed is 9.6 ± 2.0 for the control subjects and 8.5 ± 1.7 for the women with a hip fracture, a cumulative value significantly higher for the control group ($p = 0.04$), suggesting that these women have been more active physically all through their lifetime than those who later fracture a hip.

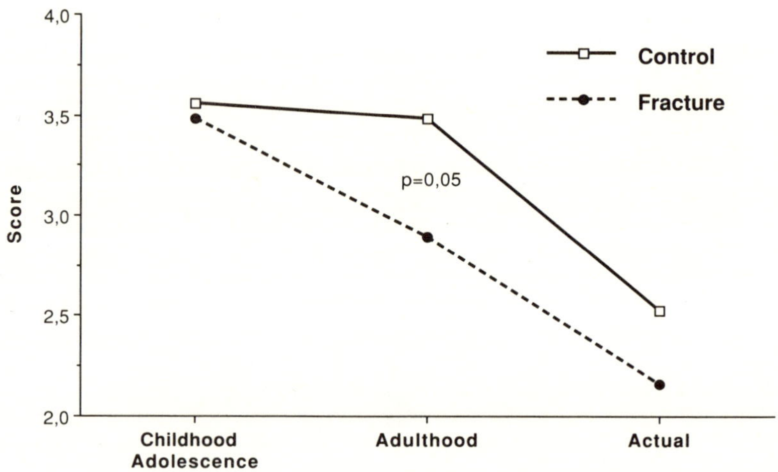

Figure 2. Retrospective assessment of leisure physical activity at different times of life, as expressed by a score, corresponding to the average intensity level of activities then practiced. In adulthood, the two groups of subjects were significantly different from each other: ($p = 0.05$).

Physical Activity Level at the Time of Study or Prior to the Fracture

To quantify better the level of leisure physical activity at the time of the study or prior to the hip fracture, frequency and duration of practice were examined. The frequency of practice was significantly greater for the control subjects, who had a score of 3.4 ± 0.8 on a maximum of 4, than for the women with a hip fracture, who scored only 2.7 ± 0.9 (p = 0.004).

The time spent each week on physical activities other than the normal activities of life is shown in Figure 3. Control subjects spent twice the time allocated by the fracture group to leisure physical activity, that is 8.0 ± 5.2 hours/week, compared to 4.6 ± 4.9, a significant difference (p = 0.002). The combination of the intensity values in METS of the different activities practiced and the hours/week of practice, yields an intensity of practice of 32 METS/week ± 22.0 for the control group and of 14.9 METS/week ± 17.0 for the women who sustained a hip fracture, a significant difference (p <0.002) (Figure 3). Introducing the weight factor, the energy expenditure (Figure 3) coming from leisure physical activity varies significantly, amounting to 1100 kJ/day (270 kcal) for the women without fracture and only 540 kJ/day (130 kcal) for the fracture group (p = 0.003).

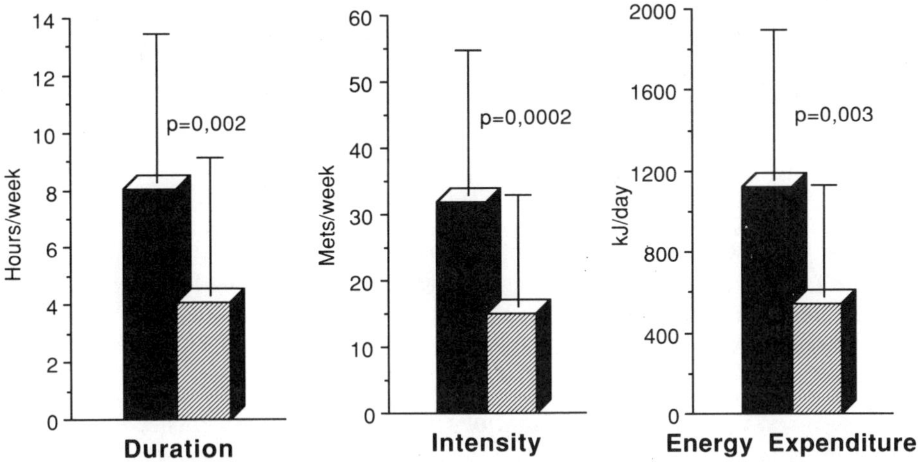

Figure 3. Assessment of physical activity level at the time of the study or just prior to the hip fracture, taking into account 1) the time spent each week for leisure physical activity, 2) the intensity in Mets of activities practiced weekly and 3) the energy expenditure in kJ/day coming from these activities. The two groups studied were significantly different from each other in each parameter, the hip fracture group (solid black vertical bars) showing consistently lower values than the control group (hatched vertical bars): 1) p = 0.002; 2) p = 0.002 and 3) p = 0.003. Vertical bars represent x ± SD.

Predictors of Hip Fracture

Some of the parameters studied were identified as significant predictors of who, among the subjects, had sustained a hip fracture. The time (hours/week) devoted to leisure physical activity came out as the best predictor P (p = 0.02), followed by the frequency of outings (p = 0.03).

DISCUSSION

This study of hip fracture in otherwise healthy postmenopausal women shows that their functional status was already impaired before the fracture when compared with control subjects of similar age and ethnic and social background who had no history of fracture. The frequency of their outings had already decreased significantly and, even though all women studied had been living independently and were labeled "autonomous," those admitted to the hospital with a hip fracture had experienced less autonomy, requiring more help for their daily activities than did the control subjects. The two groups did not differ, however, in their level of mobility, as expressed in their ability to move about, inside and outside of their homes.

When questioned retrospectively, women who fractured a hip had been less inclined to practice leisure physical activities during their adult life than had the control women, who, although coming from a similar ethnic and social background, had also maintained a higher level of physical activity in later life. This observation was also reported in a Swedish study (Åstrom et al., 1987), which found that women sustaining hip fractures had been less active physically during their fertile period than matched control subjects had been. These authors also suggested that women who were very active up to the age of 45 would probably continue to be so after that age, thus contributing to the prevention of postmenopausal osteoporosis.

At the time of the study or prior to their fracture, the two groups of women showed a marked difference in the frequency of leisure physical activities and also in the time they devoted each week to these activities, with the control women devoting twice as much time as the fracture patients, suggesting that consistency is important for gaining long-term benefits from exercise. The higher activity level of the members of the control group is also evident in its practice of more intense activities and its greater daily energy expenditure.

The results add evidence supporting the benefit of exercise in postmenopausal women to reduce the incidence of hip fracture, as suggested in previous studies (Chow et al., 1987; Cooper et al., 1988; Lau et al., 1988). The benefits of exercise might be due to a positive effect on bone mass (shown in our study by results that will be published in another paper), a lower rate of bone loss (Suominen, 1988), the maintenance of muscle function reducing the risk of falls, and/or the improvement of the neuromuscular protective responses in a fall situation (Cooper, 1989).

This study also showed that the amount of recreational exercise is an important predictor of hip fracture. A similar observation has already been made (Farmer et al., 1989), including the finding that women who reported little or no exercise in recreation were almost twice as likely to fracture a hip as were those who reported much or moderate exercise.

CONCLUSION

Based on these results, for the prevention of hip fractures, women in their adult and postmenopausal years would benefit from remaining physically active in their leisure time, and practicing sports and other activities on a regular basis. In addition, a decrease in the frequency of outings and a diminution of autonomy may signify a higher risk of sustaining a hip fracture.

ACKNOWLEDGEMENT

This study has been supported by a grant from the National Health Research and Development Program, Health and Welfare Canada, Ottawa, Canada.

REFERENCES

Åstrom J, Ahnqvist S, Beertema J, Jonsson B. Physical activity in women sustaining fracture of the neck of the femur. J Bone Joint Surg 1987;69-B:381-3.

Blair SN. How to assess exercise habits and physical fitness. In: Matarazzo JD, Miller NE, Weiss SM, eds. Behavior and Health: a Handbook of Health Enhancement and Disease Prevention. New York: John Wiley and Sons, 1984:424-47.

Chow RK, Harrison JE, Notarius C. Effect of two randomised exercise programmes on bone mass of healthy postmenopausal women. Br Med J 1987;295:1441-4.

Cooper C, Barker DPJ, Wickham C. Physical activity, muscle strength, and calcium intake in fracture of the proximal femur in Britain. Br Med J 1988; 297:1443-6.

Cooper C. Bone mass, muscle function and fracture of the proximal femur. Br J Hosp Med 1989;42:277-80.

Cummings SR, Kelsey JL, Nevitt MC, O'Dowd KJ. Epidemiology of osteoporosis and osteoporotic fractures. Epidemiol Rev 1985;7:178-208.

Delvin, EE, Imbach A, Copti M. Vitamin D nutritional status and related biochemical indices in an autonomous elderly population. Am J Clin Nutr 1988;48:373-8.

Farmer ME, Harris T, Madans JH, Wallace RB, Cornoni-Huntley J, White LR. Anthropometric indicators and hip fracture: the NHANES I epidemiologic follow-up study. J Am Ger Soc 1989;37:9-16.

Lau E, Donnan S, Barker DJP, Cooper CC. Physical activity and calcium intake in fracture of the proximal femur in Hong Kong. Br Med J 1988;297:1441-3.

Suominen H. Physical activity and bone. Ann Chir Gyn 1988;77:184-8.

Taylor HL, Jacobs DR, Schucker B, Knudsen J, Leon AS, Debacker GA. A questionnaire for the assessment of leisure time physical activities. J Chron Dis 1978;31:741-55.

Value of Complex Rehabilitative Treatment of Patients with Back Pain

Kazimiera Milanowska, M.D.

INTRODUCTION

In most cases back pain results from degeneration in intervertebral disc structure, which, having lost elasticity, becomes pathologically deformed and dislocated. These changes in the disc structure lead to multidirectional pathology of the intervertebral joints, ligaments and joint capsules of the spine, resulting in collision between bony elements and nerve roots, spinal cord and blood vessels. The damage and flaccidity of elastic elements of the spine bring about its instability, which itself is the factor causing pain. In many patients, especially in women over the age of 40, an additional factor causing back pain is osteoporosis.

With age the human spine degenerates. This normal process alters mechanical characteristics, and leads to low back problems. This physiological aging appears primarily in the cervical or lumbar spine as osteophytic formations (osteophytes) and narrowing of the joint or disc space. Osteophytes of the lumbar spine have been found in more than fifty percent of people after the fifth decade in both sexes. These changes lead to decreased overall motion.

The additional factor of back pain in postmenopausal women and elderly males is osteoporosis. Bone loss is a normal phenomenon that occurs during aging. As the life span of the adult population continues to lengthen, the clinical manifestations of osteoporosis are now clearly recognized in an ever-increasing population of senior citizens. Osteoporosis is a cause of vertebral fractures. Vertebral compression fractures or wedge fractures are estimated to occur in five to 40 percent of postmenopausal women (Kahanovitz, 1990).

REHABILITATIVE TREATMENT

The precise and full analysis of pathogenesis and pathomechanism of back pain determines the choice of the most effective treatment. The Rehabilitation Department at the University of Poznan has developed and introduced a complex, systematic rehabilitative treatment consisting of: 1) pain elimination, 2), stretching of spine to relieve compressed nerve roots, 3) strengthening of trunk muscles to form a strong "muscle corset," and 4) restoring good body posture and thus stability of the spine. The basics of treatment are: 1) gradation of the strength of pelvic traction, 2) analgesic physiotherapy, 3) systematization and gradation of kinesitherapy, 4) teaching exercises that the patient does at home, and 5) teaching the correct physical work and way of active life (Milanowska et al., 1978).

Pain Elimination

1st week. In cases of acute pain syndrome, the patient lies on a flat bed in the most comfortable and pain eliminating positions. Usually the patient lies on the back or on the side with lower extremities bent in hip and knee joints. This position lessens lumbar lordosis and loosens tension of ischio-femoral muscles. To relieve pain, analgesic electrotherapy like diadynamic currents, interferential currents (Nemectrodyn), and anode galvanization is used. During the first week, isometric exercises of trunk muscles, especially of abdominal muscles, breathing exercises and active exercises of upper extremities are introduced. These exercises are carried out in a position of the patient in which there is good pelvic stabilization and no lumbar lordosis. This means the elimination of all factors that may cause or increase pain. For example, when a patient must walk to the bathroom, he has to use crutches to eliminate overloading of the spine.

2nd week. After the disappearance of the acute pain syndrome, pelvic traction in bed with the initial load reaching 1/8 of the patient's weight (8 to 10 kg) is introduced. In cases where the patient has come to the hospital without symptoms of acute pain, traction in bed is recommended during the first week. Isometric exercises of trunk muscles are continued, followed by hot paraffin compresses and electrotherapy, and exercises that stretch and relax the spinal muscles are applied. These exercises are particularly advisable in cases of pain reflex scoliosis and strongly positive Lasaque sign.

3rd week. After a few days of traction in bed, intermittent traction on the traction table with gradual increase of load up to 1/2 of the patient's weight (30 to 40 kg) is introduced. Intermittent traction is applied after hot paraffin compresses during a period of 10 to 14 days. Directly after the traction the patient lies on his back with lower extremities bent in hip and knee joints for about one hour. Exercises that stretch spinal muscles are applied, and dynamic exercises that strengthen trunk muscles are gradually introduced.

4th - 6th week. The intensity of exercises is gradually increased, paying attention, first of all, to strengthening of abdominal, spinal, and gluteal muscles to form a strong muscle corset. Exercises aiming at obtaining proper posture of the body - mainly lessening of lumbar lordosis and forward tilt of the pelvis - are also applied. During exercises great attention is paid to the pain factor. Intensification or occurrence of pain during exercises calls for revision and analysis of applied exercises, eventual changes in exercise program or eliminating some exercises. After pain declines, in addition to performing individual exercises patients take part in group exercises with appropriately chosen exercises. They also exercise in water and swim in a pool with water temperature of 28 to 30° C.

Before the patient is discharged from the hospital, he is educated about proper care of the back. He is advised to:

1. Avoid soft beds, as these allow the spine to sag and give no support.

2. Avoid sitting on low soft chairs. Do not sit for prolonged periods. If you have to sit, avoid slouching, support the lumbar spine with a small pillow and use a high upright chair.

3. Do not lift heavy objects; if lifting is necessary, bend the knees and not the back, keeping the object as close to the body as possible (Grochmal, 1977).

4. Avoid prolonged standing.

5. Keep weight down, as obesity can contribute towards postural problems.

6. Perform trunk muscle exercises for 10 to 15 minutes every day, with the aim of strengthening abdominal, spinal and gluteal muscles.

For patients with marked degenerative changes, which are common among elderly patients, spa treatment is recommended.

Cervical Pain Syndromes

The symptoms present in cervical pain syndromes caused by spondylosis or spondyloarthrosis are mainly connected with the pressure on nerve roots. Thus, the aim of treatment in these cases is first of all decompression of the nerve roots and then stabilization of the cervical spine.

The rehabilitation treatment consisted of the following:

1) To remove pain due to stretching of cervical spine and decompression of the nerve roots, we applied: physical analgesic therapy, interferential currents, electrostimulation, physical therapy improving circulation, solux lamp, warm paraffin compresses, autotraction, traction on Glisson's loop. First, we recommend the traction of cervical spine on Glisson's loop, in sitting position with good stabilization of shoulder. The applied traction force is 6-8 kg. Before the traction, paraffin compresses of the neck are recommended if the patient tolerates warm procedures well or during the traction the solux lamp on the neck. After a few days of Glisson's loop traction, intermittent traction on a special table is introduced. This type of traction is performed in the lying position, the force applied being 8 to 14 kg.

After the traction, the patients get the orthopedic collar and lie in it for one hour. Neck massage and relaxation exercises are also recommended.

2) Main aim of treatment is, by strengthening of nape, neck and shoulder muscles, to achieve stabilization of the cervical spine. This aim was reached by systematized isometric and dynamic exercises and by application of orthopedic collars.

In order to stabilize the cervical spine, the patients perform exercises to strengthen the muscles that stabilize this segment of spine; these are exercises of upper part of trapezius muscle and neck extensor. The important stabilizing factor is the use of orthoses (orthopedic collars).

We have evaluated the degree of stabilization of the three types of collars: 1, soft; 2, partial/semistiff; 3, stiff (stabilizing with support under mandibula and occipit, and on the sternum).

Patients, especially female ones, were more willing to wear soft or partial semi-stiff collars, saying that they had less pain in them. The stiff collars made some functions difficult, although the patients stated they had a marked decrease of ailments or total disappearance of pain when wearing this type of collar (Milanowska et al., 1986).

The most common form of neck pain is caused by overstretching of ligaments due to postural stresses. This may occur when sitting with poor posture for a long time, when lying or sleeping overnight with the head in an awkward position, and when working in strained positions. In order to prevent the development of neck pain due to prolonged poor sitting it is necessary to:

1. Sit correctly - if one sits slouched with low back rounded, it is not possible to correct the posture of the neck. Therefore, it is necessary first to correct the posture of the lower back. To achieve this the use of a lumbar roll or pillow is essential. These support the lower back, counteract slouching and keep the head upright. The lumbar roll should be placed in the small of the back at the level of the belt line whenever sitting in an easy chair, car, or office chair.

2. Perform exercises to regain full mobility in the neck or as much movement as possible under the given condition. The first and most important exercise is head retraction, which means pulling the head backwards. The exercises - neck extension, flexion, and rotation and side bending of the neck - should be repeated a few times throughout the day (McKenzie, 1987).

We also recommend sleeping on the special pillow which stretches the cervical spine. The main function of the pillow is to support both head and neck. Therefore, it should fill the natural hollow in the contour of the neck between head and shoulder girdle without tilting the head or lifting it up; the head should be allowed to rest in a dish-shaped hollow.

Treatment for Vertebral Osteoporosis

In the treatment program for patients with vertebral osteoporosis a diet rich in calcium must be considered. Many elderly people do not have a sufficient dietary calcium intake. The recommended daily intake of calcium for postmenopausal and elderly patients is approximately 1,600 mg/day. In addition to the correction of dietary calcium deficiency, excessive and prolonged consumption of alcohol, tobacco, coffee, corticosteroids, and foods high in phosphorus should be discontinued (Panjabi, 1990).

Exercises and active life have a beneficial effect on bone metabolism and bone mineral content. Therefore, systematic general exercises and various physical activity must be included in the treatment of osteoporosis. Constant physical activity has a great influence on the delay and slower course of involutional changes. In order to maintain health we recommend:

1. Daily general exercises for 15 to 30 minutes

2. Proper nutrition and keeping the proper body weight

3. Weekend rest creating the possibilities for recreation and sport that are appropriate for the age and tastes.

CONCLUSION

Concluding this report on treatment and prophylaxis of back pain, it is important to stress that enriching the life style with diverse physical activity and exercises, health maintenance, fitness, and physical efficiency improves the prospects for good and healthy aging.

REFERENCES

Grochmal S. Profilaktyka zespolu bolow dolnego odcinka kregoslupa z przeciazenia praca zawodowa (Prophylactics of low back pain overloaded by work). In: Proc Symp Rehab Comm Pol Acad Sci. Warsaw: PZWL, 1977:119-24.

Kahanovitz N. Osteoporosis. In: Weinstein JM, Wiesel SW, eds. The Lumbar Spine. Philadelphia: W.B. Saunders Company, 1990:760-9.

McKenzie R. Treat Your Own Neck. Hong Kong: C Joint Printing Co./HK/Ltd., 1987:26-34.

Milanowska K, Konieczna D, Bembnista A. Leczenie usprawniajace osob z zespolem bolow dolnego odcinka kregoslupa (Rehabilitating treatment of patients with low back pain). Proc Symp Rehab Comm Pol Acad Sci. Warsaw: PZWL, 1978:50-5.

Milanowska K, Konieczna D, Szmigielska M. Ocena zastosowanego leczenia usprawniajacego w przypadkach bolow odcinka szyjnego kregoslupa (Evaluation of treatment in patient with cervical pain). Proc II Cong TWK. Warsaw: PZWL, 1986:151-4.

Panjabi MM. Degeneration, injury, and spinal instability. In: Weinstein JM, Wiesel SW. The Lumbar Spine. Philadelphia: W.B. Saunders Company, 1990: 188-94.

Tai Chi Chuan: Mind and Body in Harmony

Stephen H. Tolins, M.D., F.A.C.S.

INTRODUCTION

Tai Chi Chuan was first described about 1000 A.D. Tai Chi is translated as "grand ultimate," and Chuan means "fist" or "boxing;" metaphorically it means action (Crompton, 1986; Delza, 1961; Koh, 1981b). Since that time historians and practitioners have shown the importance of exercise in the ancient Chinese culture, the characteristics of Tai Chi and its benefits for old and young, frail and healthy.

In this article the many books on Tai Chi are discussed and the claims for preventive health and curative powers reviewed. Modern scientific reports on Tai Chi, its physiological effects and its benefits in specific conditions are summarized.

Discussion stresses the importance of exercise in aging and the relative safety, as well as efficiency, of Tai Chi as an exercise for the elderly. Suggestions for future application and study are made, such as, "does the improved balance for the Tai Chi practitioner limit the occurrence of hip fracture in the elderly?"

ORIGINS AND CHARACTERISTICS OF TAI CHI

Tai Chi had its origin some time during the Sung Dynasty (960-1279 A.D.) (Cheng, 1963) when Chang San-Feng, the famous boxer and Taoist saint, watched a snake and a crane fighting (Kauz 1974; Maisel, 1963). Chang was a master of the boxing form of the Shao-lin Temple, a form designed by a Buddhist monk in the sixth century A.D. (Galante, 1981). The crane was pecking furiously while the snake swayed gently, avoiding the thrusts. Finally, the exhausted crane was easy prey to the snake's recoil. It was the ancient Taoist philosophy of conquering the unyielding with the yielding (Cheng, 1963). This eventually became Tai Chi, the Yang long form of movements. The essential qualities of Tai Chi were and still are: slowness, lightness, clarity, balance, calmness; in other words, body and mind in harmony (Chen, 1947; Eisenberg, 1985). Tai Chi is an exercise with a "rhythmic, flowing style" and a "relaxed mental attitude" (Tegner, 1968). It has also been called "meditation in movement" (Crompton, 1986; Lewis, 1987; Koh, 1981a), and "a mental, emotional attitude of calm detachment and harmony" (Lewis, 1987). Tai Chi has been described as demanding "body control and exquisite balance" (Eisenberg, 1985); and its "movements are slow, smooth, rounded, flowing, gentle" (Tegner, 1968).

The importance of the position of the body has been described and emphasized by many (Chen, 1947; Cheng, 1963; Galante, 1981; Tegner, 1968). The head must be straight and move with the trunk; the trunk must not lean forward. The sacrum must not stick out. The knees must be bent but must not go beyond the tips of the toes. The elbows must be slightly bent. Shoulders are low and relaxed. The mouth is closed and the tongue touches the palate and the back of the upper teeth.

Breathing, of course, is important. Most authorities, however, stress that breathing should be natural, through the nostrils and with the mouth closed (Crompton, 1986; Galante, 1981; Sutherland, 1986). The breathing should not be forced, or even thought about. As the Tai Chi exerciser progresses with the form, the rhythmic breathing will blend with the slow movements (Sutherland, 1986). The breathing will be diaphragmatic with distension of the abdomen on inspiration and contraction of the abdomen on exhalation. Most upswing motions will be accompanied by inhalations and downward motions or forward pushes accompanied by exhalations.

The simplicity and effortlessness of Tai Chi make it fit for young and old (Delza, 1961; Lewis, 1987); and Wang and Zeng (1983) say it is "not too hard a task for aged or weak." Tai Chi has other benefits; no special clothing or equipment is needed (Maisel, 1963; Tegner, 1968), and only a small area, approximately three by six feet, either indoors or out, is all that is needed by the solo practitioner. And, finally, it is said of Tai Chi that it is evenly balanced and does not subject the body to sudden shearing and tearing forces that so commonly lead to injury (Woodworth, 1990b).

The early Yang long form of Tai Chi, with its some 108 to 138 positions, was modified in the late 1950's by the master Cheng Man-ch'ing, and it is this short Yang form that has become most popular both in China and in the United States, where Chen Manch'ing started teaching in the early 1960's. In many of the books on Tai Chi, published both in China and the United States in the past 31 years, there are drawings or photographs illustrating each position of the short form (Cheng, 1963; Delza, 196l; Galante, 1981; Kauz, 1974; Maisel, 1963; Tegner, 1968; Wang, 1983; Wu, 1984). Practically all of the writers, however, warn that, to learn Tai Chi properly, one must go to a qualified teacher rather than just to the books.

USAGE AND CLAIMS

In the famous Yellow Emperor's Classic of Internal Medicine, about 400 B.C., there is the advice: "A sound mind in a sound body is essential to longevity" (Zhuo, 1982). There is also the warning that "excesses and extremes were regarded as harmful to health." Activity is also encouraged by the ancient proverbs: "A door-pivot will never be worm-eaten, and flowing water will never be putrid" (Cheng, 1963).

In more recent times the health benefits of exercise in an aging society have been stressed (Larson and Bruce, 1987). Bogdonoff (1983), in his book, "Forever Fit," writes: "Men and women who are more active in organizations and who engage in more physical activity are more likely to age successfully than those in fewer organizations and activities." He advocates "energetic life style in the middle years" and states: "clearly, physical activity was crucial to good health."

Boyer and Kasch (1970) showed that moderate exercise decreased the diastolic blood pressure in hypertensive men, and stated that essential hypertension was not necessarily a contraindication to controlled exercise training.

"Controlled exercise training" is exactly what Tai Chi is, and it is not surprising that in the past 30 years it has become so popular in China and the United States. Chen, in 1947, wrote: "Tai Chi Chuan rebuilds one's spirit and body," and it "promotes deep breathing, develops the lungs to their normality, and tones up the heart. It promotes digestion and enables the stomach to absorb the nourishment from food more efficiently." (Chen, 1947). Cheng said: "Tai Chi is a sport that suits everybody - the weak, the sick, the aged, as well as children and women." (Cheng, 1963). Cheng and Smith (1967) wrote: "whoever practices Tai Chi correctly and regularly will gain the pliability of a child, the health of a lumberjack, and the peace of mind of a sage." Da Liu (1974) said: "Tai Chi Ch'uan is a bonafide adjunct to medical therapy in many hospitals, sanitariums, and convalescent homes."

In 1970, de Vries tested 112 men aged 52 to 87 on a moderate regime of calisthenics, jogging, and stretching. He found that there was improved oxygen transport capacity, muscle strength and physical work capacity, and that, even in the older subject, this moderate exercise - which Tai Chi is - was safe.

Kauz (1977), in his book, "The Martial Spirit," stresses (as did the ancient Chinese) that without exercise there is deterioration of one's health.

In the literature of Tai Chi there are personal stories of a disease cured, as well as long lists of diseases cured or improved by Tai Chi. Cheng Man-ch'ing (1963) described his cure of almost fatal tuberculosis after he took up Tai Chi.

Koh (1982) told how his ankylosing spondylitis was greatly improved by the practice of Tai Chi. Chen (1947) lists: neurasthenia, high blood pressure, anemia, tuberculosis, gastric and enteric diseases, paralysis, kidney diseases; and he ends by stating "extraordinary results will come to even those with incurable diseases."

Cheng and Smith (1967) modestly state: "There is also basis for the claim that Tai-chi can relieve, if not actually cure neurasthenia, high blood pressure, anemia, tuberculosis, and many other maladies." Delza (1961), in the earliest book on Tai Chi in the United States, puts her stamp of approval on the foregoing lists. Galante (1981) has his list of diseases improved by Tai Chi: arteriosclerosis, arthritis, asthma, bronchitis, cholecystitis, colds, constipation, diabetes, dizziness, influenza gastrointestinal disorders, heart disease, hemiparesis, high blood pressure, hypertension, insomnia, kidney malfunctions, lethargy, liver disease, loss of breath, low blood pressure, nervous disorders, neurasthenia, paralysis, rheumatism, senility, stress, tuberculosis, ulcers. Galante cites a study at First Medical Academy, Shanghai, where some of the above diseases were treated using Tai Chi, with approximately 50 percent cured and 100 percent improved. Eight of eight nervous breakdowns were cured, and four of four depressions.

Crompton (1986) quotes a study of Professor Qu Mianyu done in 1980 in which patients treated with Tai Chi had fewer electrocardiogram abnormalities, better cardiopulmonary function, fewer spinal column deformities, and less senile osteoporosis than a control group.

Woodworth (1990a) remarks on the benefits of Tai Chi in cases of arthritis and Parkinson's Disease.

Wang and Zeng (1983) reported that between 1974 and 1981 over 250,000 people in China were taught Tai Chi. Of those with chronic diseases, 90 percent had marked improvement and many returned to their jobs.

Wu (1984) states that Tai Chi is "actually beneficial to patients with high blood pressure, stomach or intestinal ulcers, heart troubles, tuberculosis and other ailments." He concludes: "a constantly active body is free from indigestion, circulatory trouble and other physical problems, just like the door hinge which is free from rot or rust."

Zhuo (1982) claimed that ischemic electrocardiogram changes were less evident in a Tai Chi group than in a control group. He stated: "In terms of a general well-being, it was found that most of the Tai Chi group showed none or few symptoms of general weakness while 50 percent of the controls had marked symptoms and sign of general weakness". Zhuo (1986) also recommends Tai Chi for mild arthritis, and states: "Tai Chi helps improve coordination and balance."

The following paragraph from Chen (1947) gives us a good picture of what we can expect if we do Tai Chi regularly: "cheeks will have a healthy red color; the temples will be full and swelling; the ears will be crimson; the hearing will be quick; the eyeballs will be brilliant and full of spirit. The voice will be loud and reach far; breathing will be regular, with no panting and hastiness. The teeth, the gums, and the jaws will be strong. The shoulders and chest will be sturdy and sleek. The abdomen will be solid and elastic like drum leather. When one is standing, the two feet will be as firm as if stuck to the ground. The step will be light. The muscles will be as soft as cotton when the intrinsic energy remains inactive; but they will be stiff when intrinsic energy is active."

MODERN SCIENTIFIC STUDIES

Studies involving Tai Chi which could be called "modern" and "scientific" are relatively few, and have been done primarily in the last decade.

Such studies fall mainly into two categories: those involving the assessing of metabolic and cardiorespiratory responses in Tai Chi practitioners, and those assessing the effects of Tai Chi exercise on specific diseases.

Gong (1981) studied 100 Tai Chi practitioners, both men and women, aged 46 to 80, who had regularly done Tai Chi four to 10 years. The heart rate peak for each age group, while doing the exercise, was an increase of 20 to 30 beats per minute, and there was no appreciable change in blood pressure. He therefore concluded that Tai Chi was a moderate exercise and that further studies were needed to understand its benefits in alleviating symptoms.

Schneider and Leung (1991) studied the cardiorespiratory responses to Tai Chi exercise and noted the moderate increase, 36.4 percent of maximum oxygen consumption, and 59.8 percent of maximum heart rate. They concluded that practice of Tai Chi should not be considered dangerous for individuals at high risk for cardiovascular disease.

Zhuo et al (1984) observed 11 healthy males, aged 24 to 35, who had practiced Tai Chi for three to eight years, while they did the long form of Tai Chi. Heart rate peak was 134, and oxygen consumption was 50 percent of maximum. The flexibility scores were outstanding. They concluded Tai Chi was an exercise of moderate intensity, good for conditions with increased tension or diminished range of joint movements, but was insufficient to improve cardiorespiratory fitness in young adults.

Plummer (1981) discussed the threefold effect Tai Chi has on man's physiology, his posture and his mind; an effect due probably to a feedback type of relationship.

Brown et al. (1989) compared the ventilatory and cardiovascular responses of Tai Chi practitioners to their responses during cycle ergometry. Six males experienced in Tai Chi were the subjects. The percentage of minute ventilation used for alveolar ventilation was significantly higher during Tai Chi than cycle ergometry. Cardiac output, stroke volume and heart rate were not significantly different at the same oxygen consumption. There was more efficient use of the ventilatory volume with Tai Chi.

Jiang (1984) studied the blood lipids and high density lipoprotein-cholesterol in a group of in-patients of Jinjishan Sanatorium who did Tai Chi daily, as compared to a control group. After a month there was a significant increase of the high density lipoprotein in the Tai Chi group. Jiang concludes that Tai Chi might be effective in the prevention of atherosclerosis.

Studies of specific diseases treated by Tai Chi are few. Maevskii (1990) followed eight bronchial asthma patients for two years who daily performed short form Tai Chi. There were six women and two men, ranging in age from 13 to 70 years. All the patients had significant improvement.

Arthritic conditions have been the subject of studies using Tai Chi as therapy. Mention has already been made of Koh's improvement of his severe ankylosing spondylitis after he began regular Tai Chi exercise (Koh, 1982).

Van Deusen (1987) studied 33 adults with rheumatoid arthritis. Seventeen had Tai Chi exercise added to the traditional exercise and occupational therapy program and 16 formed the control group. After four months, the Tai Chi group showed significantly greater upper extremity range of motion, and more enjoyment of the program than the control group. Further studies were urged by the author. Kirsteins et al. (1991) evaluated the safety of Tai Chi on rheumatoid arthritis patients. Eleven patients were given Tai Chi weekly for ten weeks and compared with nine controls. Joint tenderness, joint swelling, time to walk 50 feet, and handgrip strength were all measured and compared. There were no significant increases of joint symptoms with the Tai Chi, which appears to be safe for rheumatoid arthritis patients. Further long-term studies are urged in view of the potential of weight-bearing exercises to stimulate bone growth.

Psychiatric patients have also been introduced to Tai Chi. Yalom et al. (1977) divided 33 patients in long-term individual therapy into three weekend groups: affect-arousing, gestalt therapy and meditation - Tai Chi. After 12 weeks there were no demonstrable differences among the three groups, but only the Tai Chi group was without risk of psychological damage.

Lund (1988) (unpublished review by Richard Paul Lund, exercise physiologist) monitored eight Tai Chi instructors, 25 to 40 years of age, while they did the short form. Increased oxygen consumption and increased heart rate revealed an energy involvement roughly equivalent to walking. Lund's conclusion was that Tai Chi is safe for cardiac patients, convalescing patients, and senior citizens. Lund quotes a study from Beijing in which 33 Tai Chi instructors of 40 years experience, age 66, were compared to a control group of 56, aged 70, who did exercise and manual labor but not Tai Chi. The Tai Chi group showed increased lung capacity, wrist and back power, lower systolic blood pressure and greater ability to do step test and to touch toes. In a similar study from the Shanghai Medical Center, 80 Tai Chi instructors aged 50 to 79, were compared to 141 retired workers who did not practice Tai Chi. It was concluded that Tai Chi had a positive effect on preventing diseases related to aging as well as improving health; blood pressure was lower, lung capacity greater, muscle power stronger, reaction time faster, and vision better. The conclusion was that Tai Chi practitioners had less chance of being affected with the usual aging diseases.

DISCUSSION

Exercise, as a necessary adjunct to healthy living, has been stressed for thousands of years. After the ancient Chinese, the Greeks, and then the Romans stressed the idea of a sound mind in a sound body.

In modern times, with increased numbers of people living past 65 and even past 85, the importance of exercise for this aging population has been emphasized. Such exercise, obviously, must be suited to an elderly, frail practitioner. It must be safe, with no stress-related injuries. It must be readily accessible, with no requirements for special clothing or equipment. It must be pleasurable and calming.

Tai Chi, it has been shown, fulfills all the above requirements. It is slow and gentle, bringing calmness and improving balance. Studies have shown that Tai Chi is a moderate exercise, improving ventilation and increasing heart rate only 50 to 60 percent of maximum.

With indications in a few small studies of possible benefits of Tai Chi, it is now time to institute large-scale, long-term studies in many areas. Such studies, using the many nursing homes, senior citizen centers and retirement housing groups, could include many hundreds of people, both male and female.

One such study could be centered on patients with rheumatoid arthritis to assess the benefits to such patients and the lack of possible painful side effects from a weight-bearing exercise.

Bronchial asthma patients, in a large-scale study over several years, could be monitored for their response to Tai Chi.

Does Tai Chi really improve the high density lipoprotein ratio in the aging population? A large-scale, long-term study might give the answers as to whether Tai Chi retards the progress of arteriosclerosis and decreases strokes and myocardial infarcts.

Balance is mentioned often as improved and characteristic in Tai Chi practitioners. Will the practice of Tai Chi significantly reduce the number of hip fractures in the elderly?

Calmness and relaxed mental attitude are frequently described by the writers on Tai Chi. Would a large-scale, long-term study confirm that the use of Tai Chi is a cure for depression and stress-related symptoms?

With an increasing aging population, can Tai Chi be used as a widespread method to improve safely the general fitness of this population? Will the widespread use of Tai Chi improve the quality of life in this aging population and decrease the need for more and more nursing homes?

These questions deserve an answer.

REFERENCES

Bogdonoff MD. Forever Fit: The Exercise Program for Staying Young. New York: Little Brown & Co., 1983:6.

Boyer JL, Kasch FW. Exercise therapy in hypertensive men. JAMA 1970;211:1668-71.

Brown DD, Mucci WG, Hetzler RK, Knowlton RG. Cardiovascular and ventilatory responses during formalized Tai Chi Chuan. Res Q Exerc Sport 1989;60:246-50.

Chen YK. Tai-Chi Ch'uan its Effects and Practical Applications. Shanghai: 1947:10-11,9,12,13-14.

Cheng M-C. Tai Chi Chuan: A Simplified Method of Calisthenics for Health and Self Defense. Taipei Taiwan: Shih Chung Tai Chi Chuan Center 1963:10,30,51,52,63.

Cheng M-C, Smith RW. Tai-Chi The "Supreme Ultimate" Exercise for Health, Sport, and Self-Defense. Rutland, Vermont: Charles E. Tuttle Co., 1967:1.

Crompton P. The Tai Chi Workbook. Boston: Shambala Publications, Inc., 1986:139,9,33,134-136.

Da L. Taoist Health Exercise Book. New York: Links Books, 1974:72.

Delza S. Tai Chi Chuan Body and Mind in Harmony. North Canton, Ohio: Good News Publishing Co., 1961:4,7,9.

de Vries HA. Physiological effects of an exercise training regimen upon men aged 52 to 88. J Gerontol 1970;25:325-36.

Eisenberg D, Wright TL. Encounters with Qi: Exploring Chinese Medicine. New York: W.W. Norton and Co., 1985:41.

Galante L. Tai Chi The Supreme Ultimate. York Beach, Maine: Samuel Weiser Inc., 1981:25-27,59.

Gong L, Qian J, Zhang J, Yang Q, Jiang J, Tao Q. Changes in heart rate and electrocardiogram during Taijiquan exercise. Chi Med J 1981;94:589-92.

Jiang J. Effect of "Taijiquan" on serum high density lipoprotein - cholesterol and other lipid concentration. Chin Ath J 1984:99-104.

Kauz H. Tai Chi Handbook Exercise, Meditation, and Self-Defense. New York: Doubleday & Co., Inc., 1974:11.

Kauz H. The Martial Spirit, an Introduction to the Origin, Philosophy and Psychology of the Martial Arts. Woodstock, NY: The Overlook Press, 1977:23.

Kirsteins AE, Dietz F, Hwang S-M. Evaluating the safety and potential use of a weight-bearing exercise, Tai-Chi Chuan, for rheumatoid arthritis patients. Am J Phys Med Rehab 1991;70:136-41.

Koh TC. Chinese medicine and martial arts. Am J Chin Med 1981a;9:181-6.

Koh TC. Tai Chi Chuan. Am J Chin Med 1981b;9:15-22.

Koh TC. Tai Chi and Ankylosing Spondylitis - a personal experience. Am J Chin Med 1982;10:59-61.

Larson EB, Bruce RA. Health benefits of exercise in an aging society. Arch Intern Med 1987;147:353-6.

Lewis P. Martial Arts. New York: Gallery Books, 1987:20,16.

Maevskii AA. Experience with the Chinese therapeutic gymnastics in the complex treatment of patients with bronchial asthma. Klin Med Mosk 1990;68:71.

Maisel E. Taichi for Health. Englewood Cliffs, NJ: Prentice-Hall, Inc., 1963:182,17.

Plummer JP. Acupuncture and homeostasis; physiological, physical (postural) and psychological. Am J Chin Med 1981:9:1-4.

Schneider D, Leung R. Metabolic and cardiorespiratory responses to the performance of Wing Chun and Tai Chi Chuan exercise. Int J Sports Med 1991;12:319-23.

Sutherland JC. Tai Chi Warmups. Phys Ther Forum, May 28, 1986:7.

Tegner B. Book of Kung Fu and Tai Chi. Ventura, CA: Thor Publishing Co., 1968:89-90.

Van Deusen J, Harlowe D. The efficacy of the ROM Dance Program for adults with rheumatoid arthritis. Am J Occup Ther 1987;41:90-5.

Wang P, Zeng W. Wu Style Taijiquan. Hong Kong: Hal Feng Publishing Co., 1983:227, 221.

Woodworth B. Therapeutic Values of Tai Chi. Phys Ther Forum July 23, 1990a:7-8.

Woodworth B. Tai-Chi - possibilities for occupational therapy. Phys Ther Forum October 22, 1990b:9.

Wu V. Taijiquan in 88 Forms. Hong Kong: Hai Feng Publishing Co., 1984:2.

Yalom ID, Bond G, Bloch S, Zimmerman E, Friedman L. The impact of a weekend group experience on individual therapy. Arch Gen Psychiatry 1977;34:399-415.

Zhuo D, Shephard RJ, Plyley MJU, Davis GM. Cardiovascular and metabolic responses during Tai Chi Chuan exercises. Can J Appl Sci 1984;9:7-10.

Zhuo D. The Chinese Exercise Book. Vancouver, BC: Hartley & Marks Ltd., 1986:21.

Zhuo D. Preventive geriatrics: an overview from traditional Chinese Medicine. Am J Chin Med 1982;10:32-9.

Index

Index